Springer Texts in Statistics

Series Editors

G. Allen, Department of Statistics, Houston, TX, USA

R. De Veaux, Department of Mathematics and Statistics, Williams College, Williamstown, MA, USA

R. Nugent, Department of Statistics, Carnegie Mellon University, Pittsburgh, PA, USA

Springer Texts in Statistics (STS) includes advanced textbooks from 3rd- to 4th-year undergraduate courses to 1st- to 2nd-year graduate courses. Exercise sets should be included. The series editors are currently Genevera I. Allen, Richard D. De Veaux, and Rebecca Nugent. Stephen Fienberg, George Casella, and Ingram Olkin were editors of the series for many years.

More information about this series at http://www.springer.com/series/417

Richard A. Berk

Statistical Learning from a Regression Perspective

Third Edition

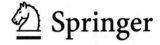 Springer

Richard A. Berk
Department of Criminology
Schools of Arts and Sciences
University of Pennsylvania
Philadelphia, PA, USA

ISSN 1431-875X   ISSN 2197-4136   (electronic)
Springer Texts in Statistics
ISBN 978-3-030-42923-2   ISBN 978-3-030-40189-4   (eBook)
https://doi.org/10.1007/978-3-030-40189-4

This Springer imprint is published by the registered company Springer Nature Switzerland AG.
The registered company address is: Gewerbestrasse 11, 6330 Cham, Switzerland

*In God we trust. All others
must have data*

(W. Edwards Deming)

In memory of Peter H. Rossi,
a mentor, colleague, and friend

Preface to the Third Edition

The preface to the third edition is very brief. There is substantial continuity with the Second Edition in aims, conventions, and style. But there are also some important differences. First, there have been useful theoretical advances and ways to rethink statistical inference for statistical learning. Consequently, some new inferential tools are available. Greater clarity for many difficult conceptual issues is another benefit. As statistical learning continues to move into the mainstream, it has become increasingly important to address the differences between statistical inference anchored in models and statistical inference anchored in algorithms. This message is prominent in the pages ahead.

Second, the development of unifying concepts continues. Despite differences in disciplinary roots and applications, fundamental commonalities across a wide range of algorithmic methods are now more apparent. These commonalities help to mute unjustified claims that some procedure is new and better. They also foster better understanding. Regularization, for example, is almost universally employed, but it can be difficult to recognize because regularization comes in so many different forms with different notation and naming conventions. Once regularization in its many incarnations is properly identified, a wide range of algorithmic operations are conceptually integrated. Often there is far less going on than meets the eye. In this edition, readers should find the overarching concepts introduced very helpful.

Third, deep learning has exploded on the scene and for the special applications on which it thrives has fundamentally changed practice. Pattern recognition for images will never be the same. Nor will the analysis of human speech. And its key role in so many applications advertised as artificial intelligence means that deep learning is at the center of current policy controversies. However, most deep learning applications are peripheral to the kinds of data and questions most central to the social, environmental, and biomedical sciences. For now, that makes deep learning somewhat of a niche player for these disciplines. Coverage in this book is designed accordingly. Nevertheless, the third edition would be remiss if deep learning were not meaningfully included.

Fourth, I continue to receive very helpful feedback from students in my machine learning classes. Many of the topics covered in the first two editions are now explained far more effectively, and identified, earlier errors have been corrected. I have also added many footnotes, partly in response to questions from students over the years and partly to elaborate points for readers who want to go a bit deeper. As a whole, I believe the third edition is a far more effective didactic enterprise.

Fifth, I have found that students generally perform better on real applications working with the material in an "active learning" setting, sometimes called a "flipped classroom." The readings are done at home and various exercises are done in class. The key is to pitch these exercises at the right technical level, using real data, so that the task is not just "make work." My lectures have generally been well received, but I suspect induce too much passivity.

Finally, the passing of Larry Brown has been deeply felt throughout the discipline of statistics, not just because of his intelligence and accomplishments, but because of his deep kindness. He is sorely missed at Penn and is irreplaceable. But I still have my other remarkable colleagues in the Department of Statistics: Andreas Buja, Ed George, Abba Kreiger, Paul Rosenbaum, Dylan Small, Adi Wyner, and Linda Zhao. My two new colleagues, Arun Kuchibhotla and Eric Tchetgen Tchetgen, have patiently and with good cheer furthered my statistical education on theoretical matters. I have also benefited enormously from working with Michael Kearns and Aaron Roth of Penn's Department of Computer and Information Sciences. Both are very smart, hardworking, and above all, sensible. Here too, it takes a village.

Philadelphia, PA, USA   Richard A. Berk

Preface to the Second Edition

Over the past 8 years, the topics associated with statistical learning have been expanded and consolidated. They have been expanded because new problems have been tackled, new tools have been developed, and older tools have been refined. They have been consolidated because many unifying concepts and themes have been identified. It has also become more clear from practice which statistical learning tools will be widely applied and which are likely to see limited service. In short, it seems time to revisit the material and make it more current.

There are currently several excellent textbook treatments of statistical learning and its very close cousin, machine learning. The second edition of *Elements of Statistical Learning* by Hastie et al. (2009) is in my view still the gold standard, but there are other treatments that in their own way can be excellent. Examples include *Machine Learning: A Probabilistic Perspective* by Kevin Murphy (2012), *Principles and Theory for Data Mining and Machine Learning* by Clarke et al. (2009), and *Applied Predictive Modeling* by Kuhn and Johnson (2013).

Yet, it is sometimes difficult to appreciate from these treatments that a proper application of statistical learning is comprised of (1) data collection, (2) data management, (3) data analysis, and (4) interpretation of results. The first entails finding and acquiring the data to be analyzed. The second requires putting the data into an accessible form. The third depends on extracting instructive patterns from the data. The fourth calls for making sense of those patterns. For example, a statistical learning data analysis might begin by collecting information from "rap sheets" and other kinds of official records about prison inmates who have been released on parole. The information obtained might then be organized so that arrests were nested within individuals. At that point, support vector machines could be used to classify offenders into those who re-offend after release on parole and those who do not. Finally, the classes obtained might be employed to forecast subsequent re-offending when the actual outcome is not known. Although there is a chronological sequence to these activities, one must anticipate later steps as earlier steps are undertaken. Will the offender classes, for instance, include or exclude juvenile offenses or vehicular offenses? How this is decided will affect the choice of statistical learning tools, how they are implemented, and how they are interpreted. Moreover, the preferred statistical learning procedures anticipated place constraints on how the offenses are coded, while the ways in which the results are likely to be used affect how the procedures are tuned. In short, no single activity should be considered in isolation from the other three.

Nevertheless, textbook treatments of statistical learning (and statistics textbooks more generally) focus on the third step: the statistical procedures. This can make good sense if the treatments are to be of manageable length and within the authors' expertise, but risks the misleading impression that once the key statistical theory is understood, one is ready to proceed with data. The result can be a fancy statistical analysis as a bridge to nowhere. To reprise an aphorism attributed to Albert Einstein: "In theory, theory and practice are the same. In practice they are not."

The commitment to practice as well as theory will sometimes engender considerable frustration. There are times when the theory is not readily translated into practice. And there are times when practice, even practice that seems intuitively sound, will have no formal justification. There are also important open questions leaving large holes in procedures one would like to apply. A particular problem is statistical inference, especially for procedures that proceed in an inductive manner. In effect, they capitalize on "data snooping," which can invalidate estimation, confidence intervals, and statistical tests.

In the first edition, statistical tools characterized as supervised learning were the main focus. But a serious effort was made to establish links to data collection, data management, and proper interpretation of results. That effort is redoubled in this edition. At the same time, there is a price. No claims are made for anything like an encyclopedic coverage of supervised learning, let alone of the underlying statistical theory. There are books available that take the encyclopedic approach, which can have the feel of a trip through Europe spending 24 h in each of the major cities.

Here, the coverage is highly selective. Over the past decade, the wide range of real applications has begun to sort the enormous variety of statistical learning tools into those primarily of theoretical interest or in early stages of development, the niche players, and procedures that have been successfully and widely applied (Jordan and Mitchell 2015). Here, the third group is emphasized.

Even among the third group, choices need to be made. The statistical learning material addressed reflects the subject-matter fields with which I am more familiar. As a result, applications in the social and policy sciences are emphasized. This is a pity because there are truly fascinating applications in the natural sciences and engineering. But in the words of Dirty Harry: "A man's got to know his limitations" (from the movie Magnum Force, 1973).[1] My several forays into natural science applications do not qualify as real expertise.

The second edition retains its commitment to the statistical programming language R. If anything, the commitment is stronger. R provides access to state-of-the-art statistics, including those needed for statistical learning. It is also now a standard training component in top departments of statistics so for many readers, applications of the statistical procedures discussed will come quite naturally. Where it could be useful, I now include the R code needed when the usual R documentation may be insufficient. That code is written to be accessible. Often there will be more elegant, or least more efficient, ways to proceed. When practical, I develop examples using data that can be downloaded from one of the R libraries. But, R is a moving target. Code that runs now may not run in the future. In the year it took to complete this edition, many key procedures were updated several times, and there were three updates of R itself. *Caveat emptor*. Readers will also notice that the graphical output from the many procedures used does not have common format or color scheme. In some cases, it would have been very difficult to force a common set of graphing conventions, and it is probably important to show a good approximation of the default output in any case. Aesthetics and common formats can be a casualty.

In summary, the second edition retains its emphasis on supervised learning that can be treated as a form of regression analysis. Social science and policy applications are prominent. Where practical, substantial links are made to data collection, data management, and proper interpretation of results, some of which can raise ethical concerns (Dwork et al. 2011; Zemel et al. 2013). I hope it works.

The first chapter has been rewritten almost from scratch in part from experience I have had trying to teach the material. It now much better reflects new views about unifying concepts and themes. I think the chapter also gets to punch lines more quickly and coherently. But readers who are looking for simple recipes will be disappointed. The exposition is by design not "point-and-click." There is as well some time spent on what some statisticians call "meta-issues." A good data analyst must know what to compute and what to make of the computed results. How to compute is important, but by itself nearly purposeless.

All of the other chapters have also been revised and updated with an eye toward far greater clarity. In many places, greater clarity was sorely needed. I now appreciate much better how difficult it can be to translate statistical concepts and notation into plain English. Where I have still failed, please accept my apology.

I have also tried to take into account that often a particular chapter is downloaded and read in isolation. Because much of the material is cumulative, working through a single chapter can on occasion create special challenges. I have tried to include text to help, but for readers working cover to cover, there are necessarily some redundancies and annoying pointers to material in other chapters. I hope such readers will be patient with me.

I continue to be favored with remarkable colleagues and graduate students. My professional life is one ongoing tutorial in statistics, thanks to Larry Brown, Andreas Buja, Linda Zhao, and Ed George. All four are as collegial as they are smart. I have learned a great deal as well from former students Adam Kapelner, Justin Bleich, Emil Pitkin, Kai Zhang, Dan McCarthy, and Kory Johnson. Finally, there are many students who took my statistics classes and whose questions got me to think a lot harder about the material. Thanks to them as well.

But I would probably not have benefited nearly so much from all the talent around me were it not for my earlier relationship with David Freedman. He was my bridge from routine calculations within standard statistical packages to a far better appreciation of the underlying foundations of modern statistics. He also reinforced my skepticism about many statistical applications in the social and biomedical sciences. Shortly before he died, David asked his friends to "keep after the rascals." I certainly have tried.

Philadelphia, PA, USA   Richard A. Berk

Preface to the First Edition

As I was writing my recent book on regression analysis (Berk 2003), I was struck by how few alternatives to conventional regression there were. In the social sciences, for example, one either did causal modeling econometric style or largely gave up quantitative work. The life sciences did not seem quite so driven by causal modeling, but causal modeling was a popular tool. As I argued at length in my book, causal modeling as commonly undertaken is a loser.

There also seemed to be a more general problem. Across a range of scientific disciplines, there was too often little interest in statistical tools emphasizing induction and description. With the primary goal of getting the "right" model and its associated p-values, the older and interesting tradition of exploratory data analysis had largely become an under-the-table activity; the approach was in fact commonly used, but rarely discussed in polite company. How could one be a real scientist, guided by "theory" and engaged in deductive model testing while at the same time snooping around in the data to determine which models to test? In the battle for prestige, model testing had won.

Around the same time, I became aware of some new developments in applied mathematics, computer science, and statistics making data exploration a virtue. And with the virtue came a variety of new ideas and concepts, coupled with the very latest in statistical computing. These new approaches, variously identified as "data mining," "statistical learning," "machine learning," and other names, were being tried in a number of natural and biomedical sciences, and the initial experience looked promising.

As I started to read more deeply, however, I was struck by how difficult it was to work across writings from such disparate disciplines. Even when the material was essentially the same, it was very difficult to tell if it was. Each discipline brought its own goals, concepts, naming conventions, and (maybe worst of all) notation to the table.

In the midst of trying to impose some of my own order on the material, I came upon *The Elements of Statistical Learning*, by Trevor Hastie, Robert Tibshirani, and Jerome Friedman (Springer-Verlag, 2001). I saw in the book a heroic effort to integrate a very wide variety of data analysis tools. I learned from the book and was then able to approach more primary material within a useful framework.

This book is my attempt to integrate some of the same material and some new developments of the past 6 years. Its intended audience is practitioners in the social, biomedical, and ecological sciences. Applications to real data addressing real empirical questions are emphasized. Although considerable effort has gone into providing explanations of why the statistical procedures work the way they do, the required mathematical background is modest. A solid course or two in regression analysis and some familiarity with resampling procedures should suffice. A good benchmark for regression is Freedman's *Statistical Models: Theory and Practice* (2005). A good benchmark for resampling is Manly's *Randomization, Bootstrap, and Monte Carlo Methods in Biology* 1997. Matrix algebra and calculus are used only as languages of exposition, and only as needed. There are no proofs to be followed.

The procedures discussed are limited to those that can be viewed as a form of regression analysis. As explained more completely in the first chapter, this means concentrating on statistical tools for which the conditional distribution of a response variable is the defining interest and for which characterizing the relationships between predictors and the response is undertaken in a serious and accessible manner.

Regression analysis provides a unifying theme that will ease translations across disciplines. It will also increase the comfort level for many scientists and policy analysts for whom regression analysis is a key data analysis tool. At the same time, a regression framework will highlight how the approaches discussed can be seen as alternatives to conventional causal modeling.

Because the goal is to convey how these procedures can be (and are being) used in practice, the material requires relatively in-depth illustrations and rather detailed information on the context in which the data analysis is being undertaken. The book draws heavily, therefore, on datasets with which I am very familiar. The same point applies to the software used and described.

The regression framework comes at a price. A 2005 announcement for a conference on data mining sponsored by the Society for Industrial and Applied Mathematics (SIAM) listed the following topics: query/constraint-based data mining, trend and periodicity analysis, mining data streams, data reduction/preprocessing, feature extraction and selection, post-processing, collaborative filtering/personalization, cost-based decision-making, visual data mining, privacy-sensitive data mining, and lots more. Many of these topics cannot be considered a form of regression analysis. For example, procedures used for edge detection (e.g., determining the boundaries of different kinds of land use from remote sensing data) are basically a filtering process to remove noise from the signal.

Another class of problems makes no distinction between predictors and responses. The relevant techniques can be closely related, at least in spirit, to procedures such as factor analysis and cluster analysis. One might explore, for example, the interaction patterns among children at school: who plays with whom. These too are not discussed.

Other topics can be considered regression analysis only as a formality. For example, a common data mining application in marketing is to extract from the purchasing behavior of individual shoppers patterns that can be used to forecast future purchases. But there are no predictors in the usual regression sense. The conditioning is on each individual shopper. The question is not what features of shoppers predict what they will purchase, but what a given shopper is likely to purchase.

Finally, there are a large number of procedures that focus on the conditional distribution of the response, much as with any regression analysis, but with little attention to how the predictors are related to the response (Horváth and Yamamoto 2006; Camacho et al. 2006). Such procedures neglect a key feature of regression analysis, at least as discussed in this book, and are not considered. That said, there is no principled reason in many cases why the role of each predictor could not be better represented, and perhaps in the near future that shortcoming will be remedied.

In short, although using a regression framework implies a big-tent approach to the topics included, it is not an exhaustive tent. Many interesting and powerful tools are not discussed. Where appropriate, however, references to that material are provided.

I may have gone a bit overboard with the number of citations I provide. The relevant literatures are changing and growing rapidly. Today's breakthrough can be tomorrow's bust, and work that by current thinking is uninteresting can be the spark for dramatic advances in the future. At any given moment, it can be difficult to determine which is which. In response, I have attempted to provide a rich mix of background material, even at the risk of not being sufficiently selective. (And I have probably missed some useful books and papers nevertheless.)

In the material that follows, I have tried to use consistent notation. This has proved to be very difficult because of important differences in the conceptual traditions represented and the complexity of statistical tools discussed. For example, it is common to see the use of the expected value operator even when the data cannot be characterized as a collection of random variables and when the sole goal is description.

I draw where I can from the notation used in *The Elements of Statistical Learning* (Hastie et al., 2001). When I am referring in general to certain kinds of variables or features, I used capital letters: X, Y, G, N, K, and so on. Thus, the symbol X is used for an input variable, or predictor in statistical parlance. When X is a set of inputs to be treated as a vector, each component (e.g., a variable) is indexed by a subscript (e.g., X_j). Quantitative outputs, also called response variables, are represented by Y, and categorical outputs, another kind of response variable, are represented by G with K categories. Sometimes these variables are treated as random variables, and sometimes not. I try to make that clear in context.

Observed values are represented in lowercase, usually with a subscript. Thus, x_i is the ith observed value for the variable X. Sometimes these observed values are nothing more than the data on hand. Sometimes they are realizations of random variables. Again, I try to make this clear in context.

Sometimes, it will be important to be explicit about definitions or operations in linear algebra notation. Then, matrices are represented in bold uppercase fonts. For example, in matrix form the usual set of p predictors, each with N observations, is an $N \times p$ matrix $\mathbf{X}$.[2] The subscript i is generally used for observations and the subscript j for variables. Bold lowercase letters are used for vectors, such as the columns of $\mathbf{X}$ or $\hat{\mathbf{y}}$ for fitted values.

If one treats Y as a random variable, its observed values y are either a random draw from a population or realizations of a stochastic process. The conditional means of the random variable Y for various configurations of $\mathbf{X}$-values are commonly referred to as "expected values" and are either the conditional means of Y for different configurations of $\mathbf{X}$-values in the population or for the stochastic process by which the data were generated. A common notation is $E(Y|\mathbf{X})$. The $E(Y|\mathbf{X})$ is also often called a "parameter." The conditional means computed from the data are often called "sample statistics," or in this case "sample means." In the regression context, the sample means are commonly referred to as the fitted values, often written as $\hat{\mathbf{y}}|\mathbf{X}$. Subscripting can follow as already described.

Unfortunately, after that it gets messier. First, I often have to decipher the intent in the notation used by others. No doubt I sometimes get it wrong. For example, it is often unclear if a computer algorithm is formally meant to be an estimator or a descriptor.

Second, there are some complications in representing nested realizations of the same variable (as in the bootstrap), or model output that is subject to several different chance processes. There is a practical limit to the number and types of bars, asterisks, hats, and tildes one can effectively use. I try to provide warnings (and apologies) when things get cluttered.

There are also some naming issues. When I am referring to the general linear model (i.e., linear regression, analysis of variance, and analysis of covariance), I use the terms classical linear regression or conventional linear regression. All regressions in which the functional forms are determined before the fitting process begins, I call parametric. All regressions in which the functional forms are determined as part of the fitting process, I call nonparametric. When there is some of both, I call the regressions semiparametric. Sometimes the lines between parametric, nonparametric, and semiparametric are fuzzy, but I try to make clear what I mean in context. Although these naming conventions are roughly consistent with much common practice, they are not universal.

All of the computing done for this book was undertaken in R. R is a programming language designed for statistical computing and graphics. It has become a major vehicle for developmental work in statistics and is increasingly being used by practitioners. A key reason for relying on R for this book is that most of the newest developments in statistical learning and related fields can be found in R. Another reason is that it is free.

Readers familiar with S or S-plus will immediately feel at home; R is basically a "dialect" of S. For others, there are several excellent books providing a good introduction to data analysis using R. Dalgaard (2002), Crawley (2007), and Maindonald and Braun (2007) are all very accessible. Readers who are especially interested in graphics should consult (Murrell 2006). The most useful R website can be found at http://www.r-project.org/.

The use of R raises the question of how much R code to include. The R code used to construct all of the applications in the book could be made available. However, detailed code is largely not shown. Many of the procedures used are somewhat in flux. Code that works 1 day may need some tweaking the next. As an alternative, the procedures discussed are identified as needed so that detailed information about how to proceed in R can be easily obtained from R help commands or supporting documentation. When the data used in this book are proprietary or otherwise not publicly available, similar data and appropriate R code are substituted.

There are exercises at the end of each chapter. They are meant to be hands-on data analyses built around R. As such, they require some facility with R. However, the goals of each problem are reasonably clear so that other software and datasets can be used. Often the exercises can be usefully repeated with different datasets.

The book has been written so that later chapters depend substantially on earlier chapters. For example, because classification and regression trees (CART) can be an important component of boosting, it may be difficult to follow the discussion of boosting without having read the earlier chapter on CART. However, readers who already have a solid background in material covered earlier should have little trouble skipping ahead. The notation and terms used are reasonably standard or can be easily figured out. In addition, the final chapter can be read at almost any time. One reviewer suggested that much of the material could be usefully brought forward to Chap. 1.

Finally, there is the matter of tone. The past several decades have seen the development of a dizzying array of new statistical procedures, sometimes introduced with the hype of a big-budget movie. Advertising from major statistical software providers has typically made things worse. Although there have been genuine and useful advances, none of the techniques has ever lived up to their most optimistic billing. Widespread misuse has further increased the gap between promised performance and actual performance. In this book, therefore, the tone will be cautious, some might even say dark. I hope this will not discourage readers from engaging seriously with the material. The intent is to provide a balanced discussion of the limitations as well as the strengths of the statistical learning procedures.

While working on this book, I was able to rely on support from several sources. Much of the work was funded by a grant from the National Science Foundation: SES-0437169, "Ensemble Methods for Data Analysis in the Behavioral, Social and Economic Sciences." The first draft was completed while I was on sabbatical at the Department of Earth, Atmosphere, and Oceans, at the Ecole Normale Supérieur in Paris. The second draft was completed after I moved from UCLA to the University of Pennsylvania. All three locations provided congenial working environments. Most important, I benefited enormously from discussions about statistical learning with colleagues at UCLA, Penn, and elsewhere: Larry Brown, Andreas Buja, Jan de Leeuw, David Freedman, Mark Hansen, Andy Liaw, Greg Ridgeway, Bob Stine, Mikhail Traskin, and Adi Wyner. Each is knowledgeable, smart, and constructive.

I also learned a great deal from several very helpful, anonymous reviews. Dick Koch was enormously helpful and patient when I had problems making TeXShop perform properly. Finally, I have benefited over the past several years from interacting with talented graduate students: Yan He, Weihua Huang, Brian Kriegler, and Jie Shen. Brian Kriegler deserves a special thanks for working through the exercises at the end of each chapter.

Certain datasets and analyses were funded as part of research projects undertaken for the California Policy Research Center, The Inter-America Tropical Tuna Commission, the National Institute of Justice, the County of Los Angeles, the California Department of Correction and Rehabilitation, the Los Angeles Sheriff's Department, and the Philadelphia Department of Adult Probation and Parole. Support from all of these sources is gratefully acknowledged.

Philadelphia, PA, USA   Richard A. Berk

Endnotes

[1] "Dirty" Harry Callahan was a police detective played by Clint Eastwood in five movies filmed during the 1970s and 1980s. Dirty Harry was known for his strong-armed methods and blunt catchphrases, many of which are now ingrained in American popular culture.

[2] A careful read would have already noticed an inconsistency. Why p and not P? P is often used to denote a probability, so in this setting p is used for clarity. These kinds of complications are also usually clear in context.

References

Berk, R. A. (2003). *Regression analysis: A constructive critique*. Newbury Park, CA.: SAGE.

Camacho, R., King, R., & Srinivasan, A. (2006). 14th international conference on inductive logic programming. *Machine Learning, 64*, 145–287.

Clarke, B., Fokoué, E, & Zhang, H. H. (2009). *Principles and theory of data mining and machine learning*. New York: Springer.

Crawley, M. J. (2007). *The R book*. New York: Wiley.

Dalgaard, P. (2002). *Introductory statistics with R*. New York: Springer.

Dwork, C., Hardt, M., Pitassi, T., Reingold, O., & Zemel, R. (2011). Fairness through awareness. arXiv:1104.3913v2 [cs.CC] 29 Nov 2011.

Hastie, T., Tibshirani, R., & Friedman, J. (2009). *The elements of statistical learning* (2nd edn.). New York: Springer.

Horváth, T., & Yamamoto, A. (2006). International conference on inductive logic programming. *Journal of Machine Learning, 64*, 3–144.

Jordan, M. I., & Mitchell, T. M. (2015). Machine learning: Trends, Perspectives, and Prospects. *Science, 349*(6234), 255–260.

Kuhn, M., & Johnson, K. (2013). *Applied predictive modeling*. New York: Springer.

Maindonald, J., & Braun, J. (2007). *Data analysis and graphics using R* (2nd edn.). Cambridge, UK: Cambridge University Press.

Murphy, K. P. (2012). *Machine learning: A probabilistic perspective*. Cambridge, Mass: MIT.

Murrell, P. (2006). *R graphics*. New York: Chapman & Hall/CRC.

Zemel, R., Wu, Y., Swersky, K., Pitassi, T., & Dwork, C. (2013). Learning fair representations. *Journal of Machine Learning Research, W & CP, 28*(3), 325–333.

Contents

Chapter 1
Statistical Learning as a Regression Problem

Summary This chapter makes four introductory points: (1) regression analysis is defined by the conditional distribution of $Y|X$, not by a conventional linear regression model; (2) different forms of regression analysis are properly viewed as approximations of the true relationships, which is a game changer; (3) statistical learning can be just another kind of regression analysis; (4) and properly formulated regression approximations can have asymptotically most of the desirable estimation properties. The emphasis on regression analysis is justified in part through a rebranding of least squares regression by some as a form of supervised machine learning. Once these points are made, the chapter turns to several key statistical concepts needed for statistical learning: overfitting, data snooping, loss functions, linear estimators, linear basis expansions, the bias–variance tradeoff, resampling, algorithms versus models, and others.

Before getting into the material, it will be useful to anticipate an ongoing theme throughout book. *Computing usually is easy. Figuring out what to compute and what the results mean can be very hard.* With modern hardware and software, all one really has learn in order to compute is how to make a data analysis procedure run. Current user interfaces typically make this rather simple to do. Some readers will be thinking that how to compute is all they need to know, and that this book can help. Although I hope this book can help in that manner, its main intent is to help data analysts compute smarter. That means understanding what is instructive to compute and how to convey what has been learned. Both can be very challenging and will usually depend substantially on subject-matter knowledge and the uses that will be made of the data analysis results. If the data analyst has sparse knowledge of either, partnering with others who can help may be a life saver.

It probably helpful to reprise and expand a bit on points made in the prefaces—most people do not read prefaces. First, there is no universally accepted term for the regression-like procedures that will be discussed. Options include machine learning, statistical learning, algorithmic modeling, nonparametric regression, pattern recog-

© Springer Nature Switzerland AG 2020

R. A. Berk, *Statistical Learning from a Regression Perspective*,

Springer Texts in Statistics, https://doi.org/10.1007/978-3-030-40189-4_1

nition, algorithmic learning, artificial intelligence, and others. These can differ in the procedures emphasized and disciplinary genealogy. The term statistical learning will be most commonly used early in the book because of an emphasis on concepts central to the discipline of statistics: uncertainty, estimation, statistical tests, and confidence intervals. These are far less visible for procedures developed in computer science. But it will be natural to gradually increase the use of terms and concepts from computer science later as the distance increases between conventional linear regression and the procedures discussed.

Second, any credible statistical analysis combines sound data collection, intelligent data management, an appropriate application of statistical procedures, and an accessible interpretation of results. This is sometimes what is meant by "analytics." More is involved than applied statistics. Most statistical textbooks focus on the statistical procedures alone, which can lead some readers to assume that if the technical background for a particular set of statistical tools is well understood, a sensible data analysis automatically follows. But as some would say, "That dog won't hunt."

Third, the coverage is highly selective. There are many excellent, encyclopedic, textbook treatments of statistical learning. Topics that some of them cover in several pages are covered here in an entire chapter. Data collection, data management, formal statistics, and interpretation are woven into the discussion where feasible. But there is a price. The range of statistical procedures covered is limited. Space constraints alone dictate hard choices. The procedures emphasized are those that can be framed as a form of regression analysis, have already proved to be popular, and have been battle tested. Some readers may disagree with the choices made. For those readers, there are ample references in which other methods are well addressed. However, it is becoming increasingly apparent that many of the procedures that properly can be treated as a regression analysis arrive at much the same results by somewhat different means. Each shiny new object that appears in the technical journals need not be mastered unless the different methods themselves are of interest.

Fourth, the ocean liner is slowly starting to turn. Over the past decade, the 50 years of largely unrebutted criticisms of conventional regression models and extensions have started to take. One reason is that statisticians have been providing useful alternatives. Another reason is the growing impact of computer science on how data are analyzed. Models are less salient in computer science than in statistics, and far less salient than in many popular forms of data analysis. Yet another reason is the growing and successful use of randomized controlled trials, which is implicitly an admission that far too much was expected from causal modeling. Finally, many of the most active and visible econometricians have been turning to various forms of quasi-experimental designs and new methods of analysis in part because conventional modeling often has been unsatisfactory. The pages ahead will draw heavily on these important trends.

Finally, there is a dirty little secret that applies to all expositions of statistical learning, including in this book. Errors are inevitable. Sometimes the author does not have a sufficient grasp of the material. Sometimes fields change rapidly and treatments become dated. Sometimes an author "misspeaks" or is at least unclear. Sometimes there are internal contradictions because claims made early in the book are forgotten by the time the last chapter is written. And sometimes it is just a matter of typos.

If there appears to be an error, there well could be an error. If the error seems important, follow up from other sources, many of which are cited below. An internet search can help. If you are a student, ask your instructor. Passive learning can be little different from no learning at all.

1.1   Getting Started

Statistical learning, especially when linked to machine learning or artificial intelligence, has been imbued by the media with near-supernatural powers. Yet, statistical learning is just a form of data analysis that can be well understood by ordinary people. As a first approximation, one can think of statistical learning as the "muscle car" version of exploratory data analysis (EDA). Just as in EDA, the data can be approached with relatively little prior information and examined in a highly inductive manner. Knowledge discovery can be a key goal. But thanks to the enormous developments in computing power and computer algorithms over the past two decades, it is possible to extract information that previously would have been inaccessible. In addition, because statistical learning has evolved in a number of different disciplines, its goals and approaches are far more varied than conventional EDA.

Statistical learning as subsequently discussed also can be usefully approached as little more than fancy variants of regression analysis. It is all about the conditional distribution of a response variable Y and a one or more predictors X; that is, $Y|X$. Researchers in statistics, applied mathematics, and computer science responsible for most statistical learning techniques often employ their own distinct jargon and have a taste for attaching cute, but somewhat obscure, labels to their products: bagging, boosting, bundling, random forests, neural networks, and others. There also is widespread use of acronyms: CART, LOESS, MARS, MART, LARS, LASSO, CNN, RNN, and many more. A regression framework provides a helpful structure in which these procedures can be more easily understood.

Beyond connections to EDA and regression analysis, statistical learning can be seen as seeking a balance between a very complex fit of the data and regularization compensating for unstable results.[1] Complex fitting of a dataset can in principle reduce statistical bias when the "truth" also is complex. Intricate patterns in the data are better captured. But, by responding to very local features of the data responsible for the complexity, information in the data can be distributed very thinly. With new data, even realized in the same fashion, the results may change dramatically because many local features of the data will differ.[2] Regularization can tamp down this volatility. All of the more effective statistical learning procedures discussed in the pages ahead are basically regularizations of regression fitting exercises that respond aggressively to complicated patterns in data.

After a discussion of how statisticians think about regression analysis, this chapter introduces several key concepts and raises broader issues that reappear in later chapters. It may be a little difficult at first reading for some readers to follow parts of the discussion, or its motivation, and some of the material intentionally will be out of step with conventional practice. However, later chapters will flow far more smoothly with some of this preliminary material introduced, and readers are encouraged to return to the chapter as needed.

1.2 Setting the Regression Context

We begin by defining regression analysis. A common conception in many academic disciplines and policy applications equates regression analysis with some special case of the generalized linear model: normal (linear) regression, binomial regression, Poisson regression, or other less common forms. Sometimes, there is more than one such equation, as with hierarchical models in which the regression coefficients in one equation can be expressed as responses within other equations, or when a set of equations is linked through their response variables. For any of these formulations, inferences are often made beyond the data to some larger finite population or a data generation process. Commonly these inferences are combined with statistical tests and confidence intervals. It is also popular to overlay causal interpretations meant to convey how the response distribution would change if one or more of the predictors were independently manipulated.

But statisticians and computer scientists typically start farther back. Regression is "just" about conditional distributions. The goal is to understand "as far as possible with the available data how the conditional distribution of some response **y** varies across subpopulations determined by the possible values of the predictor or predictors" (Cook and Weisberg 1999: 27). That is, interest centers on the distribution of the response variable Y conditioning on one or more predictors X. Regression analysis fundamentally is about conditional distributions: $Y|X$.

For example, Fig. 1.1 is a conventional scatter plot for an infant's birthweight in grams and the mother's weight in pounds.[3] Birthweight can be an important indicator of a newborn's viability, and there is a reason to believe that birthweight depends in part on the health of the mother. A mother's weight can be an indicator of her health.

In Fig. 1.1, the open circles are the observations. The filled circles are the conditional means, the likely summary statistics of interest. An inspection of the pattern of observations is by itself a legitimate regression analysis. Does the conditional distribution of birthweight vary depending on the mother's weight? If the conditional mean is chosen as the key summary statistic, one can consider whether the conditional means for infant birthweight vary with the mother's weight.

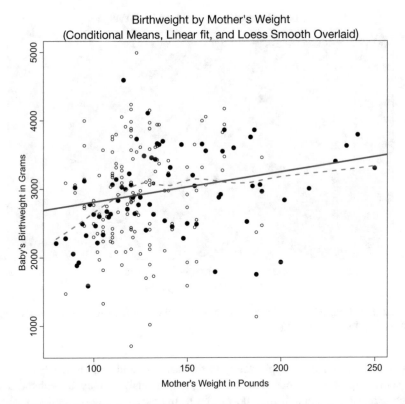

Fig. 1.1 Birthweight by Mother's weight (open circles are the data, filled circles are the conditional means, the solid line is a linear regression fit, the dashed line is a fit by a smoother. $N = 189$)

This too is a legitimate regression analysis. In both cases, however, it is difficult to conclude much from inspection alone.

The solid blue line is a linear least squares fit of the data. On the average, birthweight increases with the mother's weight, but the slope is modest (about 44 g for every 10 pounds), especially given the spread of the birthweight values. For many, this is a familiar form of regression analysis. The dashed red line shows the fitted values for a smoother (i.e., lowess) that will be discussed in the next chapter as yet another variant on regression analysis. One can see that the linear relationship breaks down when the mother weighs less than about 100 pounds. There is then a much stronger relationship in part because average birthweight can be under 2000 g (i.e., around 4 pounds). This regression analysis suggests that on the average, the relationship between birthweight and mother's weights is nonlinear.

None of the regression analyses just undertaken depend on a "generative" model; no claims are made about how the data were generated. There are also no causal claims about how mean birthweight would change if a mother's weight were altered (e.g., through better nutrition). And, there is no statistical inference whatsoever.

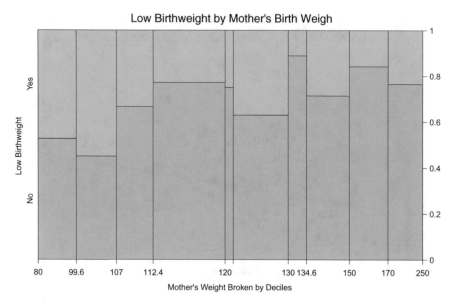

Fig. 1.2 Low Birthweight by Mother's weight with Birthweight Dichotomized (Mother's weight is binned by deciles. $N = 189$)

The regression analyses apply solely to the data on hand and are not generalized to some large set of observations. A regression analysis may be enhanced by such extensions, although they do not go to the core of how regression analysis is defined. In practice, a richer story would likely be obtained were additional predictors introduced, perhaps as "controls," but that too is not a formal requirement of regression analysis. Finally, visualizations of various kinds can be instructive and by themselves can constitute a regression analysis.

The same reasoning applies should the response be categorical. Figure 1.2 is a spine plot that dichotomizes birthweight into two categories: low and not low. For each decile of mothers' weights, the conditional proportion is plotted. For example, if a mother's weight is between 150 and 170 pounds, a little under 20% of the newborns have low birthweights. But if a mother's weight is less than 107 pounds, around 50% of the newborns have low birthweights.

The reasoning applies as well if both the response and the predictor are categorical. Figure 1.3 shows a mosaic plot for whether or not a newborn is underweight and whether or not the newborn's mother smoked. The area of each rectangle is proportional to the number of cases in the respective cell of the corresponding 2×2 table. One can see that the majority of mothers do not smoke and a majority of the newborns are not underweight. The red cell contains fewer observations than would be expected under independence, and the blue cell contains more observations than would be expected under independence. The metric is the Pearson residual for that cell (i.e., the contribution to the χ^2 statistic). Mothers who smoke are more likely to have low birthweight babies. If one is prepared to articulate a credible generative

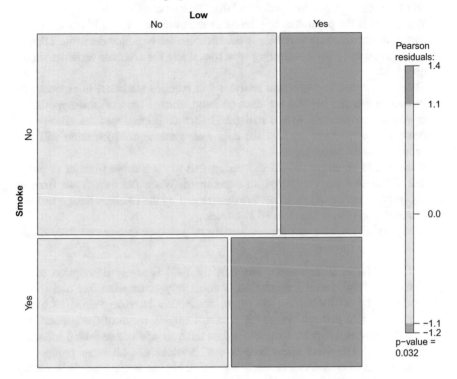

Fig. 1.3 Whether the Mother Smokes by Low Birthweight with Pearson Residuals Assuming Independence (Red indicates fewer cases than expected under independence. Blue indicates more cases than expected under independence. $N = 189$)

model consistent with a conventional test of independence, independence is rejected at the 0.03 level. Much more will be said about such assumptions later. But even without a statistical test, the mosaic represents a legitimate regression analysis.[4]

There are several lessons highlighted by these brief illustrations.

- As discussed in more depth shortly, the regression analyses just conducted made no direct use of models. Each is best seen as a *procedure*. One might well have preferred greater use of numerical summaries and algebraic formulations, but regression analyses were undertaken nevertheless. In the pages ahead, it will be important to dispense with the view that a regression analysis automatically requires arithmetic summaries or algebraic models. Once again, regression is just about conditional distributions.
- Visualizations of various kinds can be a key feature of a regression analysis. Indeed, they can be the defining feature.
- A regression analysis does not have to make conditional means the key distributional feature of interest, although conditional means or proportions dominate

current practice. With the increasing availability of powerful visualization procedures, for example, entire conditional distributions can be examined.

- Whether it is the predictors of interest or the covariates to "hold constant," the
  choice of conditioning variables is a subject-matter or policy decision. There is
  nothing in data by itself indicating what role, if any, the available variables should
  play.[5]
- There is nothing in regression analysis that requires statistical inference: estimation inferences beyond the data on hand, formal tests of null hypotheses,
  or confidence intervals. When statistical inference is employed, its validity will
  depend fundamentally on how the data were generated. Much more will said
  about this in the pages ahead.
- If there is to be cause-and-effect overlay, that too is a subject-matter or policy
  call unless one has conducted an experiment. When the data result from an
  experiment, the causal variables are determined by the research design and real
  manipulation of variables treated as causes.
- A regression analysis can serve a variety of purposes that are usefully distinguished.

  1. For a "Level I" regression analysis, the goal is solely description of the
     data on hand. Level I regression is effectively assumption-free and should
     always be on the table. Too often, description is under-valued as a data
     analysis tool perhaps because it does not employ much of the apparatus of
     conventional statistics. How can a data analysis without statistical inference
     be good? The view taken here is that p-values and all other products of
     statistical inference can certainly be useful, but are worse than useless when
     a credible rationale cannot be provided (Berk and Freedman 2003). Assume-
     and-proceed statistics is not likely to advance science or policy. Yet, important
     progress frequently can be made from statistically informed description alone.
  2. For a "Level II" regression analysis, statistical inference is the defining
     activity. Estimation is undertaken using the results from a Level I regression,
     often in concert with statistical tests and confidence intervals. Statistical
     inference forms the core of conventional statistics, but proper use with real
     data can be very challenging; real data may not correspond well to what
     the inferential tools require. For the statistical procedures emphasized here,
     statistical inference will often be overmatched. There can be a substantial
     disconnect between the requirements of proper statistical inference and
     adaptive statistical procedures such as those central to statistical learning.
     Forecasting, which will play an important role in the pages ahead, is also a
     Level II activity because projections are made from data on hand to the values
     of certain variables that are unobserved when the forecasts are made. (If the
     values were observed, there would be no need for forecasts.)
  3. For a "Level III" regression analysis, causal inference is overlaid on the
     results of a Level I regression analysis, often coupled with Level II results.
     There can be demanding conceptual issues such as specifying a sensible
     "counterfactual." For example, one might consider the impact of the death

penalty on crime; states that have the death penalty are compared to states that do not. But what is the counterfactual to which the death penalty being compared? Is it life imprisonment without any chance of parole, a long prison term of, say, 20 years, or probation? In many states the counterfactual is life in prison with no chance of parole. Also, great care is needed to adjust for the possible impact of confounders. In the death penalty example, one might at least want to control for average clearance rate in each of the state's police departments. Clearance rates for some kinds of homicides are very low, which means that it is pretty easy to get away with murder, and then the death penalty is largely irrelevant.[6] Level III regression analysis will not figure significantly in the pages ahead because of a reliance on algorithmic methods rather than model-based methods (Breiman 2001b). The important distinction between models and algorithms will be considered in depth shortly.

In summary, a focus on conditional distributions will be a central feature in all that follows. One does not require generative models, statistical inference, or causal inference. On the one hand, a concentration on conditional distribution may seem limiting. On the other hand, a concentration on conditional distributions may seem liberating. In practice, both can be true and be driven substantially by deficiencies in conventional modeling to which we now briefly turn.

Of necessity, the next several sections are more technical and more conceptually demanding. Readers with a substantial statistical background should have no problems, although some conventional ways of thinking will need to be reconsidered. There also may need to be an attitude adjustment. Readers without a substantial statistical background might be best served by skimming the content primarily to see the topics addressed, and then returning to the material as needed when in subsequent chapters those topics arise.

1.3   Revisiting the Ubiquitous Linear Regression Model

Although conditional distributions are the foundation for all that follows, linear regression is its most common manifestation in practice and needs to be explicitly addressed. For many, linear regression is the canonical procedure for examining conditional relationship, or at least the default. Therefore, a brief review of its features and requirements can be a useful didactic device to highlight similarities to and differences from statistical learning.

When a linear regression analysis is formulated, conventional practice combines a Level I and Level II perspective. Important features of the data are conceptually embedded in how the data were generated. Y is an $N \times 1$ numerical response variable, where N is the number of observations. There is an $N \times (p + 1)$ "design matrix" $\mathbf{X}$, where p is the number of predictors (sometimes called "regressors"). A leading column of 1s is usually included in $\mathbf{X}$ for reasons that will clear momentarily. Y is treated as a random variable. The p predictors in $\mathbf{X}$ are taken to be fixed. In new realizations of the data, Y can vary, but $\mathbf{X}$ cannot; the values of the predictors do not change. Some readers may not have appreciated this requirement, and it has wide ranging implications for such matters as generalizability, which will be addressed later in this chapter. Whether predictors are fixed or random is not a technical detail.

For any single observation i, the process by which the values of Y are realized then takes the form

$$y_i = \beta_0 + \beta_1 x_{1i} + \beta_2 x_{2i} + \cdots + \beta_p x_{pi} + \varepsilon_i, \tag{1.1}$$

where

$$\varepsilon_i \sim \text{NIID}(0, \sigma^2). \tag{1.2}$$

β_0 is the y-intercept associated with the leading column 1s. There are p regression coefficients and a random perturbation ε_i. One can say that for each case i, nature sets the values of the predictors, multiplies each predictor value by its corresponding regression coefficient, sums these products, adds the value of the constant, and then adds a random perturbation. Each perturbation, ε_i, is a random variable realized as if drawn at random and independently from a single distribution, often assumed to be normal, with a mean of 0.0. In short, nature behaves as if she adopts a linear model.

There are several important implications. To begin, the values of Y can be realized repeatedly for a given case because its values will vary solely because of ε_i. The predictor values never change. Thus, for a *given* high school student, one imagines that there could be a limitless number of scores on the mathematics SAT, solely because of the "noise" represented by ε_i. All else in nature's linear combination is fixed: the number of hours spent in an SAT preparation course, motivation to perform well, the amount of sleep the night before, the presence of distractions while the test is being taken, and so on. This is more than an academic formality. It is a substantive theory about how SAT scores come to be. For a given student and the student's fixed predictor values, nature stipulates that an observed SAT score can differ by chance alone in new realizations of the data.[7]

If on substantive grounds, one allows for nature to set more than one value for any given predictor and a given student (e.g., how much sleep the student got the night before the SAT was taken), a temporal process is implied, and there is systematic temporal variation to build into the regression formulation. For example, the student might take the SAT a second time several months later, in which case many predictors might be set by nature to new values. A formulation of this sort can certainly be developed, but it would be more complicated (i.e., there would be variation across students *and* over time), require that nature be even more cooperative, and for the points to be made here, adds unnecessary complexity.

From Eqs. (1.1) and (1.2), it can be conceptually helpful to distinguish between the mean function and the disturbance function (also called the variance function). The mean function is the expectation of Eq. (1.1). When in practice a data analyst specifies a conventional linear regression model, it will be "first-order correct" when the data analyst (a) knows what nature is using as predictors, (b) knows what transformations, if any, nature applies to those predictors, (c) knows that the predictors are combined in a linear fashion, and (d) has those predictors in the dataset to be analyzed. For conventional linear regression, these are the first-order conditions: the mean function applied to the data is the mean function used by nature. The only unknowns in the mean function are the values of the y-intercept and the regression coefficients. Clearly, these are daunting hurdles.

The disturbance function is Eq. (1.2). When in practice the data analyst specifies a conventional linear regression model, it will be "second-order correct" when the data analyst knows that each perturbation is realized independently of all other perturbations and that each is realized from a single distribution that has an expectation of 0.0. Because there is a single disturbance distribution, one can say that the variance of that distribution is "constant." These are the usual second-order conditions. Sometimes the data analyst also knows the functional form of the distribution. If that distribution is the normal, the only distribution unknown whose value needs to be estimated is its variance σ^2.

When the first-order conditions are met and ordinary least squares is applied to the data, estimates of the slope and y-intercept are unbiased estimates of the corresponding values that nature uses. This also applies to the fitted values, which are unbiased estimates of the conditional expectations for each configuration of x-values.

When in addition to the first-order conditions, the second-order conditions are met, and ordinary least squares is applied to the data, the disturbance variance can be estimated in an unbiased fashion using the residuals from the realized data. Also, conventional confidence intervals and statistical tests are valid, and by the Gauss–Markov theorem, each estimated β has the smallest possible sampling variation of any other linear estimator of nature's regression parameters. In short, one has the ideal textbook results for a Level II regression analysis. Similar reasoning properly can be applied to the entire generalized linear model and its multi-equation extensions, although usually that reasoning depends on asymptotics.[8]

Finally, even for a conventional regression analysis, there is no need to move to Level III. Causal interpretations are surely important when they can be justified, but they are an add-on, not an essential element. With observational data, moreover, causal inference can be very controversial (Freedman 1987, 2004).

1.3.1 Problems in Practice

There is a wide variety of practical problems with the conventional linear model, many recognized well over a generation ago, that jeopardize fundamentally all of the desirable properties of a properly specified linear regression model (e.g., Leamer 1978; Rubin 1986, 2008; Freedman 1987, 2004; Berk 2003). This is not the venue for an extensive review, and David Freedman's excellent text on statistical models

(2009a) can be consulted for an unusually cogent discussion. Nevertheless, it will prove useful later to mention now a few of the most common and vexing difficulties. These will carry over to the less familiar and more complicated procedures discussed in subsequent chapters. The linear model formulation provides convenient platform on which to build.

There is effectively no way to know whether the model specified by the analyst is the means by which nature actually generated the data. And there is also no way to know how close to the "truth" a specified model really is. One would need to know that truth to quantify a model's disparities from the truth, and if the truth were known, there would be no need to analyze any data to begin with. Consequently, all concerns about model specification are translated into whether the model is good enough.

There are three popular strategies addressing the "good enough" requirement. First, there exist a large number of regression diagnostics taking a variety of forms and using a variety of techniques including graphical procedures, statistical tests, and the comparative performance of alternative model specifications (Weisberg 2013: chapter 9). These tools can be useful in identifying problems with the linear model, but they can miss serious problems as well. Most are designed to detect single difficulties in isolation when in practice, there can be many difficulties at once. Is evidence of nonconstant variance a result of mean function misspecification, disturbances generated from different distributions, or both? In addition, diagnostic tools derived from formal statistical tests typically have weak statistical power (Freedman 2009b), and when the null hypothesis is not rejected, analysts commonly "accept" the null hypothesis that all is well. In fact, there are effectively a limitless number of other null hypotheses that would also not be rejected.[9] Finally, even if some error in the model is properly identified, there may be little or no guidance on how to fix it, especially within the limitation of the data available.

Second, reference is made to common disciplinary practices: "everyone else does it." Such justifications are actually admissions of ignorance, laziness, or cowardice. The recent controversies surrounding reproducibility in science (Open Science Collaboration 2015) help to underscore that common practice is not necessarily good practice and that because the disciplines of statistics and computer science continue to evolve, standards for sound research continue to evolve as well.

Third, claims are made on subject-matter grounds that the results make sense and are consistent with — or at least not contradicted by — existing theory and past research. This line of reasoning can be a source of good science and good policy, but also misses the point. One might learn useful things from a data analysis even if the model specified is dramatically different from how nature generated the data. Indeed, this perspective is emphasized many times in the pages ahead. But advancing a scientific or policy discourse does not imply that the model used is right, or even close.

If a model's results are sufficiently useful, why should this matter? It matters because one cannot use the correctness of the model by itself to justify the subject-matter claims made. For example, interesting findings said to be the direct product of an elaborate model specification might have surfaced just as powerfully from several scatterplots. The findings rest on a very few strong associations easily revealed by simple statistical tools. The rest is pretense.

It matters because certain features of the analysis used to bolster substantive claims may be fundamentally wrong and misleading. For example, if a model is not first-order correct, the probabilities associated with statistical tests are almost certainly incorrect. Even if valid standard errors are obtained, the relevant estimate from the data will on the average be offset by its bias. If the bias moves the estimate away from the null hypothesis, the estimated p-values will be on the average too small. If the bias moves the estimate toward the null hypothesis, the estimated p-values will on the average be too large. In a similar fashion, confidence intervals will be offset in one of the two directions.

It matters because efforts to diagnose and fix model specification problems can lead to new and sometime worse difficulties. For example, one response to a model that does not pass muster is to re-specify the model and re-estimate the model's parameters. But it is now well-known that model selection and model estimation undertaken on the same data (e.g., statistical tests for a set of nested models) lead to biased estimates even if by some good fortune the correct model happens to be found (Leeb and Pötscher 2005, 2006, 2008; Berk et al. 2010, 2014a).[10] The model specification itself is a product of the realized data and a source of additional uncertainty; with a different realized dataset, one may arrive at a different model. As a formal matter, statistical tests assume that the model has been specified *before* the data are examined.[11] This is no longer true. The result is not just more uncertainty overall, but a particular form of uncertainty that can result in badly biased estimates of the regression coefficients and pathological sampling distributions.

And finally, it matters because it undermines the credibility of statistical procedures in general. There will be times when an elaborate statistical procedure is really needed that performs as advertised. But why should the results be believed when word on the street is that data analysts routinely make claims that are not justified by the statistical tools employed?

1.4   Working with Statistical Models that are Wrong

Is there an alternative way to proceed that can be more satisfactory and help inform later chapters? The answer requires a little deeper look at conventional practice. Emphasis properly is placed on the word "practice." There are no fundamental quarrels with the mathematical statistics on which conventional practice rests.

To get things started, we focus on properties of a very large, *finite*, population with a numeric response Y and a single numeric predictor X. The finite population might be all registered voters in the United States. Far more formal detail will be provided later.

As shown in Fig. 1.4, X and Y are related in a simple but nonlinear manner. There is the population's "true response surface" (shown in red) that is comprised of the true means of Y for different values of X. These are conditional means. They will

Fig. 1.4 The true response
surface in red and population
best linear approximation for
a single predictor in blue

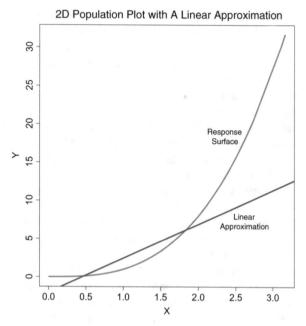

become conditional expectations or conditional probabilities later when we move
beyond finite populations. The true response surface is what one would ideally like
to estimate with data from this very large, finite population.

There is also a linear approximation of the true response surface shown in blue.
It too is comprised of means of Y for different values of X; they too are conditional
means. We will see later that the linear approximation can be the population's "best"
linear approximation of the true response surface, and that with data can be properly
estimated using linear regression. Clearly, the true response surface and the linear
approximation are different.

These ideas carry over when there is more than a single predictor. Figure 1.5
shows a two predictor setting. The plotting style is somewhat different from Fig. 1.4
to make it more accessible with the additional predictor. The population distribution
is nonlinear, actually the product of X and Y. But a plane for the two additive
predictors is shown. It can be a population's best linear approximation as well. With
more than two predictors, the best linear approximation is a hyperplane.

Now consider estimation. How does one proceed when the linear regression
model does not meet the first-order and second-order conditions? Do you push
through as if the conditions are met, perhaps offering occasional mia cuplas, or
do you do the best you can with a model that is openly acknowledged to be
misspecified?

Model misspecification is hardly a new topic, and some very smart statisticians
and econometricians have been working on it for decades. One tradition concentrates on trying to patch up models that are misspecified. The other tradition tries to

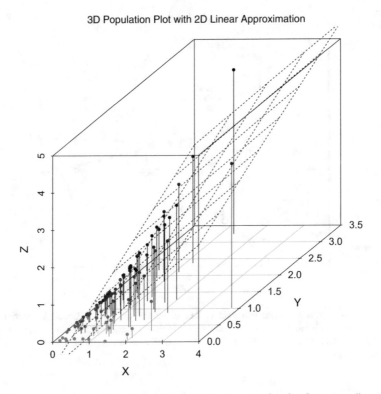

Fig. 1.5 A true response surface and population best linear approximation for two predictors (The true response surface is the product of X and Y. The linear approximation is linear least squares fit summing X and Y. Larger values of Z are in black. Smaller values of Z are in Red)

work constructively with misspecified models. We will proceed within the second tradition. For many statisticians and practitioners, this can require a major attitude adjustment.

Figure 1.6 is a highly stylized representation of the sort of practical problems that can follow for a Level II analysis when for a linear model one assumes incorrectly that the first- and second-order conditions are met. The figure is not a scatterplot but an effort to illustrate some key ideas from the relevant statistical theory "in" the population. For simplicity, but with no important loss of generality for the issues to be addressed, there is a single numeric predictor on the horizontal axis. For now, that predictor is assumed to be fixed.[12] The numeric response variable is on the vertical axis.

The red, horizontal lines in Fig. 1.6 are the true conditional means that constitute the population response surface. They are the true response surface exactly as just described, but only a few conditional means are shown for visual simplicity.

The vertical, black, dotted lines represent the distribution of y-values around each conditional mean. These distributions are also a feature of the population.

Estimation Using a Linear Function

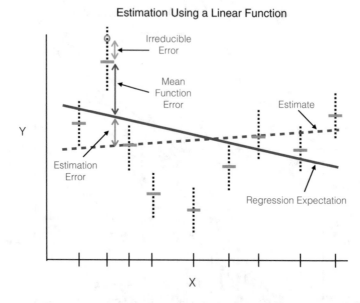

Fig. 1.6 Estimating a nonlinear response surface under the true linear model perspective (The broken line is an estimate from a given dataset, solid line is the expectation of such estimates, the vertical dotted lines represent conditional distributions of Y with the red bars as each conditional distribution's mean)

No assumptions are made about what form the distributions take, but for didactic convenience, each conditional distribution is assumed to have the same variance.

An eyeball interpolation of the true conditional means reveals an approximate U-shaped relationship but with substantial departures from that simple pattern. A data analyst is provided with values of X and Y. The red circle is one such y-value. More details will follow shortly.

A data analyst assumes the usual linear model $y_i = \beta_0 + \beta_1 x_i + \varepsilon_i$. This means that the data analysis proceeds as if the data on hand are produced exactly as the linear regression equation requires. As before, nature adopts a linear model.

With a set of *realized* y-values and their corresponding x-values (not shown), estimates $\hat{\beta}_0$, $\hat{\beta}_1$, and $\hat{\sigma}^2$ are obtained. The broken blue line shows an estimated mean function. One can imagine nature using the model to generate many (formally, a limitless number) such datasets in the same manner so that there are many mean function estimates that will naturally vary because the realized values y will change from dataset to dataset.[13] The solid blue line represents the expectation of those many estimates that can be seen as the average regression line over datasets. The regression expectation looks like it might be the population best linear approximation, but formally it is not. It is an average over many datasets, not a feature of the population.

Clearly, the assumed linear mean function is incorrect because the true conditional means do not fall on any straight line. The blue, two-headed arrow shows the bias at one value of x. The size and direction of the biases differ over the values of x because the disparities between regression expectation and the true conditional means differ. This is a key point.

The data analyst does not get to work with the expectation of the estimated regression lines. Usually, the data analyst gets to work with one such line. The random variation captured by one such line is shown with the magenta, double-headed error. Even if the broken blue line fell right on top of the solid blue line, and if both went exactly through the true conditional mean being used as an illustration, there would still be a gap between the true value of Y (the red circle) and that conditional mean (the short red horizontal line). In Fig. 1.6, that gap is represented by the green, double-headed arrow. It is sometimes called "irreducible error" because it exists even if the population response surface is known.

To summarize, the blue double-headed arrow shows the bias in the estimated regression line, the magenta double-headed arrow shows the impact of the variability in that estimate, and the green double-headed arrow shows the irreducible error. For any given estimated mean function, the distance between the estimated regression line and a realized y-value is a combination of mean function error (also called mean function misspecification), random variation in the estimated regression line caused by ε_i, and the variability in ε_i itself. Sometimes these can cancel each other out, at least in part, but all three will always be in play.

Some might claim that instrumental variables provide a way out. Instrumental variable procedures in fact can correct for some forms of estimation bias if (a) a valid instrument can be found and if (b) the sample size is large enough to capitalize on asymptotics. But the issues can be tricky (Bound et al. 1995; Freedman 1987, section 8.2). A successful instrument does not address all mean function problems. For example, it cannot correct for wrong functional forms nor multiple sources of bias. Also, it can be very difficult to find a credible instrumental variable. Even if one succeeds, an instrumental variable may remove most of the regression coefficient bias and simultaneously cause a very large increase in the variance of the regression coefficient estimate. On the average, the regression line is actually farther away from the true conditional means even though the bias is largely eliminated. One arguably is worse off.

It is a simple matter to alter the mean function. Perhaps something other than a straight line can be used to accurately represent the true conditional means. However, one is still required to get the first-order conditions right. That is, the mean function must be correct. Figure 1.7 presents the same kinds of difficulties as Fig. 1.6. All three sources of error remain: mean function misspecification, sampling variability in the function estimated, and the irreducible error. Comparing the two figures, the second seems to have on the average a less biased regression expectation, but in practice it is difficult to know whether that is true or not. Perhaps more important, it is impossible to know how much bias remains.[14]

One important implication of both Figs. 1.6 and 1.7 is that the variation in the realized observations around the fitted values will not be constant. To anticipate the formulation that will be introduced more fully shortly, suppose X is a random variable. The bias, which varies across x-values, then is incorporated in the

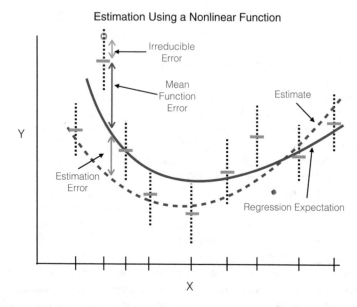

Fig. 1.7 Estimating a nonlinear response surface under the true nonlinear model perspective (The broken line is an estimate from a given dataset, solid line is the expectation of such estimates, the vertical dotted lines represent conditional distributions of Y with the red bars as each distribution's mean)

population residuals. Because X now is random, bias as traditionally defined becomes a source of nonconstant variance. To the data analyst, this can look like heteroscedasticity even if the variation in ε_i is actually constant. Conventional estimates of σ^2 will likely be incorrect. Incorrect standard errors for the intercept and slope follow, which jeopardize statistical tests and confidence intervals.

Such problems resulting from an incorrect mean function were powerfully addressed by Halbert White (1980a). His "sandwich" estimator—more on that soon—can provide asymptotically valid standard errors despite the nonconstant variance produced a misspecified mean function. However, proper standard errors do *not* lead to valid statistical tests and confidence intervals. If the estimation target is the true response surface, statistical tests will be biased (even asymptotically) and confidence intervals will not cover as they should. Estimated test statistic values will be systematically offset. They will be too large or two small. The p-values that follow will systematically be too large or too small as well. The requirement of proper mean function specification remains and is too commonly is overlooked. Sandwich standard errors with a misspecified mean function do not produce valid statistical tests and confidence intervals if the estimation target is the true response surface (Freedman 2012).

The introduction of random predictor variables may seem a diversion for a discussion of the conventional linear regression model. But, random predictors and their consequences will play big as we move forward. The next section provides an alternative approach to "wrong" models that builds on predictors as random variables.

To summarize, if one can be satisfied with a Level I regression analysis, the difficulties just described disappear. A satisfactory data analysis will depend substantially on how well instructive patterns in the data are revealed.

Alternatively one can live with at least some bias. Unbiased estimates of the nature's (true) response surface are not a prerequisite if one can be satisfied with estimates of nature's true response surface that are close on the average over realizations of the data. In particular, there can be bias, if in trade there is a substantial reduction in the variance. We will see that in practice, it can be difficult to decrease both the bias and the variance, but often there will be ways to arrive at a beneficial balance in what is called the "bias–variance tradeoff." Still, as long as any bias remains, statistical tests and confidence intervals need to be reconsidered. As for the irreducible variance, it is still irreducible.

A final option is to reformulate conventional linear regression so that the estimation task is more modest. This fundamentally changes the enterprise and requires lots of rethinking and even unlearning. It too will play well in later chapters and will be an important part of our end game. We now settle for an introduction.

1.4.1   An Alternative Approach to Regression

The material in this section is not just a useful way to reformulate linear regression, but a foundation we later need to consider statistical inference for statistical learning. The ideas are conceptually demanding and have layers. There are also lots of details. It may be helpful, therefore, to make three introductory observations. First, in the words of George Box, "All models are wrong..." (Box 1976). It follows that one must learn to work with wrong models and not proceed as if they are right. This is a large component of what follows. Second, if one is to work with wrong models, the estimation target is also a wrong model. Standard practice has the "true" model as the estimation target. In other words, one should be making correct inferences to an incorrect model rather than making incorrect inferences to a correct model. Third, these initial points set the stage for working with data analysis procedures not based on models, but based on algorithms for which, as we will consider shortly, the idea misspecification is no longer even relevant. Let us see how all this plays out.

If a data analyst wants to employ a Level II regression analysis, inferences from the data must be made to something. Within conventional conceptions, that something is the set of parameters for the linear model used by nature to generate the data. The parameters are the estimation targets. Given the values of those parameters and their fixed-x values, each y_i is realized by the linear model shown in Eqs. (1.1) and (1.2).[15]

Consider as an alternative what one might call the "joint probability distribution model." It has much the same look and feel as the "correlation model" formulated by Freedman (1981), and is very similar to a "linear approximation" perspective proposed by White (1980a). Both have important roots in the work of Huber (1967) and Eicker (1963, 1967). Angrist and Pischke (2009: section 3.1.2) provide a very accessible introduction, although it is now a bit dated.

For the substantive or policy issues at hand, one imagines that there exists a substantively relevant, joint probability distribution composed of variables represented by Z. The joint probability distribution has familiar parameters such as the mean (i.e., the expected value) and variance for each variable and the covariances between variables. No distinctions are made between predictors and responses.

Nature can realize independently a limitless number of observations from the joint probability distribution. More formally, one can say that each observation is realized IID; each realized case is generated at random, independently of all other realized cases, from the same joint probability distribution.[16] This is how the data are generated. One might call the process by which observations are realized from the joint probability distribution the "true generative model." In short, features of the joint probability distribution are the "what" to which inferences are to be made in a Level II analysis.

A conceptually equivalent "what" is to imagine a population of limitless size that represents all possible realizations from the joint probability distribution. Inferences are made from the realized data to features of this "infinite population." In some circles, that population is called a "superpopulation."

Closely related ideas can work for finite populations (Cochran 1977: chapter 7). For example, the data can be a simple random sample from a well-defined population that is in principle observable. This is the way one usually thinks about sample surveys, such as well-done political polls. The population is all registered voters, and a probability sample is drawn for analysis. In finite populations, the population variables are fixed; They are not random variables. There is a joint distribution of all the variables in the population that is essentially a multivariate histogram. Still, one can use one's frequentist imagination to extend insights about finite populations to limitless populations.

Data analysts will typically distinguish within Z between predictors X and a response Y. Some of Z may be substantively irrelevant and ignored.[17] In contrast to conventional regression analysis, *these distinctions have nothing to do with how the data are generated.* They derive from the preferences of individuals who will be analyzing the data. The difference between data generated by a linear model and data generated IID from a joint probability distribution marks a very important transition fundamental to later chapters.

Generalizing from the earlier discussion with a single predictor, for any particular regression analysis, attention then turns to a conditional distribution of Y given some $X = x$. For example, X could be predictors of longevity, and x is the predictor values for a given individual. These values might be 42 years of age, working full time, married, and no history of heart disease. The distribution of Y is thought to vary from one x to another x. Variation in the conditional mean of Y is usually the primary concern. But now, because the number of observations in the population is limitless, one should, as a formality, think about the $E[\mu(x)]$.[18]

The values for $E[\mu(x)]$ constitute a "true response surface." This true response surface determines the way the expected values of Y are actually related to X within the joint probability distribution. It is unknown. Disparities between the $E[\mu(x)]$ and the potential values of Y are the "true disturbances" and necessarily have an expectation of 0.0.[19]

Now we make another very important transition essential for later chapters. The data analyst specifies a working regression model using a conventional, linear mean function meant to characterize *another* response surface within the same joint probability distribution. Beginning in the next chapter, we will consider more flexible mean functions.

The conditional expectations of this other response surface are equal to a linear combination of predictors, in matrix notation, $X\beta$. The response y is then taken to be $X\beta + \varepsilon$, where β is an array of least squares coefficients. Conceptually, one can regard this as a least squares regression applied to the limitless number of observations that the joint probability distribution could produce. It is another theoretical construct; there are no data yet.

Continuing in this manner, because ε also is a product of least squares, it has by construction an expectation of 0.0 and is uncorrelated with X. For reasons that will be clear later, there is no requirement that ε have constant variance. Nevertheless, thanks to least squares, one can equate the conditional expectations from the working model with the population-level *best linear approximation* of the true response surface. We will see shortly that it is the best linear approximation of the true response surface that we seek to estimate, not the true response surface itself. Again, it is a feature of the joint probability distribution, not realized data.

This is a major reformulation of conventional, fixed-x linear regression. For the working model, there is no a priori determination of how the response is related to the predictors and no commitment to linearity as the truth. In addition, the chosen predictors share no special cachet. Among the random variables Z, a data analyst determines which random variables are predictors and which random variables are responses. Hence, there can be no such thing as an omitted variable that can turn a correct model into an incorrect model. *If important predictors are overlooked, the regression results are just incomplete*; the results are substantively deficient but potentially very informative nevertheless. Finally, causality need not be overlaid on the analysis. Although causal thinking may well have a role in an analyst's determination of the response and the predictors, a serious consideration of cause and effect is not required at this point. One need not ponder whether any given predictor is actually manipulable holding all other predictors constant.

Why all this attention to linear models? Looking ahead to subsequent chapters, a very similar approach will be used when the linear model is discarded. For a Level II analysis, a joint probability distribution will still be the source of all realized data. There will still be a true, unknown, response surface and in the population, an approximation of that response surface. Where possible, valid inferences will be made to that approximation, typically represented by its fitted values or forecasts. We have focused on linear models primarily as a didactic device.

Nevertheless, some readers may be wondering if we have simply traded one, convenient science fiction story for another. The linear model is fiction, but so is the joint probability distribution responsible for the data. What has been gained?

From an epistemological point of view, there is real merit in such concerns. However, in science and policy settings, it can be essential to make empirically based claims that go beyond the data on hand. For example, when a college admissions office uses data from past applicants to examine how performance in college is related to the information available when admission decisions need to be made, whatever is learned will presumably be used to help inform future admission decisions. Data from past applicants are taken to be realizations from the social processes responsible for academic success in college. Insofar as those social processes are reasonably consistent over several years, the strategy can have merit. Moreover, those social processes can be statistically captured as joint probability distribution.[20] A science fiction story? Perhaps. But if better admission decisions are made as a result, there are meaningful and demonstrable benefits. To rephrase George Box's famous aphorism, *all models are fiction, but some stories are better than others.* And there is much more to this story.

1.4.2 More on Statistical Inference with Wrong Models

Suppose a data analyst operating at Level II wants to estimate from data the best linear approximation of nature's true response surface. The estimation task can be usefully partitioned into five steps. The first requires making the case that each observation in the dataset was independently realized from a relevant joint probability distribution.[21] Much more is required than hand-waving. Required usually is subject-matter expertise and knowledge about how the data were collected. There will be examples in the pages ahead. Often a credible case cannot be made, which takes estimation off the table. Then, there will probably be no need to worry about step two.

The second step is to define the target of estimation. For linear regression of the sort just discussed, an estimation target is easy to specify. Should the estimation target be the true response surface, estimates will likely be of poor statistical quality and perhaps very misleading. Should the estimation target be the best linear approximation of the true response surface, the estimates can have good statistical properties, at least asymptotically. We will see in later chapters that defining the estimation target often will be far more difficult because there commonly will be no model in the conventional regression sense. However, one cannot sensibly proceed to step three unless there is clarity about what is to be estimated.

The third step is to select an estimator. Sometimes the best estimator will be apparent. It is common, for instance, to use "plug-in" estimators. The calculation that would in principle be undertaken with the hypothetical population of observations is actually undertaken with the dataset to be analyzed.[22] The usual least squares regression estimator is a good example. One implements ordinary least squares with the data on hand because one imagines applying ordinary least squares in the population. This may seem like the old paradigm is still in play. But the estimand has fundamentally changed, and a very different interpretation of the results follows.

But as clarified shortly, most of the procedures considered in later chapters capitalize on various forms of inductive fitting even if not quite in plain sight. Informal data snooping also is a common practice. Getting the estimator right then can be challenging. The risk is that an inappropriate estimator is used by default, justified by incorrect performance claims.

Fourth, the estimator needs to be applied to the data. This is usually the easiest step because the requisite software is often readily found and deployed without dfficulty. But there are exceptions when the data have unusual properties or the empirical questions being asked of the data are unusual. One hopes that appropriate code can be readily written, but sometimes important underlying statistical problems are unsolved. One always should be a cautious about all results unless one is confident that existing software is doing what it should.

When software is proprietary, there usually is no way to look under the hood. Marketing claims can be misleading or just plain wrong. Open source software allows for testing and evaluation, but the assessment burden can be excessive. Much more will be said about software later, but for now, suffice it to say that it can be prudent to step back from the bleeding edge. Stick with software that respected researchers have appraised and found satisfactory.

In the final step, the estimates, associated confidence intervals, and tests are interpreted. The major risk is that important, earlier steps are not properly considered. A common example is asserting asymptotic properties with far too few observations on hand. Such limitations must be acknowledged.

Let us play this through for estimates of the best linear approximation. In the absence of real data, not much can be said here about the first step. It will figure large in real applications later. The second step has already been addressed. The estimation target is the best linear approximation of the true response surface.

Important technical complications can materialize for steps three, four, and five. Consider Fig. 1.8. Suppose that in one joint probability distribution, the values of X are concentrated at smaller values. This is illustrated by Population A in Fig. 1.8. Because the nonlinear true response surface has a small positive slope in that region, the linear approximation does as well. In contrast, consider Population B. In this population, the values of X are concentrated at the larger values. Because the nonlinear true response surface has a steeper positive slope in that region, the linear approximation also does.

Conceptually, more is involved than simply getting different results from different joint probability distributions. When the linear (or any) approximation differs depending on where in the predictor space the predictor values tend to fall, one can say that the relationship is not "*well-specified*." This is a very different from "misspecification," which usually refers to violations of mean function first-order conditions. One has associations that differ depending on the *population distribution of the predictor*. The true, nonlinear, response function in Fig. 1.8 *does not change*,

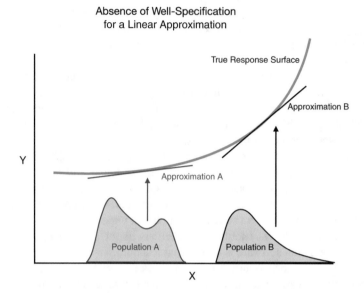

Fig. 1.8 A violation of well-specification (The gray curved line is the true response surface, the blue straight line is the best linear approximation from population A, and the black straight line is the best linear approximation from population B. The true response surface and both approximations about composed of conditional expectations for $Y|X$.)

as it would for a conventional regression interaction effect. Nevertheless, the population, best linear approximations are *not the same*.

The very similar generalization problems can materialize for a *single* joint probability distribution when the best linear approximation is not well-specified. Suppose Y is earnings, X is years of education, and another predictor is gender. Looking back at Fig. 1.8, population A is re-labeled as the female cases, and population B is re-labeled as the male cases. Even though the economic returns to education (i.e., the true response surface) are *the same* for men and women, the best linear approximations differ because in the joint probability distribution, men tend to have more years of education than women. One has the appearance of an interaction effect—men appear to have greater returns to eduction—whereas the real explanation is that on the average higher educational levels for men tend to place them at a different location in x-space where the true returns to education are larger. It is important not to forget that the population, best linear approximation is already stipulated to be misspecified. Well-specification is a different issue.

There are good diagnostics for well-specification with parametric approximations (Buja et al. 2019b), which can help enrich subject-matter interpretations, but so far at least, they have not been developed for the procedures discussed in the chapters ahead. At the same time, the role of regression coefficients will recede, making these concerns less salient. In the pages ahead, our interests will center on fitted values and prediction, not explanation.

Even with well-specification complications, when the estimation target remains that best linear approximation, rather than the true response surface, one can have asymptotically unbiased estimates of the approximation (Buja et al. 2019a,b). And despite the sources of nonconstant variance described earlier, asymptotically valid standard errors may be obtained using a sandwich estimator or a nonparametric bootstrap. (See the next section.) Asymptotically valid statistical tests and confidence intervals follow (Buja et al. 2019a,b). In practice, all one does is obtain the usual regression output but employ sandwich standard error estimates when test statistics and p-values are computed. Alternatively, one can bootstrap the regression using the nonparametric bootstrap to obtain valid standard error estimates or direct estimates of each regression coefficient's sampling distribution. In short, for best linear approximations and least squares applied to IID data, one can in principle have it all, at least asymptotically.

These results apply to nonlinear parametric approximations as well. For example, one might choose to approximate the true response surface with a cubic polynomial function of X. One would have the best (by least squares) cubic approximation of the true response surface. The conclusions also apply to the entire generalized linear model (Buja et al. 2019a,b). For example, the response might be binary and a form of binomial regression could be the estimation procedure. Because the response variable is categorical, the conditional expectations in the joint probability distribution are conditional probabilities (not conditional means), whether for the true response surface or the approximation.

There is more good news. Forecasts from a proper approximation retain the same desirable asymptotic properties (Berk et al. 2019). One can exploit asymptotically unbiased forecasts, tests, and confidence intervals as long as one appreciates that the forecasts are not made from valid estimates of the true response surface. Still more good news is that recent work from the perspective of conformal inference (Lei et al. 2018) provides several other very good inferential approaches that can apply quite generally and sometimes have excellent finite sample properties. At the same time, it cannot be overemphasized that all of this good news depends on a complete absence of data snooping. Data snooping will be addressed shortly and will be a central consideration of the procedures discussed in later chapters.

1.4.3 Introduction to Sandwich Standard Errors

Reference earlier was made to sandwich standard errors which figure centrally in statistical inference for best linear approximations. Sandwich standard errors are also used in some statistical learning applications. It may be helpful to briefly provide a few details.

Recall the requisite structure for the disturbances in the canonical linear regression model. The disturbances are realized independently at random from a single probability distribution and have an expectation of 0.0:

$$\varepsilon_i \sim \text{NIID}(0, \sigma^2). \tag{1.3}$$

The normality assumption usually is not essential.

From Eq. (1.3), the usual estimation expression for the regression coefficient variances is (Freedman 1987: 46)

$$\widehat{\text{cov}}(\hat{\boldsymbol{\beta}}|\mathbf{X}) = \hat{\sigma}^2(\mathbf{X}'\mathbf{X})^{-1}, \tag{1.4}$$

where

$$\hat{\sigma}^2 = \frac{1}{N-p} \sum_{i=1}^{N} e_i^2. \tag{1.5}$$

N is the number of observations, p is the number of predictors, e_i^2 is a squared regression residual, and variances are on the main diagonal of Eq. (1.4).

If the assumptions of Eq. (1.3) are not met, the manner in which $\hat{\sigma}^2$ is computed no longer holds. For example, if a disturbance can be drawn independently from one of two probability distributions, there could be two disturbance variances not one. In other words, nonconstant variance requires that Eq. (1.5) have a different form which, in turn, affects Eq. (1.4). This is much like the challenge provided by estimates of the best linear approximation because mean function specification error causes a form of nonconstant variance.

Each squared residual has information about the variance of its parent probability distribution. A squared residual will tend to be larger if its parent probability distribution has a greater variance. The sandwich estimate of the regression standard errors exploits that information using

$$\widehat{\text{cov}}_{sandwich}(\hat{\boldsymbol{\beta}}|\mathbf{X}) = (\mathbf{X}'\mathbf{X})^{-1}(\mathbf{X}'\hat{\mathbf{W}}\mathbf{X})^{-1}(\mathbf{X}'\mathbf{X})^{-1}, \tag{1.6}$$

where $\hat{\mathbf{W}}_{ij} = e_i^2$ if $i = j$ and 0 if $i \neq j$. Some refer to the two expressions in parentheses on the left and right as the bread and the expression in the middle parentheses as the meat. It is the meat that introduces the information contained in each residual.

This reasoning can be applied in many different settings when Eq. (1.3) does not apply, although the expression for the sandwich can change a bit. Here, the primary application will be for true response surface approximations with IID data. There also are different flavors of the sandwich that result from efforts to improve its performance in finite samples. In short, there are a number of unresolved details, but sandwich standard errors seem to perform well with best linear approximations. One simply uses a sandwich standard error instead of the conventional standard error when statistical tests and confidence intervals are needed. A wide variety of sandwich procedures can be found in the R libraries *car* and *sandwich*. However, all sandwich estimators depend on asymptotic justifications. Large N datasets are essential (e.g., several hundred degrees of freedom once the number of predictors is subtracted).[23]

1.4.4 Introduction to Conformal Inference

If one moves beyond best linear approximations, as we do in the next chapter, and focuses on forecasting, procedures under the broad umbrella of "conformal inference" are promising ways to consider uncertainty (Lei et al. 2018). One seeks valid prediction intervals for forecasts produced using an approximation of a true response surface.

Suppose a data analyst, using an approximation of a true response surface, has made a forecast. How good is that forecast compared to the true response variable value? Conformal prediction intervals can draw on variation in residuals from a model or statistical learning procedure to construct a 95% prediction interval containing the true value of the response variable with a probability of at least .95. And, there is not need for asymptotic justifications.

Consider a large number of independent investors who use, for example, misspecified linear regression models to forecast the price of a particular stock one day in advance. Each investor also computes a conformal prediction interval. If the stock prices are generated in an IID fashion, the conformal prediction intervals will contain the true stock price for 95% of the investors.

The basic idea is that the residuals provide a yardstick for variation in the disparities between true response values and fitted response values. They serve as "conformity" measures from which one can then determine the range of values in which a forecast is likely to fall. If the residuals tend to be small in absolute value, the true response value will likely fall within a relatively narrow range. If the residuals tend to be large in absolute value, the true response value will likely fall within a relatively large range. The beauty of this approach is that there are in practice no important assumptions for the procedure used to obtain the fitted values or the forecast. Because of its relative simplicity and close ties to approaches employed in later chapters, we consider the special case of "split conformal prediction sets."

One has, as before, a dataset of (x_i, y_i) values realized IID, where X can be high dimensional. Y might be income, and X might be regressors thought to be related to income. Some fitting procedure is applied such as linear regression. For a given vector of x-values (e.g., 25 years of age, 12 years of eduction, employed full time) a forecast is made. How good is that forecast? A prediction interval can help. One specifies a critical threshold α (e.g., .05) for which one computes an interval in which the true income value falls with probability $1 - \alpha$ (Geisser 1993: section 2.1.1).[24]

Here are the operational steps for a dataset realized IID and for a 95% prediction interval.

1. One constructs two random, disjoint subsets of the data, usually of equal size.
2. The first split, called the training dataset, is used to fit some procedure that can be as simple as linear regression or as complicated as deep neural networks. Once the fitting is accomplished, it becomes a given and is not revisited. The training dataset and the estimated mean function are now treated as fixed.
3. There are new x-values $\mathbf{X}^*$ realized IID from the same joint probability distribution but lacking associated values for Y. Predictions are made in the usual way. For example, $\hat{y} = \mathbf{X}^*\hat{\beta}$.
4. The second split, called test data, or the"calibration" dataset, is used to construct fitted values, also in the usual way.[25]
5. The second-split predicted values are subtracted from the second-split observed y-values to obtain residuals. In practice, the absolute values of those residuals are used. There are variants of this idea because conformity scores can take different forms.
6. The conformity scores are sorted in ascending order, and the value that corresponds to the kth case is used as to construct the prediction interval: $k = [(N/2 + 1)(1 - \alpha)]$.
7. To obtain the prediction intervals, the value of the kth quantile is alternatively added to and subtracted from each fitted value to be used as the forecast.[26]

The formal properties of split sample, conformal prediction intervals are well beyond the scope of this discussion. Lei et al., (2018) and Kuchibhotla (2020) provide excellent discussions. Also, it is important to appreciate that uncertainty in the training data, the fitting procedure itself (e.g., if cross-validation is used), and the data splitting is ignored. A prediction interval is still valid – it does what it says it does – but would likely be larger if these additional sources of uncertainty were included. This will resurface in subsequent chapters. A lot will depend on how the statistical inference is formulated.

There are a number of interesting extensions and refinements under development. Nevertheless, one has already a simple and practical tool to compute prediction intervals from statistical learning procedures when the data are IID. Illustrative code is shown in Figure 1.9.[27] The fitting function is a smoother discussed in the next chapter.

The code can be easily adopted to other fitting methods by replacing the *gam* procedure with something else. Categorical response variables are readily handled. One can allow for many different forecasts and more than one predictor. In short, the code in Figure 1.9 provides useful prediction intervals that properly can be used in practice.[28] There currently are also two conformal inference packages in R, *conformalInference* and *conformalClassification*. Both are very powerful with many options. Both also have substantial learning curves.

```
##### Split Conformal Code #####
# Get data in shape
library(car)
library(mgcv)
data(Freedman)
index<-sample(1:110,55,replace=F)
train<-Freedman[index,c(2,4)] # Split 1
test<-Freedman[-index,c(2,4)] # Split 2

# Fit gam and get CI for a single x-value
fit<-gam(crime~s(nonwhite),data=train) # A smoothing spline
resids<-abs(predict(fit,newdata=test)-test[,"crime"])
k<-ceiling(((nrow(test)/2)+1)*.95)
resord<-sort(resids)
error<-resord[k]
newd<-data.frame(nonwhite=3.5) # Forecast for this x-value
Y.hat<-predict(fit,newdata = newd)
CI<-c(Y.hat-error,Y.hat+error) # Confidence Interval

# Plot results
plot(test$nonwhite,predict(fit,newdata=test),ylim=c(500,4500),
     xlab="Percent Nonwhite",ylab="Crime Rate Per 100,000",
     main="Split Conformal Example for X = 3.5")
points(test$nonwhite,test$crime,col="blue")
abline(v=newd,col="red")
points(newd,Y.hat+error,cex=2, lwd=3)
points(newd,Y.hat-error,cex=2, lwd=3)
text(20,3250,"Fitted Values")
text(3.5,3100,"Upper Bound")
text(3.5,1800,"Lower Bound")
```

Fig. 1.9 Illustrative R code for split sample conformal prediction intervals

1.4.5   Introduction to the Nonparametric Bootstrap

The nonparametric bootstrap will figure significantly in the pages ahead when statistical inference is undertaken. It is a special case of a rich array of bootstrap procedures that, in turn, are special cases of a broad class of resampling procedures. All of these techniques are based on simulating statistical inference from a frequentist perspective using the data on hand as a stand-in for the source of those data (Efron and Tibshirani 1993; Hall 1997; Davidson 1997; Edgington and Ongehena 2007). A broad overview follows. More details will be provided later as relevant.

The nonparametric bootstrap (also the "pairs bootstrap" or "X-Y bootstrap") can be a useful tool for statistical inference, especially statistical tests and confidence

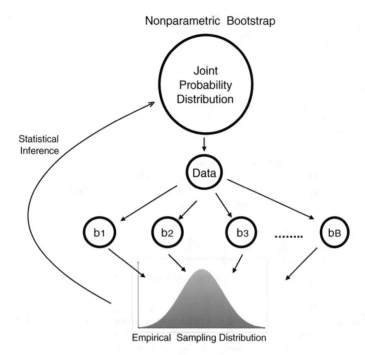

Fig. 1.10 Diagram of the nonparametric bootstrap

intervals, when conventional mathematical expressions for standard errors are unavailable or inconvenient. Figure 1.10 is a visualization of steps required.

There is a finite population or joint probability distribution from which data are realized in an IID fashion. The statistical challenge, as usual, is statistical inference from those observations back to their source. Insofar as the data are realized IID, the data can serve as a proxy for source of the data.

The IID process is simulated by drawing cases at random *with replacement* from the data on hand.[29] Conventionally, for N observations, a total of B samples is drawn, each with N observations. Depending on the application, B can range from about 50 to several thousand or more.

For each of the B "bootstrap samples," one or more estimators are applied. There are then B estimates of each specific estimand. Each set of the B estimates represents an empirical sampling distribution from which statistical inference can follow directly. For example, the distance between the 2.5th percentile and the 97.5th percentile can be an approximation of the 95% confidence interval arrived at by the "bootstrap percentile method." There are alternatives to the percentile method that arguably are more accurate (Efron and Tibshirani 1993: chapter 14), but for statistical learning applications, that may be gilding the lily.

The percentile method is easy to program and understand, although R provides a very rich package of bootstrap procedures in the *boot* library.[30] In subsequent chapters, the form taken by the nonparametric bootstrap will vary a bit depending on nature of the statistical learning procedure.

Just as for the sandwich and conformal prediction intervals, the bootstrap is only can be justified asymptotically. Large datasets are essential. There is no formal way to determine how large is large enough, but a histogram of the empirical sampling distribution usefully can be examined and a normal quantile-quantile plot constructed. If the plot passes an eyeball linearity test, data analysts will usually proceed. The empirical sampling distribution should be approximately normal.

1.4.6 Wrong Regression Models with Binary Response Variables

Up to this point, analyses with quantitative response variables have dominated the discussion, in part to make connections to conventional linear regression. The majority of subsequent chapters will introduce procedures for the analysis of categorical response variables. Some of the most interesting and useful work on statistical learning has focused such procedures, commonly called "classifiers," whose enterprise is "classification."

To help set the stage, in Fig. 1.11 again illustrates features of a joint probability distribution. There is a binary response Y coded as 1 or 0, and as before, a single numerical X. Dropping out of high school might be coded as 1, and graduating might be coded as 0. The 1s at the top and the 0s at the bottom represent potential realized values.

There is, as before, a true response surface and its population approximation. The former is shown with a red curve. The latter is shown with a blue line and is the estimation target. Both are comprised of conditional probabilities. The values from 0 to 1 on the vertical axis are the conditional probabilities for class 1. The parallel for a numeric response variable would be conditional expectations for Y. For any value of X, the conditional probability is the sole parameter for a binomial process responsible for hypothetical realized of 1s.

We need a reasoned way to get from the conditional probabilities to Y's classes. In Fig. 1.11, there are two classes. There is also a threshold shown at an illustrative value of 0.30. All conditional probabilities at or above the threshold would determine an outcome class of 1. All conditional probabilities below that threshold would determine an outcome class of 0.

The threshold formally is not a component of the binomial process and is not a feature of the joint probability distribution. It is imposed on the conditional probabilities by researchers when there is a need to get from an estimated conditional probability to one of the two outcome classes. Yet, it is sometimes helpful to think about the classes assigned by researchers as a kind of fitted value or at least as an output from the data analysis.

In Fig. 1.11, working from the true response surface compared to its approximation can affect the classes assigned. For the value of X at the black vertical line, the true response surface would assign a class of 0, but the linear approximation would assign a class of 1. In this instance, the true response surface assigns the correct class. The linear approximation assigns the incorrect class. For many other x-values, the true response surface and the linear approximation would assign the same class. With $X > 1.0$, both functions assigned the class of 1, which happens to be the correct class. The use of 0.30 as a threshold might seem strange, but we will see later that there can be principled reasons for choosing threshold values other than the intuitive value of 0.50.

If a data analyst chose to apply conventional logistic regression to the realized data, substantial structure necessarily would be imposed, ideally justified by subject-matter theory. The analyst would be working within modeling traditions. The true logistic response surface would be the estimation target. All predictors would be fixed and assumed to combine in a linear fashion. Hypothetical 1s and 0s *generated by the model* would be viewed as Bernoulli draws determined by the conditional probabilities that constitute the true response surface. Should the first- and second-order conditions for logistic regression be met, estimates of the true response surface

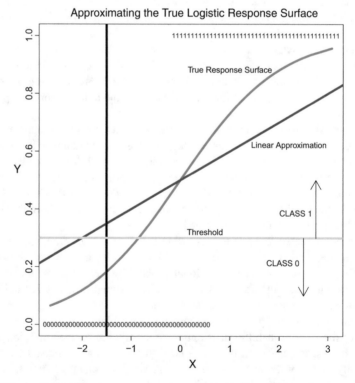

Fig. 1.11 Classification for a binary response variable in a joint probability distribution (shown in red is the true response surface, a linear approximation as a blue line, and a researcher imposed classification threshold in light blue)

(and the corresponding logistic regression parameters) would be asymptotically unbiased, and valid statistical tests and confidence intervals would follow.[31] In short, the first- and second-order conditions are essential, which means that the usual logistic regression approach is vulnerable to the same challenges as conventional linear regression. We need not repeat them.

Logistic regression, or any form of binomial regression, will not figure significantly in later chapters because one requires that first- and second-order condition be met. We will be building on the wrong model approach already described. But classification will be huge. A variety of classifiers will be considered in some depth for which the primary goal is to classify observations accurately using an acknowledged approximation of the true response surface. Figure 1.11 is provided in that spirit.[32]

1.5   The Transition to Statistical Learning

As a first approximation, statistical learning can be seen as a form of nonparametric regression in which the *search* for an effective mean function is especially data intensive. For example, one might want to capture how longevity is related to genetic and lifestyle factors. A statistical learning algorithm could be turned loose on a large dataset with no preconceptions about what the nature of the relationships might be. Fitted values from the exercise could then be used to anticipate which kinds of patients are more likely to face life-threatening, chronic diseases. Such information would be of interest to physicians and actuaries. Likewise, a statistical learning algorithm could be applied to credit card data to determine which features of transactions are associated with fraudulent use. Again, there would be no need for any preconceptions about the relationships involved. With the key relationships determined, banks that issue credit cards would be able to alert their customers when their cards were likely being misused. Government agencies can have similar needs. The U.S. Securities and Exchange Commission, for example, recently has been using a statistical learning algorithm to detect suspicious securities trading, and at least one Goldman Sachs banker will apparently serve a prison term (Bolen 2019).

So far, this sounds little different from conventional regression analyses. And in fact, there has been considerable confusion in the applications literature about the nature of statistical learning and which procedures qualify. In truth, the boundaries are fuzzy. To take an extreme example, least squares regression is usually credited to Carl Friedrich Gauss, who developed the procedure in the early nineteenth century (Stigler 1981). Yet, least squares regression is commonly included in textbooks on machine learning (e.g., Murphy 2012, Chapter 7) as if it were some shiny new object.[33]

Almost as extreme, we will see later that neural networks make use of "hidden layers" that are actually latent variables whose roots can be traced back to principal components analysis (PCA) invented by Karl Pearson in the very early twentieth century (Pearson 1901). This, in turn, became the basis for factor analysis widely used by social scientists beginning in the1950s (Rummel 1988), and has been since the 1970s an essential component of much structural equation modeling in psychology, political science, and sociology (Jöeskog 1979).

Imposing a regression perspective on statistical learning is consistent with "supervised" statistical learning, characterized by a focus on $Y|X$. There is also "unsupervised" statistical learning in which the joint distribution of X alone is the concern. Unsupervised statistical learning is more closely aligned with PCA and factor analysis than is supervised statistical learning and with procedures like multidimensional scaling and cluster analysis, both of which also have long intellectual histories (e.g., Torgerson 1958). Many machine learning textbooks include supervised and unsupervised learning, which can make it even more difficult to understand what really is novel and what is just a rebranding of existing and well-understood data analysis procedures.[34]

In the pages ahead, we will proceed with an incremental transition from regression procedures formulated before a data analysis begins to regression procedures formulated as part of the data analysis. Through that progressive transition, a conventional regression analysis becomes (supervised) statistical learning. But, because that transition is gradual, some fuzzy boundaries will remain. The difference between models and algorithms is a good place to start clarifying the issues.

1.5.1   Models Versus Algorithms

Consider again the pair of equations for the conventional linear model with a numeric response variable.

$$y_i = \beta_0 + \beta_1 x_{1i} + \beta_2 x_{2i} + \cdots + \beta_p x_{pi} + \varepsilon_i, \qquad (1.7)$$

where

$$\varepsilon_i \sim \text{NIID}(0, \sigma^2). \qquad (1.8)$$

Equations (1.7) and (1.8) are a theory of how each case i came to be. They are a generative model because they represent the data generation mechanisms. When a data analyst works with these equations, a substantial amount of thought goes into model specification. What predictors should be used? What, if any, transformations are needed? What might be done about possible dependence among the disturbances or about nonconstant disturbance variances? But once these decisions are made, the necessary computing follows almost automatically. Usually, the intent is to minimize the sum of the squared residuals, and there is a convenient closed-form solution routinely implemented. On occasion, a more robust fitting criterion is used, such as minimizing the sum of the absolute value of the residuals, and although there is no closed- form solution, the estimation problem is easily solved with linear programming.

Statistical learning allocates a data analysts' effort differently. Equations (1.7) and (1.8) sometimes can be replaced by

$$y_i = f(\mathbf{X}_i) + \varepsilon_i, \tag{1.9}$$

In contrast to some approaches, we will *not* treat Eq. (1.9) as a generative model. For a Level I analysis, $f(\mathbf{X}_i)$ is some unknown function of one or more predictors that provides a summary of how the conditional means of Y are related to $\mathbf{X}$ in the data on hand. In these data, there are residuals ε_i that are nothing more than the arithmetic difference between the observed values of Y and the fitted values of Y. They have no deeper meaning.

For a Level II analysis, Eq. (1.9) is a feature of the joint probability distribution from which the IID observations were realized. Its expectation is an acknowledged approximation of the true response surface. As before, the population residuals combine the population disparities between the true response surface and the expectation of the approximation with the irreducible random error. All that has changed is that we do not specify the functional form the mean function takes.[35] We will let an algorithm figure that out.

Very little is asked of the data analyst because no commitment to any particular mean function is required. Indeed, the only decision may be to introduce ε_i additively. There is effectively no concern about whether the mean function is right or wrong, because for all practical purposes, there is no mean function responsible in part for generating the data. In practice, the objective is to arrive at fitted values from a computed $\hat{f}(\mathbf{X}_i)$ that make subject-matter sense and that correspond as closely as possible to realized values of Y. The form that $\hat{f}(\mathbf{X}_i)$ takes to get the job done is determined inductively.

In contrast, there needs to be serious thought given to the algorithm through which the fitted values are computed. This is one reason why the methods often are called "algorithmic." A simple and somewhat stylized outline of one kind of algorithmic method proceeds as follows.

1. Specify a linear mean function of the form of Eq. (1.7) and apply least squares as usual.
2. Compute the fitted values.
3. Compute the residuals.
4. Compute a measure of fit.
5. Apply least squares again, but weigh the data so that observations with larger absolute values of the residuals are given more weight.
6. Update the fitted values obtained from the immediately preceding regression with the new fitted values weighted by their measure of fit.
7. Repeat steps 2–6 until the quality of the fit does not improve (e.g., 1000 times).
8. Output the fitted values.

In a process that has some of the look and feel of the statistical learning procedure boosting, a regression analysis is repeated over and over, each time with altered data so that hard-to-fit values of Y are given more weight. In that sense, the hard-

36   1   Statistical Learning as a Regression Problem

Fig. 1.12 A Level II black box statistical learning algorithm (W, X, and Z are predictors, Y is the response variable, and ε represents the population disturbances)

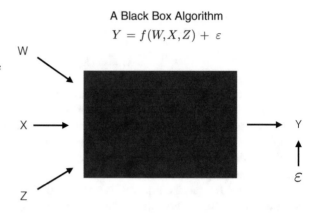

A Black Box Algorithm

$$Y = f(W, X, Z) + \varepsilon$$

to-fit observations are counted more heavily when the sum of squared residuals is computed. The final result is a single set of fitted values that is a weighted sum of the many sets of fitted values. Hard thought must be given to whether this algorithm is an effective way to link predictors to a response and whether other algorithms might do the job better.

There are also interpretative issues. In this algorithm, there can be a very large number of regressions and an even larger number of regression coefficients. For example, if there are 1000 regressions and 10 predictors, there are 10,000 regression coefficients. It is effectively impossible to make subject-matter sense of 10,000 regression coefficients. Moreover, each set is computed for data with different weights so that the fitting task is continually changing.

In the end, one has a "black box" algorithm of the form shown in Fig. 1.12. There are in Fig. 1.12 three predictors (W, X, Z), and a single response Y, connected by complicated computations that provide no information of substantive importance.[36] One can get from the predictors to the final set of fitted values. But, there is no model. The many regressions are just a computational device. In other terms, one has a *procedure* not a model.

Thinking back to the college admissions example, one can use the results of the algorithm to forecast a college applicant's freshman GPA *even though one does not know exactly how the predictors are being used to make that forecast*. In a similar fashion, one can use such methods to project the dollar value of insurance claims a given driver is likely to make over the course of a year or the total precipitation a city will receive in a particular month. When Y is binary, one can predict which parolees are likely to be rearrested or which high school students are likely to drop out of school.

There can be more interpretative information when one is able to change what inputs are used and re-run the algorithm. One could determine, for example, how the fitted values for college GPA change whether or not gender is included as an input. One could determine how much any measures of fit change as well. We will see later that there are special algorithms operating in much the same spirit that allow one to at least peek into the black box.

But one must be clear about exactly what might be learned. Suppose the association between gender and GPA operates in concert with age. The association between gender and college GPA is stronger for younger students, perhaps because male students do not mature as rapidly as female students. As a result, should the quality of the fit improve when gender is included, the improvement results from a main effect and an interaction effect. Moreover, the algorithm might have transformed age in a manner that is unknown to the data analyst. A claim that on the average gender improves the quality of the fit is technically correct, but how gender is related to college GPA remains obscure.

An extensive metaphor may help fix these ideas. Suppose one wants to bake some bread. The recipe calls for the following:

- 2 packages of yeast;
- 2 cups of warm water;
- 2 tablespoons of melted butter;
- 2 tablespoons of sugar;
- 1 tablespoon of salt; and
- 4 cups of all-purpose flour.

These ingredients are mixed and stirred until the batter is stiff, adding more flour if needed. The stiff batter is then kneaded until it is smooth and elastic, put into a greased bowl and allowed to rise for about an hour. The dough is then punched down and divided in half, placed into two greased loaf pans and again allowed to rise for about 30 min. Finally, the two loaves are baked at 400° for about 25 min.

The bread baking begins with known ingredients in specified amounts. From that point onward—the knead and baking—complicated physical and chemical processes begin that change the molecular structure of the ingredients as they are combined so that a bland watery batter can be turned into a delicious solid punctuated by air holes. The baker knows little about such details, and there is no way for the baker to document exactly how the ingredients are turned into bread. But if bread is tasty, the recipe will be repeated in the future. Looking again at Fig. 1.12, the ingredients are $\{W, X, Z\}$. The bread is Y. The black box is all of the physics and chemistry in-between.

It is possible to alter the bread recipe. For example, one might use one teaspoon of sugar rather than two. That would likely lead to changes in the bread that comes out of the oven. It might be more preferable or less. Or one might choose to substitute whole wheat flour for the all-purpose flour. It is possible therefore, to see how changing the ingredients and/or their proportions affects the quality of the bread. But the baker does not learn much about the processes by which those ingredients are transformed into bread.[37]

Why might one prefer black box algorithmic methods rather than a traditional parametric regression? If the primary goal of the data analysis is to understand how the predictors are related to the response, one would not. But if the primary goal of the data analysis is to make decisions based at least in part on information provided by fitted values, statistical learning really has no downside. It should perform at least as well as model-based methods, and often substantially better. The reasons will be considered in later chapters when particular statistical learning procedures are discussed.

What roles do estimation, statistical tests, and confidence intervals play? As before, they are effectively irrelevant for a Level I analysis. For a Level II analysis, the broader issues are the same as those already discussed. Ideally, inferences are being made to an approximation of the true, unknown response surface using the fitted values constructed from the data that one can call regression functionals.[38] The estimand is the approximation. It is the estimation target. One hopes that the fitted values obtained from the data properly can serve as estimators.[39]

However, the approximation is not model-based and is derived directly from the data. In the algorithm just summarized, for instance, each new weighted regression is altered because of the results of the earlier regressions. The algorithm is engaged in a very extensive form of automated adaptive fitting through which information in the data is being used in ways that are difficult to quantify. How many degrees of freedom have been used up in those 1000 regressions, each with recursively re-weighted data? This is an issue to which we will return many times.

Adaptive fitting is different from data snooping. In adaptive fitting, information in the data is used to arrive at a single $\hat{f}(X)$. In data snooping, different $\hat{f}(X)$s are computed and compared. The "best" $\hat{f}(X)$ is the function interpreted and used; there is a selection process at work. This can lead to even more daunting problems than adaptive fitting because the premises of conventional statistical inference are being violated fundamentally. In conventional statistical inference, the structure of the working $\hat{f}(X)$ and any null hypotheses to be tested are determined *before* the data analysis begins. This too is an issue to which we will return many times.

Forecasting remains a Level II activity. The approximation is used to compute forecasts and consequently, the forecasts will contain bias when predictions from the true response surface are the estimation targets. One hopes that the forecasts are close to the truth, but there is no way to know for sure. Statistical tests and confidence intervals are problematic. As before, one can enjoy better statistical properties when the forecasts are accepted as approximations. Legitimate prediction intervals can be constructed from approximations in many forecasting applications.

Finally, we need to briefly address what to call an algorithmic approach for linking inputs to outputs. Suppose, again, that we have a set of fitted values constructed from 1000 linear, residual-weighted regressions. Do we call the computed relationships between the inputs and the outputs a model? In statistics, the term "model" is often reserved for the "generative model." The model conveys how the data were generated. But we are proceeding for Level II applications assuming the data are generated as IID realizations from a joint probability distribution. That is not what is represented by each of the 1000 regressions. So, calling those 1000 regressions a model can be confusing.

Unfortunately, there seems to be no commonly accepted alternative term. We will proceed from here on with one of six terms: "learning algorithm," "algorithmic procedure," "statistical learning procedure," "procedure," or "learner." There should be no confusion in context, and the difference between models and algorithms is a fundamental distinction to which we will return many times. Models are algebraic theories for how the world works. Algorithms are procedures to compute quantities of interest; they inherently are not about anything.

1.6 Some Initial Concepts

Within a regression analysis framework, a wide variety of statistical learning procedures are examined in subsequent chapters. But, before going much farther down that road, a few key concepts need to be briefly introduced, largely in an intuitive manner. There are ample references for readers who want a more formal treatment.

The concepts discussed play central roles in the chapters ahead and, at this point, would benefit from some initial exposure. We return to these ideas many times, so nothing like mastery is required now. And that is a good thing. Important details can only be addressed later in the context of particular statistical learning procedures. For now, we consider what statistical learning and related concepts look like from 30,000 feet up.

1.6.1 Overall Goals of Statistical Learning

The range of procedures we examine have been described in several different ways (Christianini and Shawe-Taylor 2000; Witten and Frank 2000; Hand et al. 2001; Breiman 2001b; Dasu and Johnson 2003; Bishop 2006; Hastie et al. 2009; Barber 2012; Murphy 2012; Marsland 2014; Sutton and Barto 2018), and associated with them are a variety of names: statistical learning, machine learning, supervised learning, reinforcement learning, algorithmic modeling, and others. The term "statistical learning" as emphasized in the pages that follow is based on the following notions.

The definition of regression analysis still applies, and some statisticians favor a function estimation, modeling framework. Recall that for a numerical response,

$$Y = f(X) + \varepsilon, \tag{1.10}$$

where it is common to assume that $E(\varepsilon) = 0$ and that ε is independent of X. Therefore, the conditional distribution of Y depends on X (Hastie et al. 2009: section 2.6.1) through $f(X)$. As before, the first- and second-order conditions are in theory met. All that has really changed is the mean function is unspecified, presumably because it is unknown before the data analysis begins. Were the function known and properly implemented, first- and second-order conditions would be met.

For a categorical response, traditional practice proceeds in the spirit of binomial regression. There is no disturbance term as such because the uncertainty is captured in conditional probabilities for each of the K classes of the categorical response variable G. For example, if G is coded as 0 or 1, $E(G|X = x)$ is the conditional probability of the class coded 1 for a particular set of x-values. Should the logistic function be chosen for the $f(X)$,

$$p(G = 1|X) = \frac{1}{1 + e^{[-f(X)]}}. \tag{1.11}$$

The meaning of Eqs. (1.10) and (1.11) is unclear if one allows for the first-order and second- order conditions to be violated. For a numeric response variable, the disturbances no longer have convenient or easily understood properties. For a categorical response, the properties of the binomial distribution are unlikely to hold.[40]

Therefore, we return to the earlier approximation approach. For a Level I analysis, $f(X)$ is a mean function characterizing some associations between the response and the predictors. For Y, interest usually centers, just as before, on how the conditional means vary with X. For G, interest usually centers on how the conditional proportions vary with X.[41] The additive error term, ε, represents the residuals from the data on hand. They are just what is "left over" when the fitted values are subtracted from the observed response variable, and will incorporate any systematic relationships with the response variable not included in the mean function.

For Level II analyses, Eq. (1.10) or (1.11) each captures features of the joint probability distribution from which the observations on hand were independently realized; Y, G, and X are all random variables. The expectations of Eq. (1.10) or (1.11) are approximations of the true response surface, the former composed of conditional expectations, and the latter composed of conditional probabilities. Within the approximation perspective, ε, again represents nothing more than what is "left over." Uncertainty comes exclusively from the IID realizations.

The main goal of supervised statistical learning is to *compute an approximation of the unknown true response surface.* With no specified mean function from which to work, $f(X)$ is constructed inductively from the data—that is essentially what supervised statistical learning is all about.

When there is no interest whatsoever in a response $Y|X$ or $G|X$ and attention is limited exclusively to X, supervised statistical learning is no longer on the table. But as already mentioned, unsupervised statistical learning can be. Some kinds of cluster analysis and principal components analysis can be seen as examples of unsupervised statistical learning. Supervised statistical learning becomes unsupervised statistical learning when there is no measured response variable. In computer science terms, there is no "labeled" response. We do not consider unsupervised statistical learning because it cannot be formulated as a form of regression analysis.[42]

1.6.2 Forecasting with Supervised Statistical Learning

Because most supervised statistical learning applications focus on the fitted values that in practice often are used for prediction, it is helpful to distinguish between fitted values computed when the response values are known and fitted values computed when the response values are unknown. By "unknown," one normally means that an algorithm has already been trained on data in which Y or G is observed. A form of supervised statistical learning has been applied, and relationships between the predictors and the response approximated. Then, there is a second dataset with the same predictors, but without values for Y or G. One hopes to anticipate what the response variable values are likely to be. How this can be done will be central in later chapters.

When the response variable values in new data are unknown, there are two forms of prediction that differ in the reasons the response variable values are unavailable. The first kind of prediction is imputation. The response values exist but are not in the data. For example, can the carbon emissions from a coal-powered energy plant be approximated from information about the kind of technology the plant uses and amount of coal burned over a day? Can a student's true score in a standardized test be inferred from a pattern of answers that suggests cheating? Can the fish biomass of a tropical reef be estimated from information about the kinds of coral from which the reef is composed, the size of the reef, water temperature, and the amount of fishing allowed? In each case, the actual response variable values would be too difficult, time consuming, or costly to measure directly. Imputation is meant to fill the gap.

The second kind of analysis is forecasting: an outcome of interest is not just unknown, it has not occurred yet. What is the likely return from a given investment? What will be the top wind speed when a particular hurricane makes shore? For a certain county in Iowa, how many bushels of corn per acre can be expected in September from information available in June?

For categorical responses, one might try to impute an unknown class. For example, does a pattern of answers on a multiple choice exam indicate that the student has done the assigned reading? Does a DNA test place a given suspect at the crime scene? Do the injuries from a car crash indicate that the driver was not wearing a seat belt? But just as with quantitative responses, forecasts are commonly made as well. Will a particular prison inmate be rearrested within 2 years when later released on parole? Will a certain earthquake fault rupture in the next decade? Will a given presidential candidate win the overall popular vote when a year later the election is held?

In short, statistical learning focuses on fitted values as the primary algorithmic product. They may be used for description, especially when associations with predictors can be calculated or displayed. More important in practice, associations between predictors and a response are used to compute fitted values when the response values are unknown. The enterprise can be imputation or forecasting.

Why does the difference between imputation and forecasting matter? We will see later that statistical inference depends on how the data were generated. Datasets used for imputations can be realized differently from data used for forecasting. The former is realized in the present. The latter is realized in the future.

1.6.3   Overfitting

It is well-known that all statistical procedures are vulnerable to overfitting. The fitting procedure capitalizes on noise in the dataset as well as signal. Even if the true response surface is known, irreducible error remains. Statistical procedures will try to fit the irreducible error as well as the systematic associations between predictors and the response. This leads to overfitting.

When working with a population approximation it gets worse. Recall, that bias is folded into the irreducible error; there is an additional source of noise. This is an especially important difficulty for statistical learning when an algorithm aggressively searches the data for information with which to determine $f(X)$.

For a statistical learning Level I analysis, the result can be an unnecessarily complicated summary of relationships and the risk of misleading interpretations. For a Level II analysis, the problems are more complex and troubling. An important consequence of overfitting is that when performance of the procedure is examined with new data, even if realized from the same joint probability distribution, predictive accuracy will often degrade substantially; the error will "load" differently. If out-of-sample performance is meaningfully worse than in-sample performance, generalizing the results from original data can be badly compromised.

There is a large literature in statistics on overfitting. For example, in conventional linear regression, the greater the number of non-redundant regression coefficients whose values are to be estimated, the better the in-sample fit, other things equal. A larger number of non-redundant regression coefficients by itself can increase the complexity of $f(X)$ in a manner that can capitalize on noise as well as signal.

There have been, therefore, many attempts to develop measures of fit that adjust for this source of overfitting, typically by taking the degrees of freedom used by the procedure into account. Mallows' Cp is an example (Mallows 1973). The AIC (Akaike 1973) and BIC (Schwartz 1978) are others. In conventional regression, adjusting for the degrees of freedom used can counteract an important contributor to overfitting. Unfortunately, adjusting for degrees of freedom does not fully solve the problem, in part because a fitting algorithm cannot distinguish signal from noise in the data on hand. When in ordinary least squares the sum of the squared residuals is minimized, the minimization responds to both signal and noise in residuals.

We will see shortly that it is especially unclear how to proceed in algorithmic settings. Many algorithms are designed to search powerfully through the data in a manner that makes them particularly vulnerable to overfitting. Moreover, how does one address the degrees of freedom used when there is nothing like a linear regression model whose regression coefficients can be counted? What does one do when an algorithm sequentially implements thousands of linear regressions whose fitted values are combined? These are examples of exactly where we will be going in subsequent chapters.

1.6.4 Data Snooping

Probably the most important challenge to out-of-sample performance comes from various kinds of data snooping. By "data snooping" one loosely means revising how a data analysis is done after examining preliminary results or certain other features of the data. Consider first a very simple example.

There are 100 observations of IID data with one numeric Y and five numeric X variables. For each X, a scatterplot is constructed with Y on the vertical axis and each X, in turn, on the horizontal axis. The predictor having the strongest looking, linear association with Y is selected, and a bivariate regression analysis is performed. The output includes an intercept, a regression coefficient, and a p-value for the usual null hypothesis that in the generative joint probability distribution, the regression coefficient equals 0.0.

None of the equations responsible for output incorporate the pre-regression search for the most promising regressor. Indeed, the p-value would be the same if there was no search, and the selected regressor was the only regressor available in the dataset. Intuitively, the searching procedure seems like a form of cheating, and for statistical inference it is. All estimation, statistical tests, and confidence are likely discredited. Statistical inference after data snooping is a bit like playing a game of blackjack in which you alone are able to look at your opponents' face-down cards before placing a bet. Put another way, data analysts are trying to promote a winner before running the race.

In practice, data snooping is undertaken in a wide variety of ways, often with the best of intentions. For example, it is common to fit a regression model, look at the results and in response, revise the regression model. The aim is to build the best model possible. Yet, a winner is chosen without formally acknowledging all of the competitors that were discarded or all of the competitors that *could* have been discarded with new realizations of the dataset. It also is possible that with new realizations of the dataset, a different winner would be crowned. This too is ignored.

Data snooping has over the past several decades become a common practice as regression diagnostic techniques have been developed. For example, if evidence of nonconstant variance is found in a regression's residuals, a transformation of the response variable may be undertaken, and the regression run again. This is data snooping too, but of a more subtle kind.

This is not an argument against regression diagnostics. But once a regression model is altered because of unfavorable diagnostics, the analysis shifts from Level II to Level I. The analysis has become exploratory. The intent now is to inform *future* studies about promising model specifications. Because of data snooping, all of the usual Level II statistical tests and confidence intervals likely are compromised (Leeb and Pötscher 2005, 2006, 2008; Berk et al. 2010).

Statistical learning typically and aggressively data snoops. Powerful searches for good results usually are inherent. In addition, a learning algorithm is commonly run many times on the same data as an algorithm is "tuned." Sometimes the tuning is automated, and sometimes tuning is done by the data analyst. For example, tuning can be used to determine how complex the $\hat{f}(X)$ should be.[43] This can be analogous in stepwise regression to selecting which predictors should be retained. All of the usual statistical tests and confidence intervals are jeopardized because canonical, frequentist statistical inference assumes a known, fixed specification before the data analysis begins.

1.6.5   Some Constructive Responses to Overfitting and Data Snooping

When for a learning algorithm a sufficient amount of data is available, overfitting problems can be productively addressed with an explicit out-of-sample approach. The same applies to problems caused by data snooping, although the results are less definitive.[44] We started down this path earlier when conformal prediction intervals were introduced.

1.6.5.1   Training Data, Evaluation Data, and Test Data

The realized data to which the statistical learning procedure is initially applied are usually called "training data." Training data provide the information through which the algorithm learns but should not be used to gauge how well the algorithm performs. For an honest assessment, new data are required that played no role in the training.

There is, ideally, a second dataset, sometimes called "evaluation data," realized from the same joint probability distribution, used in the tuning process. The statistical learning procedure is tuned, not by its performance in the training data, but by its performance in the evaluation data. One uses the results from the training data to predict the response in the evaluation data. How well the predicted values correspond to the actual evaluation data outcomes provides feedback on training performance.

Finally, there is a third dataset, commonly called "test data," also realized from the same joint probability distribution, that often can be used to obtain an honest assessment of the procedure's performance in practice. Much as was done with the evaluation data, a prediction exercise can be undertaken with the test data, *conditional on the training data and algorithmic structure already obtained*; the training data and algorithmic structure are now fixed no matter what is found in the test data. The new set of fitted values from the test data can then be compared to the actual test data outcomes and honest performance measures computed uncontaminated by overfitting or data snooping. The overfitting and data snooping were sins committed with the training data, not the test data.[45]

1.6.5.2 Data Splitting

Arguably the most defensible approach is to have three datasets of sufficient size: a training dataset, an evaluation dataset, and a test dataset. "Sufficient" depends on the setting, but a minimum of about 500 cases each can be effective. All three should be IID realizations from the same joint probability distribution.

If there is only one dataset on hand that is relatively large (e.g., 2000 cases), a training dataset, an evaluation dataset, and a test dataset can be constructed as three random, disjoint subsets. Then, there can be important details to consider, such as the relative sizes of the three splits (Faraway 2014). A related issue is that most of the statistical learning procedures in later chapters are sample-size dependent. One can get different algorithmic structures depending on the number of observation analyzed. For example, the algorithmic structure obtained with N observations can differ substantially from the algorithmic structure obtained with $N/3$ observations. One result is that bias with respect to the true response surface also can be substantially smaller when the full set of observations is used for training. This will be squarely faced in the next chapter.

Another problem is that randomly splitting the data introduces a new source of uncertainty. Were the data split again, the fitted values likely would be at least somewhat different. In principle, this can be addressed by using many splits. A large number of different random splits can be constructed, and the fitted values in the test data across the different splits averaged. The main obstacle is an additional computational burden.

Despite these important challenges, split samples are increasingly employed thanks to the growing availability of big data. Using one of the splits as test data, honest performance measures can be obtained free of overfitting and data snooping. But as with "real" test data, the training data and algorithmic structure produced are taken as given whatever their problems may have been.

1.6.5.3 Cross-Validation

When only one dataset is available, and the dataset has too few observations for data splitting, there are several procedures one can use to try to approximate an out-of-sample ideal. Perhaps the most common is cross-validation, which is a fancy version of data splitting.

Consider a single IID dataset with, say, 500 observations. 500 observations are probably too few to partition into training, evaluation, and test data. Suppose the most pressing need is to select a value for a particular tuning parameter. We will see later that one such parameter can determine how complex the $\hat{f}(X)$ should be.

One can divide the data, for example, into five random, disjoint subsamples of 100 each, perhaps denoted by one of five letters A through E. For a trial value of the tuning parameter, the fitting process undertaken for the 400 cases in subsets A, B, C, D, and evaluated with the 100 hold-out cases in E. One proceeds in the same fashion until each of the five splits is used once as the hold-out subset, and each split has four opportunities to be included with three other splits when the algorithm is trained. There are then five measures of performance that are averaged.

The cross-validation is repeated in the same fashion with each potential tuning parameter value. In the end, one might compute the average of five AICs (Akaike 1973) for, say, 10 different tuning parameter values. The tuning parameter value with the best average performance over it fivefolds is selected. One has tuned using fivefold cross-validation.

The cross-validation process can be generalized to a set of values for different tuning parameters. One tries all reasonable combinations of values and chooses the one with the best average performance. In effect, one is tuning with a form of evaluation data.

Perhaps the essential conceptual point is that for each of the fivefolds, there is a legitimate set of hold-out observations not used to train the fitting procedure. Another important point is that the averaging over folds responds to uncertainty produced by the random, disjoint subsamples. Ideally, the noise cancels out. Recall that this is a problem for split samples.

Cross-validation is no doubt a clever technique for Level II analyses that might seem straightforward. It is not straightforward (Hastie et al. 2009: section 7.10). Splitting the data five ways is somewhat arbitrary. Occasionally, there are as few as three splits and often as many as ten. Also, one can treat the jackknife as "leave-one-out" cross-validation, in which case there are N splits.

And it matters. A larger number of splits means that the size of the training data relative to the evaluation data is greater. This improves performance in the training splits, but makes performance in the hold-out data less stable. The converse follows from a smaller number of splits. Common practice largely based on craft lore seems to favor either fivefold or tenfold cross-validation.

Cross-validation shares with data splitting reductions in sample size. If the statistical learning results are sample-size dependent, what does it mean to tune with a smaller sample than one ultimately uses? We will address these matters beginning in the next chapter.

Cross-validation seems to be best justified for tuning exercises. It is not clear how one should proceed once turning parameters are determined. The hold-out sample has been used as evaluation data. There is no hold-out sample to use as test data. We return to this issue in the next chapter.

Finally, formal treatments of cross-validation are complicated by the dependence between each fold. There are many common observations across the training subsets, and each evaluation subset is included in all but one of the training subsets. The strength of the dependence is dataset specific, which means that the overall properties of cross-validation are very difficult to pin down.

To summarize, for Level II analyses one should try to avoid in-sample determination of tuning parameter values and assessments of procedure performance. Having legitimate training data, evaluation data, and test data is probably the best option. Split samples are one fallback position. If interest centers on tuning alone, cross-validation can be a reasonable approach.

1.6.6 Loss Functions and Related Concepts

Equations (1.10) and (1.11) require that the $f(X)$ be learned from the data. Standard practice proceeds by finding a $\hat{f}(X)$ that minimizes some loss function. Loss functions quantifies how well the output of a statistical procedure corresponds to certain observed features of the data. As the name implies, one should favor small losses. We focus for now on numeric response variables in part because the issues are more familiar.

A very general expression for a loss function can be written as $L(Y, \hat{f}(X))$, where Y represents some feature of the data, and $\hat{f}(X)$ represents some empirical approximation of it. Often, Y is a response variable, and $\hat{f}(X)$ is the fitted values from some statistical procedure.[46]

In conventional treatments of estimation, there are loss functions that estimators minimize with respect to the data on hand. Least squares regression, for example, minimizes quadratic loss. For Poisson regression, the deviance is minimized. Quantile regression minimizes a piecewise linear loss.

On intuitive grounds, minimizing a loss functions seems reasonable. For a Level I analysis, in addition, loss functions can be sensible ways to justify the summary statistics computed. For example, least squares regression leads to fitted values for conditional means. Least absolute residual regression leads to fitted values for conditional medians. For a Level II analysis, many kinds of loss functions result in estimates that have well-known and desirable formal properties, as long as the requisite statistical assumptions are met. An absence of bias is a popular instance. Loss functions play an essential role in statistical learning for the same reasons. But as discussed in later chapters, the issues can be far more complicated in part because there is no model.

1.6.6.1 Definitions of In-Sample and Out-Of-Sample Performance

When the value of a loss function is interpreted as a summary statistic characterizing the quality of a fit (e.g., mean squared error), any conclusions are limited to the data on hand. The fitting performance is being addressed solely in-sample.

A natural Level II question is how well the $\hat{f}(X)$ performs out-of-sample. Generalization error, also called test error, is a performance metric that provides a conceptual framework (Hastie et al. 2009: 228). Suppose one has a test data denoted by (X^*, Y^*), where X^* is a set of predictors, and Y^* is the test data, numeric response variable. For the random variable Y, random variables X, and a learned algorithmic structure constructed from the training data $\mathcal{T}$, generalization error is defined as

$$\text{Err}_{\mathcal{T}} = \text{E}_{(X^*,Y^*)}[L(Y^*, \hat{f}(X^*))|\mathcal{T})]. \tag{1.12}$$

In words, the training data are treated as fixed once they are realized. A statistical learning procedure is applied to the training data to minimize some loss function in-sample. The result is a learned algorithmic structure. An example would be the result after applying the boosting-like illustration discussed earlier. Just as in many real forecasting settings, the training data and the learned structure are in the past and now do not change. Then, one may want to know how well the procedure performs with a single test data observation. One can compare Y_i^* to $\hat{f}(X_i^*)$ within a loss function such as squared error.[47]

More commonly, there is interest in average performance over realizations of the test data. $\text{E}_{(X^*,Y^*)}$ means that generalization error is the average loss over a limitless number of realized test observations, not a single observation. If one has test data, it is easy to obtain a valid estimate as well of its uncertainty—more on that later. Because generalization error treats the training data and algorithmic structure as fixed, it is a measure of fitting performance that sidesteps overfitting and data snooping.

There can also be interest in average generalization error if the training data $\mathcal{T}$ could also be realized over and over. With each realization of $\mathcal{T}$, the entire procedure represented in Eq. (1.12) is repeated. Then, *expected prediction error* (EPE) is defined as

$$\text{Err} = \text{E}_{\mathcal{T}}\text{E}_{(X^*,Y^*)}[L(Y^*, \hat{f}(X^*))|\mathcal{T})]. \tag{1.13}$$

As before, there is an expectation over realizations of the test data, but now there is also an expectation over realizations of the training data. One now has defined a second measure of out-of-sample fitting performance.

Estimating expected prediction error can be a major challenge. We will return to these issues as different algorithmic procedures are discussed. The fundamental task will be to isolate the impact of different sources of uncertainty.

1.6.6.2 Categorical Response Variables

For categorical responses, the conceptual foundations are unchanged. Generalization error can be written as

$$\text{Err}_{\mathcal{T}} = \text{E}_{(X^*,G^*)}[L(G^*, \hat{G}(X^*))|\mathcal{T})]. \tag{1.14}$$

As before, $\text{E}[\text{Err}_{\mathcal{T}}]$ is expected prediction error, and both $\text{Err}_{\mathcal{T}}$ and $\text{E}[\text{Err}_{\mathcal{T}}]$ can be of interest.

A look back at Fig. 1.11 will provide a sense of what generalization error and expected prediction error are trying to capture with $\hat{G}|X^*$. Suppose there are two actual response categories coded as 1 or 0. There are fitted values in the metric of proportions. A natural in-sample measure of loss is the deviance. There are also fitted classes depending on where a given proportion falls in relation to the classification threshold. A natural in-sample measure of loss is the proportion of cases for which the fitted class differs from the actual class. Some very powerful statistical learning procedures classify without the intermediate step of computing proportions, but disparities between the actual class and the fitted class are still central.

The estimation options and challenges for out-of-sample performance are much the same as for numerical response variables. Test data can help. There are many examples ahead.

1.6.6.3   Asymmetric Loss

The loss functions considered so far are symmetric. For a numerical response variable, a fitted value that is too large by some specific amount makes the same contribution to the loss function as a fitted value that is too small by that same amount. Consider, for example, the number of homeless in a census tract as the response variable, and predictors that are features of census tracts. Overestimating the number of homeless individuals in a census tract can have very different policy implications from underestimating the number of homeless individuals in a census tract (Berk et al. 2008). In the first instance, costly social services may be unnecessarily allocated to certain census tracts. In the second instance, those services may not be provided in census tracts that really need them. Yet, a symmetric loss function would assume that in the metric of costs, their consequences are exactly the same. One needs a loss function that properly takes the asymmetric costs into account so that the homeless estimates are responsive to how they will be used in practice.

Symmetric loss functions also dominate when the response variable is categorical. Suppose there are K exhaustive and mutually exclusive classes. Any misclassification—the fitted class is the wrong class—is given the same weight of 1.0. In a forecasting application, for instance, the error of predicting that a high school student will drop out when that student will not given the same weight as predicting that a high school student will not drop out when that student will. (Correct classifications are given a value of 0.0.)

Once again, one must ask if symmetric costs are reasonable. Are the costs really the same, or even close? In the case of the potential high school dropout, are the costs of interventions for a student who needs no interventions the same as failing to provide interventions for a student who needs them? A lot depends on the content of those interventions (e.g., academic tutoring, counseling). Especially in policy settings where decision-makers will be using the statistical learning results, symmetric costs may not be reasonable. Some mistakes are much worse than others, and the asymmetric costs must be allowed to affect how the statistical learning procedure performs. In later chapters, this will be a central concern.

1.6.7 The Bias–Variance Tradeoff

Before we move into more of the nuts and bolts of estimation, we need to revisit a bit more the bias–variance tradeoff. Recall that the bias–variance tradeoff is a Level II problem that arises when the true response surface is explicitly an estimation target. The goal is to produce an estimate of the true response surface that is as close as possible to the truth. In principle, this can be achieved by a judicious tradeoff between the bias of the estimates and the variance in those estimates.

If the estimation target is the *approximate* response surface, one hopes there is no bias, at least asymptotically, but a closely related tradeoff can be in play. When the focus is on generalization error, for example, the goal is to impute or forecast as accurately as possible even though one explicitly is using an approximation of the true response surface. That is, the actual estimation target is the potential response variable values in the joint probability distribution responsible for the data. We will see that in practice there will often be interest in both the properties of the population approximation and generalization error when the approximation is used for forecasting. For example, there can be interest in the size of the generalization error and in the predictors that are most strongly related to variation in the forecasts derived from the approximation.

To illustrate, using an asymptotically unbiased estimate of the mean function approximation linking daily ozone concentrations in a city and emergency room visits for respiratory distress, one might want to forecast a day or two in advance how many such visits there might be. Many factors affect emergency room visits, so one is clearly working with a mean function approximation. Bias in the projected number of emergency room visits might be reduced by using a different approximation; the approximation could be made more complex. Thinking in parametric terms for the moment, a 4th degree polynomial might be used instead of a second degree polynomial. But with a more complex parametric approximation, the effective degrees of freedom will be larger (more on that shortly). Other things equal, an increase in the effective degrees of freedom will increase the variance in fitted values as estimates. Hence, there is a potential tradeoff.

The tradeoff can be especially dicey with statistical learning because of the inductive nature of the procedures and the routine use of tuning. One problem is that the meaning and calculation of the effective degrees of freedom can be a challenge (Janson et al. 2015; Kaufman and Rosset 2014). We return to this issue shortly.

In practice, the bias–variance tradeoff primarily is used to think about how a learning algorithm is tuned or about the choice between different algorithms. There is usually no formal mathematics. A range of bias–variance tradeoffs is evaluated using some measure of in-sample performance. One might compare, for example, training data mean squared error for polynomial regressions of different order. Often, one goes with the approach that performs the best. Implicitly, a good bias–variance tradeoff has been made. The best formulation is then applied to test data.[48]

1.6.8   Linear Estimators

Level II statistical learning can capitalize on a wide variety of estimators. Linear estimators are often preferred because they can be seen as variants of conventional linear regression and are easily shown to have good statistical properties. Recall the hat matrix from conventional, fixed-x linear regression:

$$\hat{\mathbf{y}} = \mathbf{X}\boldsymbol{\beta} = \mathbf{X}(\mathbf{X}^T\mathbf{X})^{-1}\mathbf{X}^T\mathbf{y} = \mathbf{H}\mathbf{y}. \tag{1.15}$$

The hat matrix $\mathbf{H}$ transforms the y_i in a linear fashion into $\hat{y}_i$.[49] A smoother matrix is a generalization of the hat matrix.

Suppose there is a training dataset with N observations, a single fixed predictor X, and a single value of X, x_0. Generalizations to more than one predictor are provided in a later chapter. The fitted value for $\hat{y}_0$ at x_0 can be written as

$$\hat{y}_0 = \sum_{j=1}^{N} \mathbf{S}_{0j} y_j. \tag{1.16}$$

$\mathbf{S}$ is an N by N matrix, conventionally treated as fixed weights and is sometimes called a "smoother matrix."[50] $\mathbf{S}$ can be a product of a statistical learning procedure or some other nonparametric procedure. The subscript 0 denotes the row corresponding to the case whose fitted value of y is to be computed. The subscript j denotes the column in which the weight is found. In other words, the fitted value $\hat{y}_0$ at x_0 is a linear combination of all N values of y_i, with the weights determined by $\mathbf{S}_{0j}$. In many applications, the weights decline with the distance from x_0. Sometimes the declines are abrupt, as in a step function. In practice, therefore, a substantial number of the values in $\mathbf{S}_{0j}$ can be zero.

Consider the following cartoon illustration in matrix format. There are five observations constituting a time series. The goal is to compute a moving average of three observations going from the first observation to the last. In this setting, a moving average is a smoother, which some characterize as a form of machine learning. For simplicity, the middle value is given twice the weight of values on either side. Endpoints are often a complication in such circumstances and here, the first and last observations are just taken as is. The leftmost matrix is $\mathbf{S}$. It is post multiplied by the vector $\mathbf{y}$ to yield the fitted values $\hat{\mathbf{y}}$.

$$
\begin{pmatrix}
1.0 & 0 & 0 & 0 & 0 \\
0.25 & 0.50 & 0.25 & 0 & 0 \\
0 & 0.25 & 0.50 & 0.25 & 0 \\
0 & 0 & 0.25 & 0.50 & 0.25 \\
0 & 0 & 0 & 0 & 1.0
\end{pmatrix}
\begin{pmatrix}
3.0 \\
5.0 \\
6.0 \\
9.0 \\
10.0
\end{pmatrix}
=
\begin{pmatrix}
3.00 \\
4.75 \\
6.50 \\
8.50 \\
10.00
\end{pmatrix}. \tag{1.17}
$$

For a Level II analysis, one has a linear estimator of the conditional means of $\mathbf{y}$. It is a linear estimator because with $\mathbf{S}$ fixed, each value of y_i is multiplied by a constant before the y_i are added together; $\hat{y}_0$ is a linear combination of the y_i. Linearity can make it easier to determine the formal properties of an estimator, which are often highly desirable. Unbiasedness is a primary example.

When one views the data as generated from a joint probability distribution, X is no longer fixed. For the smoother matrix, with the hat matrix as a special case, one still has a linear estimator (Rice 2007, section 14.6). But getting the right standard errors requires a nonlinear estimator, and for the procedures in subsequent chapters, many of the estimators are nonlinear. It then can be very difficult to determine an estimator's properties and when there is success, asymptotics are usually required.

1.6.9 Degrees of Freedom

Woven through much of the discussion of Level II analyses has been the term "degrees of freedom." Its conceptual foundations are currently being re-evaluated. We need to do some of that too.

Recall that, loosely speaking, the degrees of freedom associated with an estimate is the number of observations that are free to vary, given how the estimate is computed. In the case of the mean, if one knows the values of $N - 1$ of those observations, and one knows the value of the mean, the value of the remaining observation can be easily obtained. Given the mean, $N - 1$ observations are free to vary. The remaining observation is not. So, there are $N - 1$ degrees of freedom associated with the estimator of the mean, and one degree of freedom is used up when the mean is calculated.

This sort of reasoning carries over to many common statistical procedures including those associated with linear regression analysis. The number of degrees of freedom used when the fitted values are computed is the number of regression parameters whose values need to be obtained (i.e., the intercept plus the regression coefficients). The degrees of freedom remaining, often called the "residual degrees of freedom," is the number of observations minus the number of these parameters to be estimated (Weisberg 2013: 26).

One of the interesting properties of the hat matrix is that the sum of its main diagonal elements (i.e., the trace) equals the number of regression parameters estimated. This is of little practical use with parametric regression because one can arrive at the same number by simply counting all of the regression coefficients and the intercept. However, the similarities between $\mathbf{H}$ and $\mathbf{S}$ (Hastie et al. 2009: section 5.4.1) imply that for linear estimators, the trace of $\mathbf{S}$ can be interpreted as the degrees of freedom used. Its value is sometimes called the "effective degrees of freedom" and can roughly be interpreted as the "equivalent number of parameters" (Ruppert et al. 2003: Sect. 3.13). That is, the trace of $\mathbf{S}$ can be thought of as capturing how much less the data are free to vary given the calculations required for $\mathbf{S}$. One can also think of the trace as qualifying "*optimism* of the residual sum of squares as an estimate of the out-of-sample prediction error" (Janson et al. 2015: 3).[51] As already noted several times, when more degrees of freedom are used (other things equal), in-sample fit will provide an increasingly unjustified, optimistic impression of out-of-sample performance.[52]

There are other definitions of the degrees of freedom associated with a smoother matrix. In particular, Ruppert and his colleagues (2003: Sect. 3.14) favor

$$df_{\mathbf{S}} = 2\mathrm{tr}(\mathbf{S}) - \mathrm{tr}(\mathbf{SS}^T). \tag{1.18}$$

In practice, the two definitions of the smoother degrees of freedom will not often vary by a great deal, but whether the two definitions lead to different conclusions depends in part on how they are used. If used to compute an estimate of the residual variance, their difference can sometimes matter. If used to characterize the complexity of the fitting function, their differences are usually less important because one smoother is compared to another applying the same yardstick. The latter application is far more salient in subsequent discussions. Beyond its relative simplicity, there seem to be interpretive reasons for favoring the first definition (Hastie et al. 2009: Sect. 5.4.1). Consequently, for linear estimators we use the trace of $\mathbf{S}$ as the smoother degrees of freedom.

Unfortunately, there are substantial complications. Consider a conventional linear regression. When there is model selection (e.g., using stepwise regression), more degrees of freedom are being used than the number of non-redundant regression parameters in the final model chosen. The same issues arise in supervised statistical learning, although often less visibly. Tuning requires even more degrees or freedom. How does one take this into account?

Efron's early work on prediction errors (1986) allows us to takes a step back to reformulate the problem. Effective degrees of freedom used boils down to how well the data are fit in training data compared to how well the data are fit in test data. Other things equal, the larger the gap, the larger the effective degrees of freedom used. Drawing from Efron (1986), Kaufman and Rosset (2014), and Janson and colleagues (2015), the effective degrees of freedom can be defined as

$$\mathrm{EDF} = \mathrm{E}\left[\sum_{i=1}^{N}(y_i^* - \hat{y}_i)^2\right], \tag{1.19}$$

where y_i^* is a realized y-value in test data, and $\hat{y}_i$ is a fitted value computed from the training data. The vector of x-values for case i does not change from realization to realization. Thus, one imagines two, fixed-x realizations of the response for each case. One is included in the training data and used to construct a fitted value. The other is included in the test data. The effective degrees of freedom is the expectation of the summed (over N), squared disparities between the two. The greater the average squared disparities between the fitted values from the training data and the new, realized values of Y, the greater the EDF employed. The EDF captures how much the degrees of freedom used by the fitting procedure by itself inflates the quality of the fit.

When the fitted values are constructed from a procedure with IID, finite, variance disturbances, one has

$$\text{EDF} = \frac{1}{\sigma^2} \sum_{i=1}^{N} \text{Cov}(y_i, \hat{y}_i). \tag{1.20}$$

The covariance for each case i is defined over realizations of Y with the predictor values fixed, and σ^2 is the variance of the disturbances as usual. Equation (1.20) is a standardized representation of similarity between the realized values of Y and the fitted values of Y. The greater the standardized linear association between the two, the larger the effective degrees of freedom.

In practice, neither definition is operational. But there are important special cases for which estimates of the EDF can be obtained. One of the most useful is when the estimator for the fitted values is linear (e.g., for a smoother matrix $\mathbf{S}$), and there is no data snooping. However, current thinking about the EDF appears to be limited to the fixed-x case, whereas statistical learning usually conceives both Y and X as random variables. How to formulate the EDF with random X is apparently unsolved. Indeed, the concept of EDF might usefully be abandoned and replaced by formulations for unjustified optimism. In a very wide set of circumstances, this could be addressed with training and test data in ways discussed later.

1.6.10 Basis Functions

Another consideration in thinking about effective degrees of freedom is that the procedures discussed in subsequent chapters commonly do not work directly with the given set of predictors. Rather, the design matrix in a Level I or Level II analysis can be comprised of linear basis expansions of X. Linear basis expansions allow for a more flexible fitting function, typically by increasing the number of columns in the design matrix. A set of p predictors becomes a set of predictors much greater than p. This can allow the fitted values to be more responsive to the data.

Consider first the case when there is a single predictor. X contains two columns, one column with the values of that single predictor and one column solely of 1s for the intercept. The $N \times 2$ matrix is sometimes called the "basis" of a bivariate regression model. This basis can be expanded in a linear fashion as follows:

$$f(X) = \sum_{m=1}^{M} \beta_m h_m(X). \tag{1.21}$$

There are M transformations of X, which can include the untransformed predictor, and typically a leading column of 1s is included (allowing for a y-intercept) as well. β_m is the weight given to the mth transformation, and $h_m(X)$ is the mth transformation of X. Consequently, $f(X)$ is a linear combination of transformed values of X.

One common transformation employs polynomial terms such as 1, x, x^2, x^3. Each term does not have to be a linear transformation of x, but the transformations are *combined* in a linear fashion. Then, Eq. (1.21) takes the form

$$f(X) = \beta_0 + \beta_1 x + \beta_2 x^2 + \beta_3 x^3. \tag{1.22}$$

When least squares is applied, a conventional hat matrix follows, from which fitted values may be constructed.

Another popular option is to construct a set of indicator variables. For example, one might have predictor z, transformed in the following manner.

$$f(Z) = \beta_0 + \beta_1(I[z > 5]) + \beta_2(I[z > 8 | z > 5]) + \beta_3(I[z < 2]). \tag{1.23}$$

As before, fitting by least squares leads to a conventional hat matrix from which the fitted values may be constructed.[53]

Equation (1.21) can be generalized so that $p > 1$ predictors may be included:

$$f(X) = \sum_{j=1}^{p} \sum_{m=1}^{M_j} \beta_{jm} h_{jm}(X). \tag{1.24}$$

There are p predictors, each denoted by j, and each with its own M_j transformations. All of the transformations for all predictors, each with its weight β_{jm}, are combined in a linear fashion. For example, one could combine Eqs. (1.22) and (1.23) with both X and Z as predictors. It is also possible, and even common in some forms of statistical learning, to define *each* basis function as a complicated function of two or more predictors. For example, recall that the usual cross-product matrix so central to linear regression is $\mathbf{X}^T \mathbf{X}$. As we will see later, "kernels" broadly based on $\mathbf{X}\mathbf{X}^T$ can be constructed that serve as very effective linear basis expansions.

Linear basis expansions are no less central to many forms of classification. Figure 1.13 provides a visual sense of how. Decisions boundaries are essentially fitted values from some procedure that separate one class from another, and can then be used to decide in which class a new case belongs. In Fig. 1.13, there are two classes represented by either a red circle or a blue circle. There are two predictors, X_1 and X_2. Figure 1.13 is a 3-dimensional scatterplot.

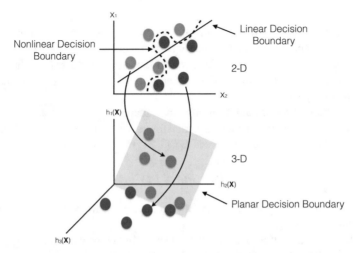

Fig. 1.13 Reductions in classification errors using linear basis expansions (The *red filled circles* and the *blue filled circles* represent different classes. The *top figure* shows how classification errors can be reduced with a nonlinear decision boundary. The *bottom figure* shows how classification errors can be reduced by including a third predictor dimension)

The upper plot shows in 2-D predictor space a linear decision boundary. All cases falling above the linear boundary are classified as red circles, because red circles are the majority. All cases falling below the linear boundary are classified as blue circles because blue circles are the majority. The linear decision boundary produces three classification errors. There is one blue circle above the decision boundary and two red circles below the decision boundary. Separation between the two classes is imperfect, and in this illustration, no linear decision boundary can separate the two classes perfectly. However, also shown is a nonlinear decision boundary that can. The trick would be to find transformations of the two predictors from which such a decision boundary could be constructed.

Sometimes there is an effective way to proceed. The lower plot in Fig. 1.13 shows the same binary outcomes in 3-D space. A third dimension has been added. The two curved arrows show how the locations for two illustrative points are moved. As just noted, new dimensions can result from transformations when there is a basis expansion. Here, the three transformation functions are shown as h_1, h_2, and h_3. Within this 3-D predictor space, all of the blue circles are toward the front of the figure, and all of the red circles are toward the back of the figure. The plane shown is a *linear* decision boundary that leads to perfect separation. By adding a dimension, perfect separation can be obtained, and one can work in a more congenial linear world. In 3-D, one has in principle an easier classification problem. Then if one wishes, the 3-D predictor space can be projected back to the 2-D predictor space to

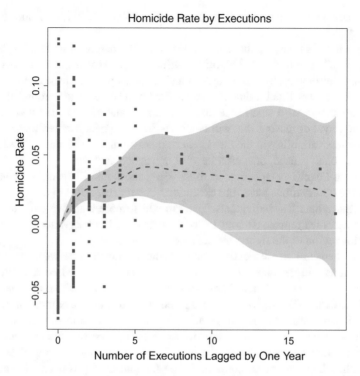

Fig. 1.14 The homicide rate per 1000 as a function of the number of executions lagged by 1 year (The homicide rate is on vertical axis, and the number of executions 1 year earlier is on the horizontal axis. The blue dots are residuals. The broken line represents the fitted values, and the gray region shows the error band)

view the results as a function of the two original predictors. Back in 2-D predictor space, the decision boundary can then be nonlinear, often very nonlinear.

But if Eq. (1.24) is essentially multiple regression, where does statistical learning come in? The answer is that statistical learning procedures often "invent" their own linear basis expansions. That is, the linear basis expansions are inductively constructed as a product of how the algorithmic procedure "learns." Alternatively, a data analyst may provide the algorithm with far too many basis expansions terms, sometimes more terms than there are observations, and the algorithm decides inductively which are really needed.

Figure 1.14 provides an illustration. The observational units are all 50 states each year from 1978 to 1998, for a total of 1000 observations. For each state each year, the homicide rate and the number of executions for capital crimes the previous year were recorded. Data such as these have been central in debates about the deterrent value of the death penalty (Nagin and Pepper 2012).

Executions lagged by 1 year is on the horizontal axis. It is the only predictor and is included as a numeric variable. The homicide rate per 1000 people is on the vertical axis. It too is numeric. Perhaps executions 1 year affect homicides the next year.

No position is taken by the data analyst about the nature of its relationship; the values "as is" are input to the algorithm. Linear basis expansions and transformations were introduced by the algorithm and hidden inside a black box. The blue, dashed line shows fitted values centered at zero. The residuals around the fitted values are shown with small blue dots. The error band around the fitted values is shown in gray. For reasons that will be discussed in the next chapter, the error band only captures variability in the fitted values; there are no confidence intervals. Still, if the error band is used, one has a Level II regression analysis.

Within a Level I perspective, in most years, most states execute no one. Over 80% of the observations have zero executions. A very few states in a very few years execute more than five individuals. Years in which more than five individuals in a state are executed represent about 1% of the data (i.e., 11 observations out of 1000) and in this region of the figure, the data are very sparse.

When there are five executions or less, the relationship between the number of executions and the homicide rate 1 year later is positive. More executions are followed 1 year later by more homicides. Thus, there is a positive association for 99% of the data. When a given state in a given year executes six or more individuals, the relationship appears to turn negative. With more executions, there are fewer homicides 1 year later. But there are almost no data supporting the change in sign, and from a Level II perspective, the error band around that portion of the curve implies that the relationship could easily be flat and even positive.[54] In short, for 99% of the data, the relationship is positive and for the atypical 1%, one really cannot tell. (For more details, see Berk 2005.)

Figure 1.14 provides a visualization of how a response of great policy interest and a single predictor of great policy interest are related. There is no model in the conventional regression sense. The fitted values shown were arrived at inductively by a statistical learning algorithm. Had a linear mean function been imposed, the few influential points to the far right of the figure would have produced a negative regression coefficient. One might incorrectly conclude that on the average, there is evidence for the deterrent effect of executions. In practice, of course, the potential role of confounders would need to be considered. We are working with an approximation of the true response surface.

In summary, linear basis expansions can be an important, and even essential, feature of statistical learning. Many statistical learning algorithms can be seen as instruments in service of finding linear basis expansions that facilitate prediction. Where the algorithms differ is in exactly how they do that.

1.6.11 The Curse of Dimensionality

Linear basis expansions increase the dimensionality of a dataset. As just described, this is often a good thing. In this era of "Big Data" it is also increasingly common

Fig. 1.15 Some consequences of high dimensional data (The predictor space spaced needed to be filled with data increases as power function of the number of dimensions, and the observations tend to move toward the outer edges)

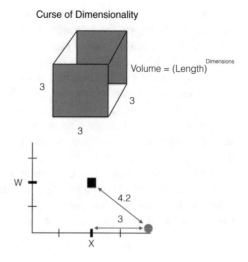

to have access to data not just with a very large number of observations, but with a very large number of variables. For example, the IRS might merge its own records with records from Health and Human Services and the Department of Labor. Both the number of observations (N) and number of dimensions (p) could be enormous. Except for data management concerns, one might assume that bigger data are always better than smaller data. But it is not that simple.

One common and vexing complication is called "the curse of dimensionality:" the number of variables exceeds the support available in the data. Figure 1.15 shows two especially common difficulties that can arise in practice. The cube at the top illustrates that as the number of dimensions increases linearly, the volume of the resulting space increases as a power function of the number of dimensions. Hence, the 3 by 3 square has 9 units of space to fill with data, whereas the 3 by 3 by 3 cube has 27 units of space to fill with data. For a dataset with a fixed number of observations, the distribution of the observations can become very sparse. The space is less adequately covered so that the sample size per unit of space decreases. A data analysis one might like to do can become impractical. In particular, key regions of a nonlinear $f(\mathbf{X})$ may be very poorly estimated for lack of sufficient data.

Unless more observations can be obtained, some simplifications need to be imposed by the data analyst. A popular approach introduces (untestable) assumptions requiring that the true response surface is relatively smooth. In effect, the smoother surface substitutes for data when for particular regions of the predictor space there are very few observations.

Alternatively, one can try to reduce the dimensionality of the data using variable selection procedures, shrinkage, an incomplete Cholesky decomposition, or principal components. But each of these comes with their own challenges. For example, if principle components analysis is used, one must determine how many of the principle components to include. In practice, there is rarely an easy answer.

The bottom figure illustrates a second complication. With an increase in the number of dimensions, the data move farther from the center of the space. For a very large p, the data can be concentrated toward the edges of the space. In the figure, a distance of 3 units in one dimension can become a distance of 4.2 in two dimensions. Thus, a hypercube with 5 sides of 3 units each has a maximum Euclidian distance of 6.7 units, whereas a hypercube with 10 sides of 3 units each has a maximum Euclidian distance of 22.3 units. The problem for a data analysis is that the region toward the center of the space becomes especially sparse. In that region, it will be very difficult to estimate effectively an approximate response surface, especially if it is complicated. Once again, the data analyst must simplify how the estimation is undertaken or reduce the number of dimensions.

In short, higher dimensional data can be very useful when there are more associations in the data that can be exploited. And at least ideally, a large p comes with a large N. If not, what may look like a blessing can actually be a curse.

1.7 Statistical Learning in Context

Data analysis, whatever the tools, takes place in a professional setting that can influence how the analysis is undertaken. Far more is involved than formal technique. Although we cannot consider these matters at any length, a few brief observations are probably worth mention.

- *It is Important to Keep Humans in the Loop*—With the increasing processing power of computers, petabytes of storage, efficient algorithms, and a rapidly expanding statistical toolbox, there are strong incentives to delegate data analyses to machines. At least in the medium term, this is a huge mistake. Humans introduce a host of critical value judgements, intuitions, and context that computers cannot. Worse than a statistical bridge to nowhere is a statistical bridge to the wrong place. A better formulation is a structured computer–human partnership on which there is already interesting work in progress (Michelucci and Dickinson 2016).
- *Sometimes There is No Good Solution*—The moment one leaves textbook examples behind, there is a risk that problems with the data and/or the statistical procedures available will be insurmountable. That risk is to be expected in the real world of empirical research. There is no shame in answering an empirical question with "I can't tell." There is shame in manufacturing results for appearance's sake. Assume-and-proceed statistical practice can be a telling example. In later chapters, we will come upon unsolved problems in statistical learning where, in the words of Shakespeare's Falstaff, "The better part of valor is discretion" (Henry the Fourth, Part 1, Act 5, Scene 4).
- *The Audience Matters*—Results that are difficult to interpret in subject-matter terms, no matter how good the statistical performance, are often of little use. This will sometimes lead to another kind of tradeoff. Algorithmic procedures that

perform very well by various technical criteria may stumble when the time comes to convey what the results mean. Important features of the data analysis may be lost. It will sometimes be useful, therefore, to relax the technical performance criteria a bit in order to get results that effectively inform substantive or policy matters. One implication is that an effective data analysis is best done with an understanding of who will want to use the results and the technical background they bring. It can also be important to anticipate preconceptions that might make it difficult to "hear" what the data analysis has to say. For example, it can be very difficult to get certain academic disciplines to accept the results from algorithmic procedures because those disciplines are so steeped in models.

- *Decisions That Can Be Affected*—Knowing your audience can also mean knowing what decisions might be influenced by the results of a data analysis. Simply put, if one's goal is to bring information from a data analysis to bear on real decisions, the data analysis must be situated within the decision-making setting. This can mean making sure that the inputs and outputs are those that decision-makers deem relevant and that the details of the algorithmic procedures comport well with decision-maker needs. For example, if forecasting errors lead to asymmetric losses, asymmetric costs should be built into the algorithmic procedure.

- *Differences That Make No Difference*—In almost every issue of journals that publish work on statistical learning and related procedures, there will be articles offering some new wrinkle on existing techniques, or even new procedures, often with strong claims about superior performance compared to some number of other approaches. Such claims are often data-specific but even if broadly true, rarely translate into important implications for practice. Often the claims of improved performance are small by any standard. Some claims of improved performance are unimportant for the subject-matter problem being tackled. But even when the improvements seem to be legitimately substantial, they often address secondary concerns. In short, although it is important to keep up with new developments, the newest are not necessarily important.

- *Software That Makes No Difference (or is actually worse)*—The hype can apply to software as well. While this edition is being written, the world is buzzing with talk of "deep learning," "big data", "analytics," and "artificial intelligence." Not surprisingly, there are in response a substantial number of software purveyors claiming to offer the very latest and very best tools, which perform substantially better than the competition. *Caveat emptor.* Often, information on how the software runs is proprietary and no real competitive benchmarks are provided. Much like for the Wizard of Oz, there may be little behind a slick user interface. That is one reason why in this book we exclusively use the programming language R. It is free, so there are no sales incentives. The source code can be downloaded. If one wants to make the effort, it is possible to determine if anyone is hiding the ball. And with access to the source code, changes and enhancements in particular procedures can be written.

- *Data Quality Really Matters*—Just as in any form of regression analysis, good data are a necessary prerequisite. If there are no useful predictors, if the data are sparse, if key variables are highly skewed or unbalanced, or if the key variables are poorly measured, it is very unlikely that the choice of one among several statistical learning procedures will be very important. The problems are bigger than that. It is rare indeed when even the most sophisticated and powerful statistical learning procedures can overcome the liabilities of bad data. A closely related point is that a substantial fraction of the time invested in a given data analysis will be spent cleaning up the data and getting it into the requisite format. These tasks can require substantial skill only tangentially related to conventional statistical expertise.

- *The Role of Subject-Matter Expertise*—Subject-matter expertise can be very important in the following:

  1. Framing the empirical questions to be addressed;
  2. Defining a data generation mechanism;
  3. Designing and implementing the data collection;
  4. Determining which variables in the dataset are to be inputs and which are to be outputs;
  5. Settling on the values of tuning parameters; and
  6. Deciding which results make sense.

But none of these activities is necessarily formal or deductive, and they leave lots of room for interpretation. If the truth be told, subject-matter theory plays much the same role in statistical learning as it does in most conventional analyses. But in statistical learning, there is often far less posturing.

Demonstrations and Exercises

The demonstrations and exercises in the book emphasize data analysis, not the formalities of mathematical statistics. The goal is to provide practice in learning from data. The demonstrations and exercises for this chapter provide a bit of practice doing regression analyses by examining conditional distributions without the aid of conventional linear regression. It is an effort to get back to first principles unfiltered by least squares regression. Another goal is to show how data snooping can lead to misleading results. Commands in R are shown in italics. However, as already noted several times, R and the procedures in R are moving targets. What runs now may not run later, although there will almost certainly be procedures available that can serve as adequate substitutes. Often, examples of relevant code in R be found in the empirical examples provided in each chapter.

Set 1

Load the R dataset "airquality" using *data(airquality)*. Learn about the dataset using *help(airquality)*. Attach the dataset "airquality" using *attach(airquality)*. If you do not have access to R, or choose to work with other software, exercises in the same spirit can be easily undertaken. Likewise, exercises in the same spirit can be easily undertaken with other datasets.

1. Using *summary* take a look at some summary statistics for the data frame. Note that there are some missing data and that all of the variables are numeric.
2. Using *pairs*, construct of a scatterplot matrix including all of the variables in the dataset. These will all be joint (bivariate) distributions. Describe the relationships between each pair of variables. Are there associations? Do they look linear? Are there outliers?
3. Using *boxplot*, construct separate side-by-side boxplots for ozone concentrations conditioning on month and ozone concentrations conditioning on day. Does the ozone distribution vary by month of the year? In what way? What about by day?
4. Construct a three-dimensional scatterplot with ozone concentrations as the response and temperature and wind speed as predictors. This will be a joint distribution. Try using *cloud* from the *lattice* package. There are lots of slick options. What patterns can you make out? Now repeat the graphing but condition on month. What patterns do you see now? (For ease of readability, you can make the variable month a factor with each level named. For really fancy plotting, have a look at the library *ggplot2*. For 3D plots, recent and powerful plotting methods are provided in the library *plot3D* and in library *scatterplot3d*.)
5. From the *graphics* library, construct a conditioning plot using *coplot* with ozone concentrations as the response, temperature as a predictor, and wind speed as a conditioning variable. How does the conditioning plot attempt to hold wind speed constant?

    (a) Consider all the conditioning scatterplots. What common patterns do you see? What does this tell you about how ozone concentrations are related to temperature with wind speed held constant?
    (b) How do the patterns differ across the conditioning scatterplots? What does that tell you about interaction effects: the relationship between ozone concentrations and temperature can differ for different wind speeds?

6. Construct an indicator variable for missing data for the variable Ozone. (Using *is.na* is a good way.) Applying *table*, cross-tabulate the indicator against month. What do you learn about the pattern of missing data? How might your earlier analyses using the conditioning plot be affected? (If you want to percentage the table, *prop.table* is a good way.)
7. Write out the parametric regression model that seems to be most consistent with what you have learned from the conditioning plot. Try to justify all of the assumptions you are imposing.

8. Implement your regression model in R using *lm* and examine the results. Look at the regression diagnostics using *plot*. What do the four plots tell you about your model? How do your conclusions about the correlates of ozone concentrations learned from the regression model compare to the conclusions about the correlates of ozone concentrations learned from the conditioning plot?

Set 2

The purpose of this exercise is to give you some understanding about how the complexity of a fitting function affects the results of a regression analysis and how test data can help.

1. Construct the training data as follows. For your predictor: $x = rep(1:30, times = 5)$. This will give you 150 observations with values 1 through 30. For your response: $y=rnorm(150)$. This will give you 150 random draws from the standard normal distribution. As such, they are on the average independent of x. This is the same as letting $y = 0 + 0x + \varepsilon$, which is nature's data generation process.
2. Plot the response against the predictor and describe what you see? Is what you see consistent with how the data were generated?
3. Apply a bivariate regression using *lm*. Describe what overall conclusions you draw from the output. The linear functional form is the "smoothest" possible relationship between a response and a predictor.
4. Repeat the linear regression with the predictor as a factor. Apply the same R code as before but use *as.factor(x)* instead of x. This is a linear basis expansion of x. The set of indicator variables for x (one for each value of x) when used as predictors leads to the "roughest" possible relationship between a response and a predictor. (Technically, you now doing a multiple regression.) Each value of the predictor can have its own estimate of the conditional mean. (In this case, you know that those conditional means are 0.0 in nature's "generative process.") Compare the R^2 and the adjusted R^2 from the *lm* output and to the output from #3. What can you say about overfitting. Is there evidence of it here?
5. Construct 1/0 indicator variables for x-indicator variables whose t-values are greater than 1.64. (The *ifelse* command is a good way to do this.) Apply *lm* again including only these indicator variables as predictors. What do you find? (By chance, it is possible—but unlikely—that there is still nothing that is "statistically significant." If so, go back to step #1 and regenerate the data. Then pick up at step $3.)
6. Construct test data by repeating step #1. Because x is treated as fixed, you only need to regenerate y. Regress the new y on the subset of indicator variables you used in the previous step. What do you find? The results illustrate the important role of test data.

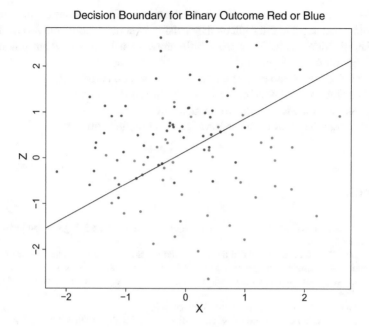

Fig. 1.16 For predictors X and Z, and a binary response coded as blue or red, an overlaid decision boundary derived from a logistic regression (N = 100: 45 Reds and 55 Blues)

Set 3

The purpose of this exercise is to get you thinking about decision boundaries for classification problems. Figure 1.16 shows a decision boundary for a binary response coded as red or blue. The predictors are X and Z. The overlaid straight line is a decision boundary based on a logistic regression and values of X and Z for which response odds are $0.5/(1 - 0.5) = 1.0$.

1. Should the observations above the decision be classified as blue or red? Why?
2. Should the observations below the decision be classified as blue or red? Why?
3. Suppose there were observations with a z-value of 1 and an x-value of -1, but with an unknown response. What would be your best guess: red or blue? Why?
4. Suppose there were observations with a z-value of -1.5 and an x-value of 0.5, but with an unknown response. What would be your best guess: red or blue? Why?
5. Why do you think the decision boundary was located at an odds of 1.0?
6. How many red observations are misclassified? (For purposes of this exercise, points that seem to fall right on the decision boundary should not be considered classification errors. They are a little above or a little below, but you cannot really tell from the plot.)

7. How many blue observations are misclassified? (For purposes of this exercise, points that seem to fall right on the decision boundary should not be considered classification errors. They are a little above or a little below, but you cannot really tell from the plot.)
8. What fraction of the blue observations is classified correctly?
9. What fraction of the red observations is classified correctly?
10. Which outcome is classified more accurately?
11. What fraction of all of the observations is classified correctly?

Endnotes

[1] Regularization will have a key role in much of the material ahead. It goals and features will be addressed as needed.

[2] "Realized" here means produced through a random process. Random sampling from a finite population is an example. Data generated by a correct linear regression model can also be said to be realized. After this chapter, we will proceed almost exclusively with a third way in which data can be realized.

[3] The data, *birthwt*, are from the MASS package in R.

[4] The χ^2 test assumes that the marginal distributions of both variables are fixed in repeated realizations of the data. Only the distribution of counts within cells can change. Whether this is a plausible assumption depends on how the data were generated. If the data are a random sample from a well-defined population, the assumption of fixed marginal distributions is not plausible. Both marginal distributions would almost certainly change in new random samples. The spine plot and the mosaic plot were produced using the R package *vcd*, which stands for "visualizing categorical data." Its authors are Meyer et al. (2007).

[5] Although there are certainly no universal naming conventions, "predictors" can be seen as variables that are of subject-matter interest, and "covariates" can be seen as variables that improve the performance of the statistical procedure being applied. Then, covariates are not of subject-matter interest. Whatever the naming conventions, the distinction between variables that matter substantively and variables that matter procedurally is important. An example of the latter is a covariate included in an analysis of randomized experiments to improve statistical precision.

[6] A crime is "cleared" when the perpetrator is arrested. In some jurisdictions, a crime is cleared when the perpetrator has been identified, even if there has been no arrest.

[7] But nature can certainly specify different predictor values for different students.

[8] By "asymptotics," one loosely means what happens to the properties an estimate as the number of observations increases without limit. Sometimes, for example, bias in the estimate shrinks to zero, which means that in sufficiently large samples, the bias will likely be small. Thus, the desirable estimation properties of logistic regression only materialize asymptotically. This means that one can get very misleading results from logistic regression in small samples if one is working at Level II.

[9] This is sometimes called "the fallacy of accepting the null" (Rozeboom 1960).

[10] Model selection in some disciplines is called variable selection, feature selection, or dimension reduction. These terms will be used interchangeably.

[11] Actually, it can be more complicated. For example, if the predictors are taken to be fixed, one is free to examine the predictors alone. Model selection problems surface when associations with the response variable are examined as well. If the predictors are taken to be random, the issues are even more subtle.

[12] If one prefers to think about the issues in a multiple regression context, the single predictor can be replaced by the predictor adjusted, as usual, for its linear relationships with all other predictors.

[13] Recall that x is fixed and does not change from dataset to dataset. The new datasets result from variation around the true conditional means.

[14] We will see later that by increasing the complexity of the mean function estimated, one has the potential to reduce bias with respect to the true response surface. But an improved fit in the data on hand is no guarantee that one is more accurately representing the true mean function. One complication is that greater mean function complexity can promote overfitting.

[15] The next several pages draw heavily on Berk et al. (2019) and Buja et al. (2019a,b).

[16] Each case is composed of a set (i.e., vector) of values for the random variables that are included.

[17] The notation may seem a little odd. In a finite population, these would be matrices or vectors, and the font would be bold. But the population is of limitless size because it constitutes what could be realized from the joint probability distribution. These random variables are really conceptual constructs. Bold font might have been more odd still. Another notational scheme could have been introduced for these statistical constructs, but that seems a bit too precious and in context, unnecessary.

[18] For exposition, working with conditional expectations is standard, but there are other options such as conditional probabilities when the predictor is categorical. This will be important in later chapters.

[19] They are deviations around a mean, or more properly, an expected value.

[20] For example, experiences in the high school years will shape variables such as the high school GPA, the number of advanced placement courses taken, the development of good study habits, an ability to think analytically, and performance on the SAT or ACT test, which, in turn, can be associated the college grades freshman year. One can easily imagine representing these variables in a joint probability distribution.

[21] We will see later that some "weak" forms of dependence are allowed.

[22] This intuitively pleasing idea has in many settings solid formal justification (Efron and Tibshirani 1993: chapter 4).

[23] There is no formal way to determine how large is large enough because such determinations are dataset specific.

[24] Technically, a prediction interval is not a confidence interval. A confidence interval provides coverage for a parameter such as a mean or regression coefficient. A prediction interval provides coverage for a response variable value. Nevertheless, prediction intervals are often called confidence intervals.

[25] The use of split samples means that whatever overfitting or data snooping that might result from the fitting procedure apply to the first split and do not taint the residuals from the second split. Moreover, there will typically be no known or practical way to do proper statistical inference that includes uncertainty from the training data and fitting procedure when there is data snooping.

[26] This works because the data are assumed to be IID, or at least exchangeable. Therefore, it makes sense to consider the interval in which forecasted values fall with a certain probability (e.g., .95) in limitless IID realizations of the forecasting data.

[27] Because of the random split, the way some of the labels line up in the plot may not be quite right when the code is run again. But that is easily fixed.

[28] The use of split samples can be a disadvantage. As discussed in some detail later, many statistical learning are sample-size dependent when the fitting is undertaken. Smaller samples lead to fitted values and forecasts that can have more bias with respect to the true response surface. But in trade, no additional assumptions need be made when the second split is used to compute residuals.

[29] If the sampling were without replacement, the existing data would simply be reproduced unless the sample size was smaller than N. More will be said about this option in later chapters based on work by Buja and Stuetzle (2006).

[30] The *boot* procedures stem from the book by Davidson (1997). The code is written by Angelo Canty and Brian Ripley.

[31] The second-order conditions differ substantially from conventional linear regression because the 1s and 0s are a product of Bernoulli draws (McCullagh and Nelder 1989: Chapter 4). It follows

that unlike least squares regression for linear models, logistic regression depends on asymptotics to obtain desirable estimation properties.

[32] Some treatments of machine learning include logistic regression as a form of supervised learning. Whether in these treatments logistic regression is seen as a model or an algorithm is often unclear. But it really matters, which will be more apparent shortly.

[33] As a categorial statement, this is a little too harsh. Least squares itself is an algorithm that in fact can be used on some statistical learning problems. But regression analysis formulated as a linear model incorporates many addition features that have little or nothing to do with least squares. This will be more clear shortly.

[34] There is also "semisupervised" statistical learning that typically concentrates on $Y|X$, but for which there are more observations for the predictors than for the response. The usual goal is to fit the response better using not just set of observations for which both Y and X are observed, but also using observations for which only X is observed. Because an analysis of $Y|X$ will often need to consider the joint probability distribution of X as well, the extra data on X alone can be very useful.

[35] Recall that because we treat the predictors that constitute $\mathbf{X}$ as random variables, the disparities between the approximation and the truth are also random, which allows them to be incorporated in ε.

[36] Some academic disciplines like to call the columns of X "inputs," and Y an "output" or a "target." Statisticians typically prefer to call the columns of X "predictors" and Y a "response." By and large, the terms predictor (or occasionally, regressor) and response will be used here except when there are links to computer science to be made. In context, there should be no confusion.

[37] In later chapters, several procedures will be discussed that can help one consider the "importance" of each input and how inputs are related to outputs.

[38] A functional is a function that takes one or more functions as arguments.

[39] An estimand is a feature of the joint probability distribution whose value(s) are primary interest. An estimator is a computational procedures that can provide estimates of the estimand. An estimate is the actual numerical value(s) produced by the estimator. For example, the expected value of a random variable may be the estimand. The usual expression for the mean in an IID dataset can be the estimator. The value of the mean obtained from the sample is the estimate. These terms apply to Level II, statistical learning but with more a complicated conceptual scaffolding.

[40] Should a linear probability model be chosen for binomial regression, one could write $G = f(X) + \varepsilon$, which unlike logistic regression, can be estimated by least squares. However, it has several undesirable properties such as sometimes returning fitted values larger than 1.0 or smaller than 0.0 (Hastie et al. 2009: section 4.2).

[41] The term "mean function" can be a little misleading when the response variable is G. It would be more correct to use "proportion function" or "probability function." But "mean function" seems to be standard, and we will stick with it.

[42] Clustering algorithms have been in use since the 1940s ((Cattell 1943)), long before there was the discipline of computer science was born. When rebranded as unsupervised learning, these procedures are just old wine in new bottles. There are other examples of conceptual imperialism, many presented as a form of supervised learning. A common instance is logistic regression, which dates back to at least the 1950s (Cox 1958). Other academic disciplines also engage in rebranding. The very popular difference-in-differences estimator claimed as their own by economists (Abadie 2005) was initially developed by educational statisticians a generation earlier (Linn and Slinde 1977), and the associated research design was formally proposed by Campbell and Stanley (1963).

[43] Tuning is somewhat like setting the dials on a coffee grinder by trial and error to determine how fine the grind should be and how much ground coffee should be produced.

[44] For linear models, several in-sample solutions have been proposed for data snooping (Berk et al. 2014a,b; Lockhart et al. 2014; Lei et al. 2018), but they are not fully satisfactory, especially for statistical learning.

[45] The issues surrounding statistical inference are more complicated. The crux is that uncertainty in the training data and in the algorithm is ignored when performance is gauged solely with test data. This is addressed in the chapters ahead.

[46] Loss functions are also called "objective functions" or "cost functions".

[47] In R, many estimation procedures have a prediction procedure that can easily be used with test data to arrive at test data fitted values.

[48] As noted earlier, one likely would be better off using evaluation data to determine the order of the polynomial.

[49] The transformation is linear because the $\hat{y}_i$ are a linear combination of the y_i. This does not mean that the *relationships* between $\mathbf{X}$ and $\mathbf{y}$ are necessarily linear.

[50] This is a carry-over from conventional linear regression in which $\mathbf{X}$ is fixed. When $\mathbf{X}$ is random, Eq. (1.16) does not change. There are, nevertheless, important consequences for estimation that we have begun to address. One may think of the $\hat{y}_i$ as estimates of population approximation, not of the true response surface.

[51] Emphasis in the original.

[52] The residual degrees of freedom can then be computed by subtraction (see also Green and Silverman 1994: Sect. 3.3.4).

[53] The symbol I denotes an indicator function. The result is equal to 1 if the argument in brackets is true and equal to 0 if the argument in brackets is false. The 1s and 0s constitute an indicator variable. Sometimes indicator variables are called a dummy variables.

[54] To properly employ a Level II framework, lots of hard thought would be necessary. For example, are the observations realized independently as the joint probability distribution approach requires? And if not, then what?.

References

Abadie, A. (2005). Semiparametric difference-in-differences estimators. *Review of Economic Studies 72*(1), 1–19.

Akaike, H. (1973). Information theory and an extension to the maximum likelihood principle. In B. N. Petrov & F. Casaki (Eds.), *International symposium on information theory* (pp. 267–281). Budapest: Akademia Kiado.

Angrist, J. D., & Pischke, J. (2009). *Mostly harmless econometrics*. Princeton: Princeton University.

Barber, D. (2012). *Bayesian reasoning and machine learning*. Cambridge: Cambridge University.

Berk, R. A. (2003). *Regression analysis: A constructive critique*. Newbury Park, CA.: SAGE.

Berk, R. A. (2005). New claims about executions and general deterrence: Déjà Vu all over again? *Journal of Empirical Legal Studies, 2*(2), 303–330.

Berk, R. A., & Freedman, D. A. (2003). Statistical assumptions as empirical commitments. In T. Blomberg & S. Cohen (Eds.), *Law, punishment, and social control: Essays in honor of Sheldon Messinger*. Part V (pp. 235–254). Aldine de Gruyter, November 1995, revised in second edition, 2003.

Berk, R. A., Kriegler, B., & Ylvisaker, D. (2008). Counting the homeless in Los Angeles county. In D. Nolan & S. Speed (Eds.), *Probability and statistics: Essays in honor of David A. Freedman*. Monograph series for the institute of mathematical statistics.

Berk, R. A., Brown, L., & Zhao, L. (2010). Statistical inference after model selection. *Journal of Quantitative Criminology, 26*, 217–236.

Berk, R. A., Brown, L., Buja, A., Zhang, K., & Zhao, L. (2014a). Valid post-selection inference. *Annals of Statistics, 41*(2), 802–837.

Berk, R. A., Brown, L., Buja, A., George, E., Pitkin, E., Zhang, K., et al. (2014b). Misspecified mean function regression: Making good use of regression models that are wrong. *Sociological Methods and Research, 43*, 422–451.

Berk, R. A., Buja, A., Brown, L., George, E., Kuchibhotla, A. K., Su, W., et al. (2019). Assumption lean regression. *The American Statistician*. Published online, April 12, 2019.

Bishop, C. M. (2006). *Pattern recognition and machine learning*. New York: Springer.

Bolen, C. (2019). *Goldman banker snared by AI as U.S. Government Embraces New Tech.* Bloomberg Government. Posted July 8, 2019.

Bound, J., Jaeger, D. A., & Baker, R. M. (1995). Problems with instrumental variables estimation when the correlation between the instruments and the endogenous explanatory variable is weak. *Journal of the American Statistical Association, 90*(430), 443–450.

Box, G. E. P. (1976). Science and statistics. *Journal of the American Statistical Association, 71*(356), 791–799.

Breiman, L. (2001b). Statistical modeling: Two cultures (with discussion). *Statistical Science, 16*, 199–231.

Buja, A., & Stuetzle, W. (2006). Observations on bagging. *Statistica Sinica, 16*(2), 323–352.

Buja, A., Berk, R., Brown, L., George, E., Pitkin, E., Traskin, M., et al. (2019a). Models as approximations—Part I: A conspiracy of random regressors and model deviations against classical inference in regression. *Statistical Science, 34*(4), 523–544.

Buja, A., Berk, R., Brown, L., George, E., Kuchibhotla, A. K., & Zhao, L. (2019b). Models as approximations—Part II: A general theory of model-robust regression. *Statistical Science, 34*(4), 545–565.

Campbell, D. T., & Stanley, J. C. (1963). *Experimental and quasi-experimental designs for research*. Boston: Cengage Learning.

Cattell, R. B. (1943). The description of personality: Basic traits resolved into clusters. *Journal of Abnormal and Social Psychology, 38*(4), 476–506.

Christianini, N, & Shawe-Taylor, J. (2000). *Support vector machines* (Vol. 93(443), pp. 935–948). Cambridge, UK: Cambridge University.

Cochran, W. G. (1977) *Sampling techniques* (3rd edn.). New York: Wiley.

Cook, D. R., & Weisberg, S. (1999). *Applied regression including computing and graphics*. New York: Wiley.

Cox, D. R. (1958). The regression analysis of binary sequences (with discussion). *Journal of the Royal Statistical Society, Series B, 20*(2), 215–242.

Dasu, T., & Johnson, T. (2003). *Exploratory data mining and data cleaning*. New York: Wiley.

Davidson, A. C. (1997). *Bootstrap methods and their application*. Cambridge, UK: Cambridge University Press.

Edgington, E. S., & Ongehena, P. (2007). *Randomization tests* (4th edn.). New York: Chapman & Hall.

Efron, B. (1986). How Biased is the apparent error rate of Prediction rule?. *Journal of the American Statistical Association, 81*(394), 461–470.

Efron, B., & Tibshirani, R. (1993). *Introduction to the Bootstrap*. New York: Chapman & Hall.

Eicker, F. (1963). Asymptotic normality and consistency of the least squares estimators for families of linear regressions. *Annals of Mathematical Statistics, 34*, 447–456.

Eicker, F. (1967). Limit theorems for regressions with unequal and dependent errors. In *Proceedings of the fifth Berkeley symposium on mathematical statistics and probability* (Vol. 1, pp. 59–82).

Faraway, J. J. (2014). Does data splitting improve prediction? *Statistics and Computing, 26*(1–2), 49–60.

Freedman, D. A. (1981). Bootstrapping regression models. *Annals of Statistics, 9*(6), 1218–1228.

Freedman, D. A. (1987). As others see us: A case study in path analysis (with discussion). *Journal of Educational Statistics, 12*, 101–223.

Freedman, D. A. (2004). Graphical models for causation and the identification problem. *Evaluation Review, 28*, 267–293.

Freedman, D. A. (2009a). *Statistical models* Cambridge, UK: Cambridge University.

Freedman, D. A. (2009b). Diagnostics cannot have much power against general alternatives. *International Journal of Forecasting, 25*, 833–839.

Freedman, D. A. (2012). On the so-called 'Huber sandwich estimator' and 'Robust standard errors.' *The American Statistician, 60*(4), 299–302.

Geisser, S. (1993). *Predictive inference: An introduction*. New York: Chapman & Hall.

Green, P. J., & Silverman, B. W. (1994). *Nonparametric regression and generalized linear models*. New York: Chapman & Hall.

Hall, P. (1997) *The Bootstrap and Edgeworth expansion*. New York: Springer.

Hand, D., Manilla, H., & Smyth, P. (2001). *Principles of data mining*. Cambridge, MA: MIT Press.

Hastie, T., Tibshirani, R., & Friedman, J. (2009). *The elements of statistical learning* (2nd edn.). New York: Springer.

Huber, P. J. (1967). The behavior of maximum likelihood estimates under nonstandard conditions. In *Proceedings of the Fifth Symposium on Mathematical Statistics and Probability* (Vol I, pp. 221–233).

Janson, L., Fithian, W., & Hastie, T. (2015). Effective degrees of freedom: A flawed metaphor. *Biometrika, 102*(2), 479–485.

Jöeskog, K. G. (1979). *Advances in factor analysis and structural equation models*. Cambridge: Abt Books Press.

Kaufman, S., & Rosset, S. (2014). When does more regularization imply fewer degrees of freedom? Sufficient conditions and counter examples from the Lasso and Ridge regression. *Biometrica, 101*(4), 771–784.

Leamer, E. E. (1978). *Specification searches: AD HOC inference with non-experimental data*. New York: Wiley.

Leeb, H., & Pötscher, B. M. (2005). Model selection and inference: Facts and fiction. *Econometric Theory, 21*, 21–59.

Leeb, H., & Pötscher, B. M. (2006). Can one estimate the conditional distribution of post-model-selection estimators? *The Annals of Statistics, 34*(5), 2554–2591.

Leeb, H., Pötscher, B. M. (2008). Model selection. In T. G. Anderson, R. A. Davis, J.-P. Kreib, & T. Mikosch (Eds.), *The handbook of financial time series* (pp. 785–821). New York, Springer.

Lei, J., G'Sell, M., Rinaldo, A., Tibshirani, R. j., & Wasserman, L. (2018). Distribution-free predictive inference for regression. *Journal of the American Statistical Association, 113*(523), 1094–1111.

Linn, R. L., & Slinde, J. A. (1977). The determination of the significance of change between pre- and post-testing periods. *Review of Educational Research, 47*, 121–150.

Lockhart, R., Taylor, J., Tibshirani, R. J., & Tibshirani, R. (2014). A significance test for the lasso (with discussion). *Annals of Statistics, 42*(2), 413–468.

Mallows, C. L. (1973). Some comments on CP. *Technometrics, 15*(4), 661–675.

Marsland, S. (2014). *Machine learning: An algorithmic perspective* (2nd edn.). New York: Chapman & Hall

McCullagh, P., & Nelder, J. A. (1989). *Generalized linear models* (2nd edn.). New York: Chapman and Hall.

Meyer, D., Zeileis, A., & Hornik, K. (2007). The Strucplot framework: Visualizing multiway contingency tables with VCD. *Journal of Statistical Software, 17*(3), 1–48.

Michelucci, P., & Dickinson, J. L. (2016). The power of crowds: Combining human and machines to help tackle increasingly hard problems. *Science, 351*(6268), 32–33.

Murdock, D., Tsai, Y., & Adcock, J. (2008). P-values are random variables. *The American Statistician, 62*, 242–245.

Murphy, K. P. (2012). *Machine learning: A probabilistic perspective*. Cambridge, Mass: MIT Press.

Nagin, D. S., & Pepper, J. V. (2012). *Deterrence and the death penalty*. Washington, D.C.: National Research Council.

Open Science Collaboration (2015). Estimating the reproducibility of psychological science. *Science, 349*(6251), aas4716-1–aas4716-8.

Pearson, K. (1901). On lines and planes of closest fit to systems of points in space. *Philosophical Magazine, 2*(11), 559–572.

Rice, J. A. (2007). *Mathematical statistics and data analysis* (3rd edn.). Belmont, CA: Duxbury Press.

Rozeboom, W. W. (1960). The fallacy of null-hypothesis significance tests. *Psychological Bulletin, 57*(5), 416–428.

Rubin, D. B. (1986). Which Ifs have causal answers. *Journal of the American Statistical Association, 81*, 961–962.

Rubin, D. B. (2008). For objective causal inference, design trumps analysis. *Annals of Applied Statistics, 2*(3), 808–840.

Rummel, R. J. (1988). *Applied Factor Analysis*. Northwestern University Press.

Ruppert, D., Wand, M. P., & Carroll, R. J. (2003). *Semiparametric regression*. Cambridge, UK: Cambridge University.

Schwartz, G. (1978). Estimating the dimension of a model. *Annals of Statistics, 6*, 461–464.

Stigler, S. M. (1981). Gauss and the invention of least squares. *The Annals of Statistics, 9*(3), 465–474.

Sutton, R. S., & Barto, A. G. (2018). *Reinforcement learning* (2nd edn.). A Bradford Book.

Torgerson, W. (1958). *Theory and methods of scaling*. New York: Wiley.

Weisberg, S. (2013). *Applied linear regression* (4th edn.). New York: Wiley.

White, H. (1980a). Using least squares to approximate unknown regression functions. *International Economic Review, 21*(1), 149–170.

Witten, I. H., & Frank, E. (2000). *Data mining*. New York: Morgan and Kaufmann.

Chapter 2
Splines, Smoothers, and Kernels

Summary This chapter launches a more detailed examination of statistical learning within a regression framework. Once again, the focus is on conditional distributions. How does the conditional mean or conditional proportion vary with different predictor values? The intent is to begin with procedures that have much the same look and feel as conventional linear regression and gradually move toward procedures that do not. Many of the procedures can be viewed as forms of nonparametric regression. Penalized fitting is also introduced. Regression coefficients will in each case play an important computational role but typically have no useful subject-matter interpretation.

2.1 Introduction

Fitted values for most of the procedures in this chapter can, under the right circumstances, be seen as the computational product of a linear regression. Those circumstances are an absence of data snooping. It then follows that the approximation perspective from the previous chapter can apply. We will still require IID data, or a close approximation, and when that case can be made, valid asymptotic statistical inference can be undertaken. The new inferential challenge is how to properly proceed when there *is* data snooping—data snooping is built into most of the procedures discussed. Legitimate test data can help.

2.2 Regression Splines

A "spline" is a thin strip of wood that can be easily bent to follow a curved line (Green and Silverman 1994: 4). Historically, it was used in drafting for drawing

© Springer Nature Switzerland AG 2020   73
R. A. Berk, *Statistical Learning from a Regression Perspective*,
Springer Texts in Statistics, https://doi.org/10.1007/978-3-030-40189-4_2

smooth curves. Regression splines, a statistical translation of this idea, are a way to represent nonlinear, but unknown, mean functions.

Regression splines are not used a great deal in empirical work as stand alone procedures. As we show later, there are usually better ways to proceed. Nevertheless, it is important to consider them, at least briefly. They provide an instructive transition between conventional parametric regression and the kinds of smoothers commonly seen in statistical learning settings. They also introduce concepts and concerns that will be relevant throughout this chapter and in subsequent chapters.

Recall the general expression for function estimation with a numeric response variable Y.

$$Y = f(X) + \varepsilon, \tag{2.1}$$

where X is a set of predictors, $f(X)$ is not specified, and ε can represent nothing more than dataset residuals or nothing less than a traditional disturbance term depending, respectively, on whether a Level I or Level II regression is being implemented. If Level II, treating ε as a traditional disturbance term means that first-order conditions are being met for $f(X)$ and second-order condition are being met for ε.

However, we have already jettisoned this approach, favoring analyses capitalizing on population approximations of the true response surface. Then, ε stands for population residuals, whose properties depend on how the population approximation would be (hypothetically) computed. For example, if the linear approximation is computed by least squares, the population residuals *by construction* have an expectation of 0.0, a covariance of 0.0 with each predictor. In other words, for a Level II analysis, the population residuals from the approximation of the true response surface have analogous descriptive properties to those of the empirical residuals if the same procedures were applied to the data.

2.2.1   Piecewise Linear Population Approximations

Suppose that the approximation relationship between the conditional mean of a numeric Y and a collection of predictors is "piecewise linear." One then can employ piecewise linear basis expansions in X. The population approximation becomes broken or hyperplane such that at each break point the left-hand edge meets the right-hand edge. When there is a single predictor, for instance, the fit is a set of straight line segments, connected end to end. *Given a particular linear basis expansion*, one can still think of the population approximation as a product of ordinary least squares. This implies that the hypothetical population calculations are the same as the calculations undertaken with the IID data. Under these circumstances, some would call the calculations with the data a "plug-in" estimator. All of the good asymptotic properties discussed in Chap. 1 follow.[1]

Consider as an example a wonderfully entertaining paper that (Zelterman 2014) documents associations by state in the United States between the number of internet references to zombies and census features for those states. The number of zombie references was determined through a "Google search" state by state. Like Zelterman, we let Y be the number of zombie references by state per 100,000 people. We let X be the average in each state of minutes per day spent watching cable TV. The values used here for both variables are total fabrications constructed for didactic purposes.

Figure 2.1 shows an example of a piecewise linear function constructed in three steps.[2] The first step is to decide where the break points on the empirical x will be. Based on prior market research, suppose there are known tipping points at 90 and 180 min of TV watching a day. At 90 min a day, viewers often become fans of zombies on TV and shows with related content. At 180 min a day, zombie saturation is reached. Break points are defined at $x = a$ and $x = b$ (with $b > a$) so that in Fig. 2.1, $a = 90$ and $b = 180$. Such break points are often called "knots."

The next step is to define two indicator variables to represent the break points. The first, I_a, is equal to 1 if x is greater than 90 and equal to 0 otherwise. The second, I_b, is equal to 1 if x is greater than 180 and equal to 0 otherwise. Both are step functions in x. We let x_a be the value of x at the first break point, and x_b be the value of x at the second break point (i.e., 90 and 180, respectively).

The final step is to define the mean function that allows for changes in the slope and the intercept:

$$f(x_i) = \beta_0 + \beta_1 x_i + \beta_2 (x_i - x_a) I_a + \beta_3 (x_i - x_b) I_b. \quad (2.2)$$

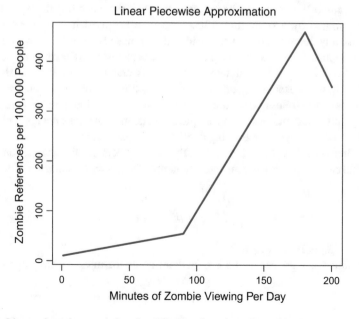

Fig. 2.1 Linear piecewise mean function (The first knot is at $X = 90$, the second knot is at $X = 180$. $\beta_0 = 10$, $\beta_1 = 0.5$, $\beta_2 = 4.0$, $\beta_3 = -10.0$)

Looking back at how linear basis expansions are defined in Eq. 1.24, it is apparent that there are four transformations of x ($m = 1, 2, \ldots, 4$), each denoted by $h_m(X)$, in which the first function of x is a constant. One has a set of predictors constructed as a linear basis expansion of X. Equation 2.2 is, therefore, the mean function for a conventional multiple regression with coefficient values that could be obtained from ordinary least squares.

Equation 2.2 is *not* a model representing how the data were generated. But, it can be used as a mean function in a least squares regression to help find fitted values that summarize associations in data. Going no farther, this can result in a Level I analysis through which relationships in the data are described.

For a Level II analysis, Eq. 2.2 can play two related roles. First, it can represent the mean function to be estimated. Equation 2.2 is the expression for the piecewise linear function that is a feature of a joint probability distribution, but as before, with no claims made about its correspondence to the truth. When embedded in the population least squares formulation, it can be viewed as a best (i.e., by least squares), piecewise linear approximation of the true response surface and an appropriate estimation target.[3] Second, used as the mean function in a least squares procedure applied to data, it is an estimator. As such, it is a plug-in estimator and again, all of the desirable asymptotic properties hold.

However, when the placement of the knots is determined as part of the data analysis (e.g., by trial and error), one has engaged in data snooping. One is picking the best regression equation and relying solely on that equation going forward. A Level II analysis cannot be formally justified, even if one has IID training data. But if one has test data, the mean function specification arrived at with training data can produce valid estimates using the test data. It is as if the mean function specification was determined by a prior study. Test data then are used just as one ordinarily would use any dataset to obtain asymptotically unbiased estimates of the regression parameters and the fitted values. Proper statistical tests and confidence intervals follow. We will apply this strategy often in this chapter and the next. However, just as in our discussion of conformal predictive inference, this strategy ignores uncertainty in the training data, and, therefore, is valid but incomplete. One can get a falsely optimistic impression of statistical precision if one does not appreciate that there is conditioning on the training data and fitting structure.

Whether for a Level I or Level II analysis, the piecewise linear function can be decomposed into its constituent line segments. The mean function for x less than a is

$$f(x_i) = \beta_0 + \beta_1 x_i. \tag{2.3}$$

In Fig. 2.1, β_0 is 10, and β_1 is 0.5.

For values of x greater than a but smaller than b, the mean function becomes

$$f(x_i) = (\beta_0 - \beta_2 x_a) + (\beta_1 + \beta_2)x_i. \tag{2.4}$$

For a $\beta_1 = 0.5$ and $\beta_2 = 4.0$, the line beyond $x = a$ is steeper because the slope is $(\beta_1 + \beta_2)$. The intercept is lower because of the second term in $(\beta_0 - \beta_2 x_a)$. This too is consistent with Fig. 2.1. If β_2 were negative, the reverse would apply.

For values of x greater than b, the mean function becomes

$$f(x_i) = (\beta_0 - \beta_2 x_a - \beta_3 x_b) + (\beta_1 + \beta_2 + \beta_3)x_i. \qquad (2.5)$$

$\beta_3 = -10$. For these values of x, the slope is altered by adding β_3 to the slope of the previous line segment. The intercept is altered by subtracting $\beta_3 x_b$. The sign and magnitude of β_3 determines whether the slope of the new line segment is positive or negative and how steep it is. The intercept will shift accordingly. In Fig. 2.1, β_3 is negative and large enough to make the slope negative. The intercept is increased substantially.

Expressions like Eq. 2.2 are all one needs for a Level I regression analysis. For a Level II regression analysis, a credible data generating process also must be articulated. As before, we will generally employ a joint probability distribution as the population from which each observation is realized as a random, independent draw. Often this approach is reasonable. But each Level II regression analysis must be considered on a case-by-case basis. For example, if time is a predictor (e.g., month or year), there can be important conceptual complications, as we will now see.

Whether a Level I or II analysis, the main intent for piecewise linear splines is to output fitted values that can be studied visually to comprehend how a single predictor is related to a numeric response. Consider Fig. 2.2, which shows a three-piecewise linear regression spline applied to water use data from Tokyo over a period of 27 years.[4] The data were collected as part of a larger research project motivated by concerns about the provision of potable water to large metropolitan areas as human-induced climate change proceeds. Residential water use in 1000s of cubic feet is on the vertical axis. Year is on the horizontal axis. The locations of the break points were chosen before the analysis began using subject-matter expertise about residential water use in Japan. There was no data snooping. The R code is shown in Fig. 2.3.

For a Level I analysis, it is clear that water use was flat until about 1980, increased linearly until about 1992, and then flattened out again. The first break point may correspond to a transition toward much faster economic and population growth. The second break point may correspond to the introduction of more water-efficient technology. But why the transitions are so sharp is mysterious. One possibility is that the break points correspond in part to changes in how the water use data were collected or reported.

In Fig. 2.2, the end-to-end connections between line segments work well, as they often do with processes that unfold over time. But there is nothing about linear regression splines requiring that time be a predictor. For example, the response could be crop production per acre, and the sole predictor could be the amount of phosphorus fertilizer applied to the soil. Crop production might increase in approximately a linear fashion until there is an excess of phosphorus causing of

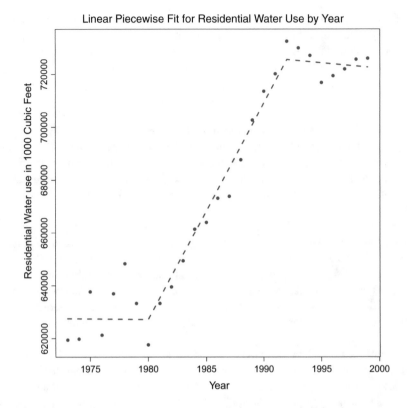

Fig. 2.2 A piecewise linear basis approximation applied to water use in Tokyo by year

```
xa<-ifelse(year>1980,1,0)
xb<-ifelse(year>1992,1,0)
x1<-(year-1980)*xa
x2<-(year-1992)*xb
working<-data.frame(hhwater,year,xa,xb,x1,x2)
out1<-lm(hhwater~year+x1+x2,data=working)
plot(year,hhwater,xlab="Year",ylab="Residential
        Water use in 1000 Cubic Feet", main="Linear
        Piecewise Fit for Residential Water Use by Year",
        col="blue",pch=19)
lines(year,out1$fitted.values, lty="dashed",col="blue",lwd=3)
```

Fig. 2.3 R code for piecewise linear fit of the Tokyo water data

metabolic difficulties for the crops. At that point, crop yields might decline in
roughly a linear manner.

Fitting end-to-end line segments to data provides an example of smoothing a scatterplot, or applying a *smoother*. Line segments are used to summarize how X and Y are related. The intent is to highlight key features of any association while removing unimportant details. This can often be accomplished by constructing fitted values in a manner that makes them more homogeneous than the set of conditional means of Y computed for each unique value of X or binned values of X.[5]

Imagine a scatterplot in which the number of observations is large enough so that for each value of X there are at least several values of Y. One could compute the mean of Y for each X-value. If one then drew straight lines between adjacent conditional means, the resulting smoother would be an *interpolation* of the conditional means and as "rough" as possible. At the other extreme, imposing a single linear fit on all of the means at once would produce the "smoothest" fit possible. Figure 2.2 falls somewhere in-between. How to think about the degree of smoothness more formally is addressed later.

For a piecewise linear basis, one can simply compute mean functions such as Eq. 2.2 with ordinary least squares. With the regression coefficients in hand, fitted values are easily constructed. Indeed, many software packages compute and store fitted values on a routine basis. Also widely available are procedures to construct the matrix of regressors, although it is not hard to do so one term at a time using common transformation capabilities (See Fig. 2.3.). For example, the R library *splines* has a procedure *bs* that constructs a B-spline basis (discussed later) that can be easily used to represent the predictor matrix for piecewise linear regression. As already noted, for a Level II analysis the estimation target is the same mean function approximation in the population or joint probability distribution. With IID data and an absence of data snooping, the estimator is a conventional linear regression. The best linear approximation approach from Chap. 1 applies, and there are convenient extensions to forecasting (Berk et al. 2019a).

But in contrast to the zombie example, these data are longitudinal. As a cautionary exercise, we re-examine some features of the approximation approach when the study units are temporal or spatial. A lot depends on how the data were collected and for the Tokyo data, the full details are unclear.

Stepping back a bit, residential accounts come and go because of households moving in and out of Tokyo, the breaking up of exiting households, and the formation of new households. Therefore, in any given year, the set of residential accounts might be seen as IID draws from the population of potential residential accounts. And important complication as an analysis undertaken is that the set up hypothetical accounts will tend to be dominated by more stable household but for any given year, the realizations can still be seen as IID.

Each account comes with its total yearly water consumption that is summed over all residential accounts. It is these year by year sums that are to be analyzed, and it is apparent from Fig. 2.2 that these year to year sums are related. But that is a consequence of the factors shaping residential water use, not a feature of how the accounts themselves are realized.

Perhaps the major message is that although the IID framework is quite general, each application must be thought through. An "assume-and-proceed" approach is usually misguided. There also will be inferential settings that currently are beyond existing technical procedures or at least depend on highly provisional approaches.

For example, temporal dependence that declines with distance is not an insurmountable problem (Kuchibhotla et al. 2018). Imagine data generated by tweets on the internet. One possible characteristic of a collection of realized tweets is that later realized tweets are in part generated as responses to earlier tweets. But as the time between any pair of tweets increases, the later tweets are less likely to be a response to earlier tweets. In other words, the realization dependence dissipates. This can be handled within our IID framework. But one would still need to determine the population of tweets to which inference is being made. Exactly, what set of social processes are in play and for whom?

Suppose the tweets of interest come from students at a particular high school. If one student from that high school tweets, and is recognized as being a student in that high school, it increases the chances that other students from the high school will tweet. The IID assumption is undermined. Statistical inference in such circumstances can be very difficult to handle. Usually additional structural assumptions are required.[6]

There are even more difficult complications if the placement of knots is chosen through data snooping. For example, there is data snooping if the scatterplot for water consumption by year was examined to choose the best knot locations. Those locations then become features of the regression specification itself so that the mean function specification could well be different with new realizations of the data (Leeb and Pötscher 2005, 2006, 2008). Look again at Fig. 2.2. Inference, even to the population approximation, is no longer asymptotically correct.[7] More will be said later in this chapter about approaches that could work.

Perhaps the major lesson from the analysis of the water use data is that moving beyond a Level I analysis often requires a conceptual reformulation of our simple IID data generation process. Temporal and/or spatial data can present special challenges. However, when the data are still IID, good things follow. On both statistical and subject-matter grounds, the form that the fitting algorithm takes may, nevertheless, need to incorporate the role of time and space.

2.2.2 Polynomial Regression Splines

Smoothing a scatterplot using a piecewise linear basis has the great advantage of simplicity in concept and execution. And by increasing the number of break points, very complicated relationships can be approximated. However, in most applications there are good reasons to believe that the underlying relationship is not well represented with a set of straight line segments. Another kind of approximation is needed.

Greater continuity between line segments can be achieved by using polynomials in X for each segment. Cubic functions of X are a popular choice because they strike a nice balance between flexibility and complexity. When used to construct regression splines, the fit is sometimes called "piecewise cubic." The cubic polynomial serves as a "truncated power series basis" in X, and is another example of a linear basis expansion.

Unfortunately, simply joining polynomial segments end to end is unlikely to result in a visually appealing fit where the polynomial segments meet. The slopes of the two lines will often appear to change abruptly even when that is inconsistent with the data. Far better visual continuity usually can be achieved by constraining the first and second derivatives on either side of each break point to be the same.

One can generalize the piecewise linear approach and impose the continuity requirements. Suppose there are K interior break points, usually called "interior knots." These are located at $\xi_1 < \cdots < \xi_K$ with two boundary knots added at ξ_0 and ξ_{K+1}. Then, one can use piecewise cubic polynomials in the following mean function exploiting, as before, linear basis expansions of X:

$$f(x_i) = \beta_0 + \beta_1 x_i + \beta_2 x_i^2 + \beta_3 x_i^3 + \sum_{j=1}^{K} \theta_j (x_i - x_j)_+^3, \qquad (2.6)$$

where the "+" indicates the positive values from the expression inside the parentheses, and there are $K + 4$ parameters whose values need to be computed. This leads to a conventional regression formulation with a matrix of predictor terms having $K + 4$ columns and N rows. Each row would have the corresponding values of the piecewise cubic polynomial function evaluated at the single value of x for that case. There is still the same underlying, single predictor, but now there are $K + 4$ basis functions in a linear regression structure. Equation 2.6 represents a best linear approximation of the true response surface that one properly can estimate with ordinary least squares.

The output for the far-right term in Eq. 2.6 may not be apparent at first. Suppose the values of the predictor are arranged in order from low to high. For example, $x = [1, 2, 4, 5, 7, 8]$. Suppose also that x_j is located at an x-value of 4. Then, $(x - x_j)_+^3 = [0, 0, 0, 1, 27, 64]$. The knot-value of 4 is subtracted from each value of x, the negative numbers set to 0, and the others cubed. All that changes from knot to knot is the value of x_j that is subtracted. There are K such knots and K such terms in the regression approximation .

Figure 2.4 shows the water use data again, but with a piecewise cubic polynomial overlaid that imposes the two continuity constraints. The code is shown in Fig. 2.5. Figure 2.4 reveals a good eyeball fit, which captures about 95% of the variance in water use. But, in all fairness, the scatterplot did not present a great challenge. The point is to compare Figs. 2.2, 2.3 and 2.4 and note the visual difference. The linear piecewise fit also accounted for about 95% of the variance. Which plot would be more instructive in practice would depend on the use to be made of the fitted values and on prior information about what a sensible $f(X)$ might be.

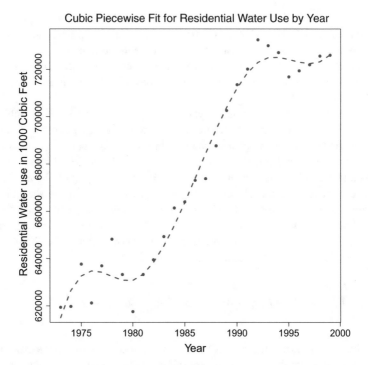

Fig. 2.4 A piecewise cubic basis approximation applied to water use in Tokyo by year

```
library(splines)
cubic<-bs(year,knots=c(1980,1992))
out2<-lm(hhwater~cubic)
plot(year,hhwater,xlab="Year",ylab="Residential Water use
        in 1000 Cubic Feet", main="Cubic Piecewise Fit for
        Residential Water Use by Year",col="blue",pch=19)
lines(year,out2$fitted.values,lty="dashed",col="blue",lwd=3)
```

Fig. 2.5 R code for piecewise cubic fit

The regression coefficients ranged widely and, as to be expected, did not by themselves add any useful information. Any story was primarily in the fitted values. The issues for a Level I and Level II analysis are essentially the same as for a piecewise linear approach.

2.2.3   Natural Cubic Splines

Fitted values for piecewise cubic polynomials near the boundaries of x can be
unstable because they fall at the ends of polynomial line segments where there
are no continuity constraints, and where the data may be sparse. By "unstable"
one means that a very few observations, which might vary substantially over
random realizations of the data, could produce rather different fitted values near
the boundaries of x. As a result, the plot of the fitted values near the boundaries
might look somewhat different from sample to sample.

Sometimes, constraints for behavior at the boundaries are added to increase
stability. One common constraint imposes linearity on the fitted values beyond the
boundaries of x. This introduces a bit of bias because it is very unlikely that if
data beyond the current boundaries were available, the relationship would be linear.
However, the added stability is often worth it. When these constraints are added, the
result is a "natural cubic spline." Once again, there is a best linear approximation
that can be properly estimated with ordinary least squares.

Figure 2.6 shows again a plot of the water use data on year, but now with a
smoother constructed from natural cubic splines. The code can be found in Fig. 2.7.
One can see that the fitted values near the boundaries of x are somewhat different

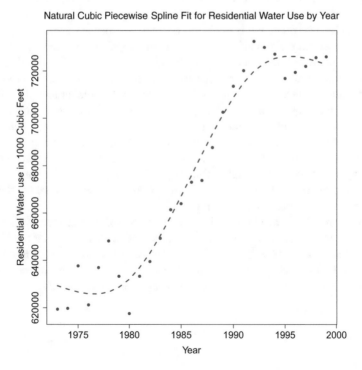

Fig. 2.6 A natural cubic piecewise basis applied to water use in Tokyo by year

```
library(splines)
Ncubic<-ns(year,knots=c(1980,1992))
out3<-lm(hhwater~Ncubic)
plot(year,hhwater,xlab="Year",ylab="Residential Water use
        in 1000 Cubic Feet", main="Natural Cubic Piecewise
        Fit for Residential Water Use by Year",col="blue",pch=19)
lines(year,out3$fitted.values,lty="dashed",col="blue",lwd=3)
```

Fig. 2.7 R code for natural piecewise cubic fit

from the fitted values near the boundaries of x in Fig. 2.4. The fitted values in Fig. 2.6 are smoother, which is the desired result. There is one less bend near both boundaries, but the issues for a Level I or Level II analysis have not changed.[8]

In a Level II setting, the option of including extra constraints to help stabilize the fit provides an example of the bias–variance tradeoff discussed in the previous chapter, but for piecewise cubic polynomials and natural cubic splines, the degree of smoothness is primarily a function of the number of interior knots. In practice, the smaller the number of knots, the smoother are the fitted values. A smaller number of knots means that there are more constraints on the pattern of fitted values because there are fewer end-to-end, cubic line segments used in the fitting process. Consequently, less provision is made for a complex response surface.

Knot placement matters too. Ideally, knots should be placed where one believes, before looking at the data, the $f(X)$ is changing most rapidly. But it will often be very tempting to data snoop. In some cases, inspection of the data, coupled with subject-matter knowledge, can be used to determine the number and placement of knots. Alternatively, the number and placement of knots can be approached as a conventional model selection problem. This option will be considered later. In both cases, however, the data snooping will have its usual price for proper statistical inference. At the same time, absent subject-matter information, knot placement has been long known to be a difficult technical problem, especially when there is more than one predictor (de Boors 2001). The fitted values are related to where the knots are placed in a very complicated manner.

In summary, for Level II regression splines of the sort just discussed, there is no straightforward way to empirically arrive at the best tradeoff between the bias and the variance because there is no straightforward way to determine the number and location of knots. Addressing these complications by eyeball data snooping can be a bad idea. Fortunately, there are extensions of regression splines discussed shortly that can help substantially especially when there are training data, evaluation data, and test data.

A broader point is that we have begun the transition from models to black box algorithms. As the substantive role for fitted values has become more prominent, the substantive role for regression coefficients has become less prominent. How one thinks about regression results should change accordingly.

.

2.2.4 B-Splines

In practice, data analyses using piecewise cubic polynomials and natural cubic splines are rarely constructed directly from polynomials in X. They are commonly constructed using a B-spline basis, largely because of computational convenience. We are considering another kind of linear basis expansion.[9] A serious discussion of B-splines would take us far afield and accessible summaries can be found in Gifi (1990: 366–370) and Hastie et al. (2009: 186–189). Nevertheless several observations are worth making even if they are a bit of a detour. Perhaps the primary message is that B-splines do not represent a model. They are strictly a computational device. The same applies to all splines.

B-splines are computed in a recursive manner from very simple functions to more complex ones.[10] Consider a single predictor X. For a set of knots, usually including some beyond the upper and lower boundaries of X, a recursion begins with indicator variables for each neighborhood defined by the knots. If a value of X falls within a given neighborhood, the indicator variable for that neighborhood is coded 1, and coded 0 otherwise. For example, if there is a knot at an x-value of 2 and the next knot is at an x-value of 3, the x-values between them constitute a neighborhood with its own indicator variable coded 1 if the value of x falls in that neighborhood (e.g., $x = 2.3$). Otherwise, the coded value is 0. In the end, there is a set of indicator variables, with values of 1 or 0, depending on the neighborhood. These indicator variables constitute a B-spline expansion of degree zero.

Figure 2.8 is an illustration with interior knots at -2, -1, 0, 1, and 2. With five interior knots, there are four neighborhoods and four indicator variables. Using indicator variables as regressors will produce a step function when Y is regressed on X; they are the linear basis expansion for a step function fit. The steps will be located at the knots and for this example, the mean function specification will allow for four levels, one for each indicator variable. With a different set of knots, the indicator variables will change.

As usual, one of the indicator variables is dropped from any regression analysis that includes an intercept. The deleted indicator becomes the baseline. In R, the procedure *lm* automatically drops one of the indicator variables in a set if an intercept is included.

Next, a transformation can be applied to the degree zero B-spline expansion (See Hastie et al. 2009: 186–189). The result is a one degree B-spline expansion. Figure 2.9 shows a degree one B-spline derived from the indicator variables shown in Fig. 2.8. The triangular shape is characteristic of a degree one B-spline and

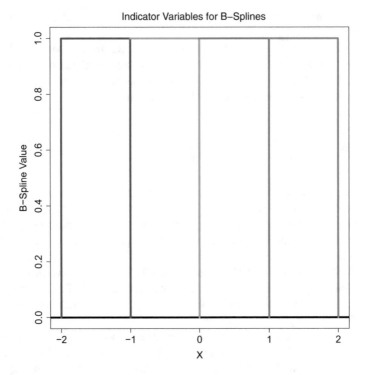

Fig. 2.8 Example of zero degree B-spline with five knots

indicates that the values are no longer just 0 or 1, but proportions in-between as well.

In Fig. 2.9, each new basis component is color coded. Starting from the left, the blue line maps X onto a set of B-spline values. From x-values of -2 to -1, the B-spline values decline from 1 to 0 but are 0 for the rest of the x-values. These B-spline values would be the first column in a new predictor matrix. For x-values between -2 and 0, the green upside down V indicates that the B-spline values are between 0 and 1, but equal to 0 otherwise. These B-spline values would be the second column in a new predictor matrix. The same reasoning applies to the purple and red upside down Vs and to the yellow line. In the end, there would be six columns of B-spline values with the sixth column coded to have no impact because it is redundant, given other five columns. That column is not shown inasmuch as it has B-spline values that are 0 for all x-values.

Degree one B-splines are the basis for linear piecewise fits. In this example, regressing a response on the B-spline matrix would produce a linear piecewise fit with four slopes and four intercepts, one for each neighborhood defined by the indicator variables. For different numbers and locations of knots, the piecewise fit would vary as well.

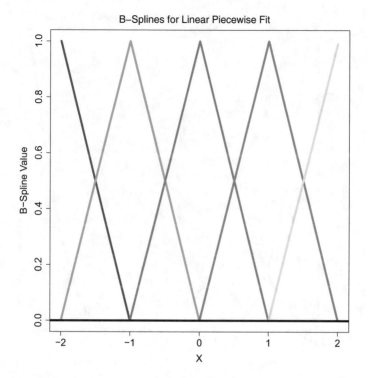

Fig. 2.9 Example of one degree B-spline with five knots

A transformation of the same form can now be applied to the degree one B-spline basis. This leads to a degree two B-spline basis. A set of such B-spline components is shown in Fig. 2.10. As before, each new basis element is color coded, and the shapes are characteristic. For this illustration, there is now a matrix having seven columns with one redundant column coded as all 0s. Should the B-spline matrix be used in a regression analysis, a piecewise quadratic fit would be produced. There would be one quadratic function for each neighborhood defined by the indicator variables.

The same kind of transformation can then be applied to the degree two B-spline basis. The result is a degree three B-spline basis. Figure 2.11 shows the set of degree three color-coded elements, whose shapes are, once again, characteristic. The regressor matrix now contains eight columns with one redundant column coded as all 0s. When these are used as regressors, there will be one cubic function for each neighborhood defined by the original indicator variables.

All splines are linear combinations of B-splines; B-splines are a basis for the space of all splines. They are also a well-conditioned basis because they are not highly correlated, and they can be computed in a stable and efficient manner. For our purposes, the main point is that B-splines are a computational device used to construct cubic piecewise fitted values. No substantive use is made of the

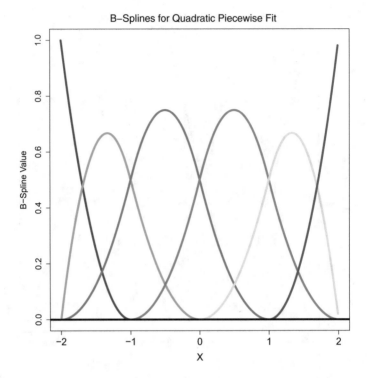

Fig. 2.10 Example of two degree *B*-spline with five knots

associated regression coefficients because they too are just part of the computational machinery. Our trek toward black box algorithms continues.

2.3   Penalized Smoothing

We return to the knot-related problems introduced in the discussion of regression splines. The placement of knots, the number of knots, and the degree of the polynomial are subject to manipulation by a data analyst. For a Level I regression analysis, the goal is to arrive at an instructive fit of the data. Is one learning what one can about associations in the data? For a Level II regression analysis, the goal is to estimate a useful approximation of the true response surface.

Whether for a Level I or Level II analysis, the data analyst is engaged in a form of "tuning." Therefore, the placement of knots, the number of knots, and the degree of the polynomial can be seen as "tuning parameters." Unlike the usual parameters of a regression model, they typically are of little substantive interest. More like dials on a piece of machinery, they are set to promote good performance.

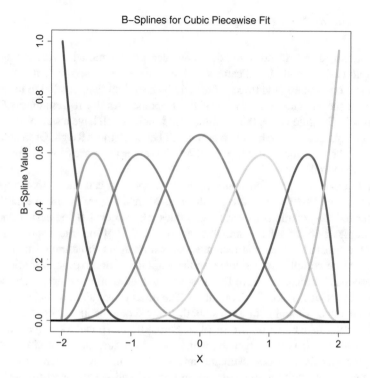

Fig. 2.11 Example of three degree *B*-spline with five knots

There are at least two problems with the tuning parameters for regression splines. First, there are at least three of them so that the tuning process can be quite complicated. For example, should one increase the number of knots or the degree of the polynomial? Usually, the only guidance is sketchy craft lore. Second, there is little or no formal theory to justify the tuning. For many, the tuning process feels like a "hack." The entire process is at least inelegant.

A useful alternative is to alter the fitting process itself so that the tuning is accomplished automatically, guided by clear statistical reasoning. One popular approach is to combine a mathematical penalty with the loss function to be optimized. The penalty imposes greater losses as an empirical mean function becomes more complicated. For greater complexity to be accepted, the fit must be improved by an amount that is larger than the penalty. The greater complexity has to be "worth it." This leads to a very popular approach called "penalized regression."[11]

Penalized regression can be a variant of the linear approximation approach discussed in the previous chapter. We turn to that next. It will seem like a bit of a diversion, but illustrates in a familiar setting how regression coefficients can be altered in search of a useful balance for the bias–variance tradeoff. Because in the background regression coefficients can be a vital part of smoothing procedures, a discussion of penalized regression can be instructive. The lessons learned will be useful in moving forward.

2.3.1   Shrinkage and Regularization

To get a feel for penalized regression, consider a conventional regression analysis with a numeric Y and an indicator variable as the sole regressor. If its regression coefficient equals zero, the fitted values will be a straight line, parallel to the x-axis, located at the unconditional mean of the response. As the regression coefficient increases in absolute value, the resulting step function will have a step of increasing size. In language we have begun to use, the fit becomes more rough. Or in still other language, the fit is more complex. In short, the larger the regression coefficient the rougher the fitted values.

For a Level I regression analysis, less complexity can mean that important features of the fitted values are overlooked. More complexity unnecessarily can complicate interpretations of the fitted values. For a Level II regression analysis, less complexity means that a smoother approximation of the true response surface is being estimated, which can increase bias with respect to nature's true response surface. More complexity can increase the variance of approximation estimates of that response surface. We have the bias–variance tradeoff once again, and we are once again seeking a Goldilocks solution. The fitted values should not be too rough. The fitted values should not be too smooth. They should be just right.

Two kinds of estimation are in play. Formally, the population *approximation* is the estimand. It is the target for which one can under the right circumstances get asymptotically unbiased estimates and valid asymptotic standard errors. More on that soon. In addition, one can use an approximation estimate as a potentially useful window on the true response surface features. It is here that the bias–variance tradeoff is directly relevant, and it is here that we seek a Goldilocks solution.

Popular Goldilocks strategies are sometimes called "shrinkage" (Hastie et al. 2009: section 3.4) and sometimes called "regularization" (Hastie et al. 2009: Chapter 5). In the context of statistical learning, both are tools for trying to address the bias–variance tradeoff. But it can be helpful to think of shrinkage as a special case of regularization in which the loss function for a conventional linear regression is altered to include a penalty for complexity. The values of the regression coefficients are shrunk toward 0.0. We will see in later chapters that regularization can apply to a much wider range of procedures and take many different forms. For now, we focus on shrinkage.

A number of proposals have been offered for how to control the complexity of the fitted values by constraining the magnitude of regression coefficients. (See Ruppert et al. 2003: section 3.5 for a very accessible discussion.) Two popular suggestions are:

1. constrain the sum of the absolute values of the regression coefficients to be less than some constant C (sometimes called an L_1-penalty); or
2. constrain the sum of the squared regression coefficients to be less than some constant C (sometimes called an L_2-penalty).[12]

The smaller the value of C, the smaller the sum. The smaller the sum, the smaller is the typical magnitude of the regression coefficients. The smaller the typical magnitude of the regression coefficients, the smoother the fitted values. In part because the units in which the regressors are measured will affect how much each regression coefficient contributes to the sum, it can make sense for fitting purposes to work with standardized regressors. For example, 3.2 additional years of age may count the same as smoking 8.4 additional cigarettes a day. Both values may be equal to one standard deviation above the mean of their respective predictors. Standardization can make little subject-matter sense, but that will be irrelevant if the primary goal is constructing a useful set of fitted values.[13] The intercept does not figure in either constraint and is usually addressed separately.

For a Level I analysis, both constraints can impose different amounts of smoothness on the fitted values. Description of the relationships between the response and the predictors can be affected. For a Level II analysis, both constraints lead to shrinkage methods. The regression coefficients can be "shrunk" toward zero, making the fitted values more homogeneous. The population approximation is altered in the same fashion. When the intent is to characterize the true response surface, one may be prepared to introduce a small amount of bias into the estimated regression coefficients in trade for a substantial reduction in their variance; the same applies to the fitted values.

One also can recast some measures of fit discussed in the last chapter within a shrinkage framework. The total number of regression coefficients to be estimated can serve as a constraint and is sometimes called an L_0-penalty. Maximizing the adjusted R^2, for example, can be seen as minimizing the usual error sum of squares subject to a penalty for the number of regression coefficients in the model (Fan and Li 2006).

Shrinkage methods can be applied with the usual regressor matrix or with smoother matrices of the sort introduced earlier. For didactic purposes, we begin within a conventional multiple regression framework and p predictors.

2.3.1.1 Ridge Regression

Suppose that for a conventional fixed X regression, one adopts the constraint that the sum of the p squared regression coefficients is less than C. This constraint leads directly to ridge regression. The task is to obtain values for the regression coefficients so that

$$\hat{\beta} = \min_{\beta} \left[\sum_{i=1}^{n} (y_i - \beta_0 - \sum_{j=1}^{p} x_{ij} \beta_j)^2 + \lambda \sum_{j=1}^{p} \beta_j^2 \right]. \tag{2.7}$$

In Eq. 2.7, the usual expression for the error sum of squares has a new component. That component is the sum of the squared regression coefficients multiplied by a constant λ. When Eq. 2.7 is minimized in order to obtain $\hat{\beta}$, the sizes of the squared regression coefficients, excluding β_0, are taken into account. This is an L_2-penalty.

For a given value of λ, the larger the $\sum_{j=1}^{p} \beta_j^2$, the larger the increment to the error sum of squares. $\sum_{j=1}^{p} \beta_j^2$ can be thought of as the penalty function. For a given value of $\sum_{j=1}^{p} \beta_j^2$, the larger the value of λ, the larger the increment to the error sum of squares; λ determines how much weight is given to the penalty. In short, $\sum_{j=1}^{p} \beta_j^2$ is what is being constrained, and λ imposes the constraint. C is inversely related to λ. The smaller the value of C, the larger is the value of λ. The larger the values of λ, the more the regression coefficients are moved toward 0.0.

It follows that in matrix notation the ridge regression estimator is

$$\hat{\beta} = (\mathbf{X}^T \mathbf{X} + \lambda \mathbf{I})^{-1} \mathbf{X}^T \mathbf{y}, \tag{2.8}$$

where $\mathbf{I}$ is a $p \times p$ identity matrix. The column of 1s for the intercept is dropped from $\mathbf{X}$. β_0 is estimated separately.

In Eq. 2.8, λ plays the same role as in Eq. 2.7, but can now be seen as a tuning parameter. It is not a feature of a finite population, a joint probability distribution, or a stochastic process. Its role is to help provide an appropriate fit to the data and can be altered directly by the data analyst. As such, it has a different status from the regression coefficients, whose values are determined through the minimization process itself, *conditional* upon the value of λ.

The value of λ is added to the main diagonal of the cross-product matrix $\mathbf{X}^T \mathbf{X}$, which determines how much the estimated regression coefficients are "shrunk" toward zero (and hence, toward each other). A λ of zero produces the usual least squares result. As λ increases in size, the regression coefficients approach zero, and the fitted values are smoother. In effect, the variances of the predictors are being increased with no change in the covariances between predictors and the response variable.

In ridge regression, the regression coefficients and fitted values obtained will differ in a complicated manner depending on the units in which the predictors are measured. It is common, therefore, to standardize the predictors before the estimation begins. However, standardization is just a convention and does not solve the problem of the scale dependent regression coefficients. There also can be some issues with exactly how the standardization is done (Bring 1994). In practice, the standardized regression coefficients are transformed back into their original units when time comes to interpret the results, but that obscures the impact of the standardization on Eq. 2.7. The penalty function has the standardized coefficients as its argument.

In whatever manner the value of λ is determined, a valid Level I analysis may be undertaken. What varies is the smoothness of the fitted values from which descriptive summaries are constructed. For a Level II analysis, if the value of λ is determined before the data analysis begins, one can try to resurrect a conventional "true model" approach. For reasons already addressed, that approach seems like a bad idea. Moreover, the shrinkage is a new source of bias. Using the "wrong model" perspective, one can estimate in an asymptotically unbiased manner a best linear approximation of the true response surface for the a priori chosen value of λ. More commonly, the value of λ is determined as part of the data analysis. Then there are significant complications for Level II analysis even if an approximation is the estimand. Data snooping is in play.

Ideally, there are training data, evaluation data, and test data as described in the last chapter. Using the training data and the evaluation data, one option is trial and error. Different values of λ are tried with the training data until there is a satisfactory fit in the evaluation data by some measure such as mean squared error. With modern computing power, a very large number of potential values can be searched very quickly. Once a value for λ is determined, a Level II analysis properly can be undertaken with the test data; for the test data, the value of λ is determined before the data analysis begins.[14]

If there are no evaluation and test data, and the dataset is too small to partition, there are Level II fallback options noted in the last chapter, such as cross-validation. The value of λ is chosen to maximize some cross-validation measure of fit. For example, if 50 different values of λ are tested, each with a tenfold cross-validation, the ridge model is fit and its fit statistic is computed 500 times. There are 50 averaged measures of fit. The value of λ with the best average fit measure is chosen. Clearly, there is a lot a data reuse, which contradicts any clean separation between training data, evaluation data, and test data. But once λ is determined, estimation of the regression coefficients can proceed using the full dataset.

One must be clear that no claims can be made that once the value of λ has been determined, one has met the linear regression first- and second-order conditions. Even if the true response surface is linear and additive, and one has in hand all of the required regressors (both unlikely), the bias–variance tradeoff means that almost certainly some bias has been introduced. The usual first- and second-order conditions, therefore, are violated.

2.3.1.2 A Ridge Regression Illustration

Perhaps an example will help fix these ideas. The data come from a survey of 95 respondents in which a key question is how various kinds of social support may be related to depression.[15] There are 19 predictors and for this illustration, we will work with three: (1) "emotional"—a "summary of 5 questions on emotional support availability," (2) "affect"—a "summary of 3 questions on availability of affectionate support sources," and (3) "psi"—a "summary of 3 questions on availability of positive social interaction." The response "BDI," which stands for Beck depression inventory, is a 21-item inventory based on self-reports of attitudes and symptoms characteristic of depression (Beck et al. 1961).

For didactic purposes, we will for now treat the data as random realizations from the relevant joint probability distribution so that the predictors and the response are random variables. One would have to know a lot more about how the data were collected to provide a fully informed determination one way or the other. For example, some of these individuals may have been referred by the same clinician. In addition, the model is probably severely misspecified. We provisionally adopt, therefore, the best linear approximation approach. The usual linear regression output from *lm* takes the following form.

```
Call:
lm(formula = BDI ~ emotional + affect + psi, data =
socsupport)

Residuals:
    Min      1Q  Median      3Q     Max
-14.141  -5.518  -0.764   3.342  32.667

Coefficients:
             Estimate Std. Error t value Pr(>|t|)
(Intercept)  31.5209     5.0111   6.290 1.09e-08 ***
emotional     0.2445     0.3458   0.707  0.48133
affect       -0.4736     0.4151  -1.141  0.25693
psi          -1.6801     0.5137  -3.270  0.00152 **
---
Signif. codes:  0 *** 0.001 ** 0.01 * 0.05 . 0.1  1

Residual standard error: 8.6 on 91 degrees of freedom
Multiple R-squared:  0.216, Adjusted R-squared:  0.1901
F-statistic: 8.355 on 3 and 91 DF,  p-value: 5.761e-05
```

Consider first a Level I analysis. The predictors "affect" and "psi" are negatively related to depression, and "emotional" is positively related to depression. As is often the case with constructed scales, it is difficult to know how substantively important the regression coefficients are. How big is big, and how small is small? For example, psi ranges from 5 to 15, and BDI ranges from 0 to 48. For each additional psi point, the average of the depression scale is about 1.7 points smaller. Even over the range of psi, the full range of BDI is not covered. Moreover, how does one translate variation in any of the variables into *clinical* importance? How many points make a clinical difference?

For Level II analysis, one has in principle an estimate of a best linear approximation of the true response surface as a property of the joint probability distribution responsible for the data. Proper estimation, confidence tests, and statistical tests can follow with sandwich estimates of the standard errors and an asymptotic justification. In this case, one would again reject the null hypothesis of 0.0 for the psi regression coefficient but not for the other regression coefficients. Still, with only 91 residual degrees of freedom it is not clear if one can count on the asymptotics.[16]

The conventional least squares estimates provide a benchmark for ridge regression results. Using the same mean function, Fig. 2.12 shows how the regression coefficients change as the ridge penalty is given more weight. When the ridge penalty is ignored, one has the ordinary least squares estimates. But as the ridge penalty gets larger, all three coefficients are shrunk toward zero in a proportional manner. The larger the coefficient, the greater the shrinkage. For λ values greater than about 1100 (i.e., approximately e^7), all three coefficients are effectively zero,

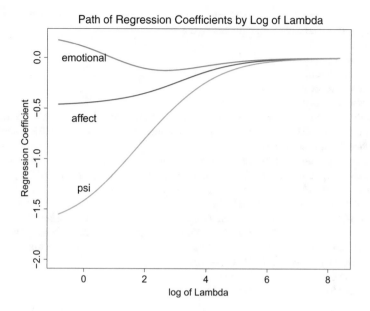

Fig. 2.12 Ridge regression coefficient shrinkage in their original units as λ increases

and all three arrive at zero together. This is a characteristic of ridge regression. The code is provided in Fig. 2.13.

But what value of λ should be used? Figure 2.14 shows with the red dotted line how the average mean squared error from a tenfold cross-validation changes with the log of λ. The "canned" code from *glmnet* was used much as in the R documentation.

The band around the average mean squared error is constructed as plus or minus two standard deviations computed from the 10 cross-validation folds. The blue vertical line shows the value of the log of λ for which the average mean squared error is the smallest. A logged value of λ equal to 1 does about as well as one can do. Looking back at Fig. 2.12, the regression coefficient for psi is shrunk from about −1.6 to about −1.0, the regression coefficient for affect is shrunk from about −0.5 to about −0.4, and the regression coefficient for emotional support is shrunk from about 0.25 to near 0.0. The regression coefficients and, consequently, the fitted values, have been regularized. But none of the regression coefficients are shrunk to exactly 0.0. The sequence of 3s across the top of the graph means that for each value of the log of λ, no predictors are dropped; all three predictors are retained in the regression.[17]

Now what? The Level I ordinary least squares analysis stands. For a Level II analysis, there can be at least two interpretations. First, the estimand can be true response surface with the three shrunken regression coefficients estimates of those in the joint probability distribution. As a tuning parameter, λ make no appearance. The regression coefficients by design are probably biased estimates because of the

```
### Get Data and Ridge Software
library(DAAG)
library(glmnet)
data(socsupport)
attach(socsupport)
### Least Squares
X<-as.matrix(data.frame(emotional,affect,psi)) #  Needs a matrix
out1<-lm(BDI~emotional+affect+psi,data=socsupport) # OLS results
### Ridge Regression
out2<-glmnet(X,BDI,family="gaussian",alpha=0) # Ridge results
plot(log(out2$lambda),out2$beta[2,],ylim=c(-2,.2),type="l",
 col="blue",lwd=3,xlab="log of Lambda",
 ylab="Regression Coef?cient",
 main="Path of Regression Coef?cients by  Log of Lambda")
lines(log(out2$lambda),out2$beta[1,],type="l",col="red",lwd=3)
lines(log(out2$lambda),out2$beta[3,],type="l",col="green",lwd=3)
text(0,0,"emotional",cex=1.5)
text(0,-.6,"affect",cex=1.5)
text(0,-1.3,"psi",cex=1.5)
```

Fig. 2.13 R code for the analysis of the Beck depression inventory

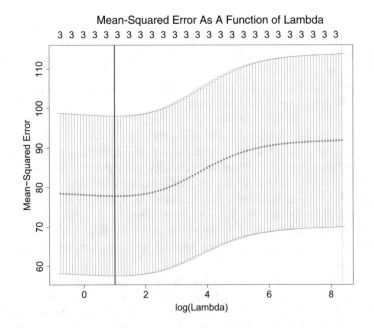

Fig. 2.14 Choosing λ by fit quality

bias–variance tradeoff. Statistical tests and confidence intervals are, therefore, not valid, even if valid standard errors are computed.

Second, the three variable linear regression altered by the value of λ chosen can be seen as a best penalized linear approximation. One could then proceed much as we did in Chap. 1. However, with the focus on the regression coefficients, it is not apparent why one should not more simply return to the original, ordinary least squares approach. Any penalized Level II interpretation must confront the model selection complications produced by the large number of cross-validation exercises undertaken (i.e., the default is 100) from which a single "best" value of λ was chosen. That value of λ, in turn, determined the "best" model.

Perhaps the major take-home message is that ridge regression showcases some importance concepts and tools, but will not likely to be a useful data analysis procedure. We need to do better.

2.3.1.3 The Least Absolute Shrinkage and Selection Operator (LASSO)

Suppose that one proceeds as in ridge regression but now adopts the constraint that the sum of the *absolute values* of the regression coefficients is less than some constant. Just like for ridge regression, all of the predictors usually are standardized for the calculations, but the regression coefficients are transformed back into their original units when time comes to interpret the results. The L_1 constraint leads to a regression procedure known as the lasso[18] (Tibshirani 1996) whose estimated regression coefficients are defined by

$$\hat{\beta} = \min_{\beta} \left[\sum_{i=1}^{n} (y_i - \beta_0 - \sum_{j=1}^{p} x_{ij}\beta_j)^2 + \lambda \sum_{j=1}^{p} |\beta_j| \right]. \tag{2.9}$$

Unlike the ridge penalty, the lasso penalty leads to a nonlinear estimator, and a quadratic programming solution is needed. As before, the value of λ is a tuning parameter, typically determined empirically, usually through some measure of fit or prediction error. Just as with ridge regression, a λ of zero yields the usual least squares results. As the value of λ increases, the regression coefficients are shrunk toward zero.

2.3.1.4 A Lasso Regression Illustration

Using the same data as for the ridge regression analysis, Fig. 2.15 shows that in contrast to ridge regression, the regression coefficients are not shrunk proportionately. (The code is provided in Fig. 2.16.) The regression coefficients are shrunk by a constant factor λ (Hastie et al. 2009: 71) so that some are shrunk relatively more than others as λ increases. But for a sufficiently large λ, all are shrunk to 0.0. This is a standard result that allows (Hastie et al. 2009: section 3.4.5) to place ridge

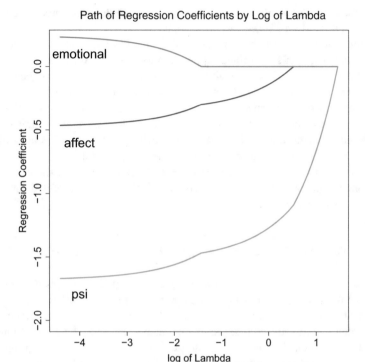

Fig. 2.15 Lasso regression results as a function of the log of the lasso penalty λ for each of the three predictors

```
### lasso Results
out3<-glmnet(X,BDI,family="gaussian",alpha=1)  # lasso
plot(log(out3$lambda),out3$beta[2,],ylim=c(-2,.2),type="l",
    col="blue",lwd=3,xlab="log of Lambda", ylab="Regression
    Coefficient", main="Path of Regression Coefficients by
    Log of Lambda")
lines(log(out3$lambda),out3$beta[1,],type="l",col="red",lwd=3)
lines(log(out3$lambda),out3$beta[3,],type="l",col="green",lwd=3)
text(-4,.1,"emotional",cex=1.5)
text(-4,-.6,"affect",cex=1.5)
text(-4,-1.8,"psi",cex=1.5)
```

Fig. 2.16 Using cross-validation to choose the value of λ in lasso regression

regression and the lasso in a larger model selection context. The lasso performs in a manner that has some important commonalities with model selection procedures used to choose a subset of regressors. When a coefficient value of 0.0 is reached, that predictor is no longer relevant and can be dropped.

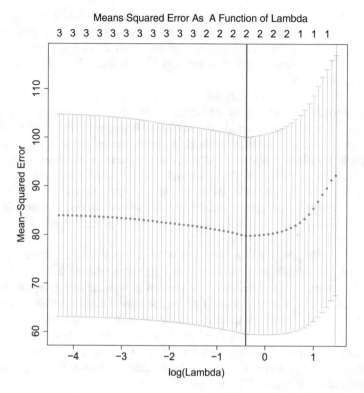

Fig. 2.17 Using cross-validation to choose the value of λ in lasso regression

Figure 2.17 shows how. We learn that a logged value for λ of about −0.4 leads to the smallest average mean squared error in the tenfold cross-validation. Looking back at Fig. 2.15, the predictor emotional has been shrunk to 0.0 and plays no role in the fitted values. On the top margin of the plot, one can see that the number of predictors has been reduced from three to two. A form of model selection has been implemented. The other two predictors remain active with psi still dominant. As the logged value of λ reaches about 0.5, the affect predictor is dropped as well. In practice, one would likely settle on the two predictors that are not shrunk to 0.0 and then use them in an ordinary least squares analysis. That is, the lasso chooses the predictors, but the analysis meant to inform subject-matter concerns is done with conventional least squares regression. Once a preferred set of regressors is chosen, the motivation for a fitting penalty is far less compelling.

Unfortunately, the lasso does not solve any of the Level II difficulties that undermined the Level II analysis with ridge regression. The main difference is in the use of an L_1-penalty rather than an L_2 can make the lasso a useful, variable selection tool. But as before, this creates very difficult problems for estimation, confidence intervals, and statistical tests.

Were one just going to make use of the fitted values, logged $\lambda = -0.4$ would produce the best performing results according to the cross-validation mean squared error and ideally, by the true generalization error that it is meant to approximate. There would be no need to revert to ordinary least squares. But all of the Level II problems remain.

Although the lasso is certainly a very slick technique, it is unlikely in practice to find the "correct" mean function. At the very least, all of the regressors responsible for nature's true response function would have to be in the dataset (how would you know?) and in the real world, combined as the regression mean function specifies (i.e., as a linear combination). In addition, there can be empirical obstacles such as high correlations among the predictors and whether some predictors that should be included contribute sufficiently to the fit after covariance adjustments to be retained. In effect, the predictors that survive are just those having a sufficiently large partial correlation with the response, given the set of predictors being empirically considered.

The lasso has generated an enormous amount of interest among statisticians. Rosset and Zhu (2007) consider the path that the regression coefficients take as the value of λ changes, place the lasso in a class of regularization processes in which the solution path is piecewise linear, and then develop a robust version of the lasso. Wang et al. (2007) combine quantile regression with the lasso to derive another robust model selection approach. Zou (2006) has proposed an adaptive version of the lasso when correlations between predictors are high so that unimportant coefficients are shrunk more aggressively. Zou and Hastie (2005) combine the ridge and lasso penalties and call the results "elastic net." Thus,

$$\hat{\beta} = \min_{\beta} \left[\sum_{i=1}^{n}(y_i - \beta_0 - \sum_{j=1}^{p} x_{ij}\beta_j)^2 + \lambda_1 \sum_{j=1}^{p} |\beta_j| + \lambda_2 \sum_{j=1}^{p} \beta_j^2 \right]. \tag{2.10}$$

Elastic net can earn its keep in settings where the lasso stumbles: when the number of predictors is larger than the number of observations (which is common with microarray data) and when there are high correlations between predictors. Elastic net is a feature of *glmnet* in R, and there are some promising extensions available in the R procedure *c060* (Sill et al. 2014).

But, much of the work on the lasso has been directed toward model selection as an end in itself (Fan and Li 2006; Ran and Lv 2008; Meinshausen and Bühlmann 2006; Bühlmann and van de Geer 2011; Lockhart et al. 2014). There are a host of complications associated with model selection briefly noted in the last chapter. There are also many unsolved problems that can make real applications problematic. But perhaps most important here, a discussion model selection as a freestanding enterprise would take us far afield. Our emphasis will continue to be how to get good fitted values.[19]

In summary, ridge regression and lasso regression introduce the very important idea of penalized fitting and show some ways in which shrinkage can work. As the value of λ is increases, the regression coefficients are shrunk toward 0.0, and the fitted values become less rough. In the process, bias can be traded against variance with the hope of reducing generalization error in the fitted values. But with our focus on a set of inputs and their fitted values, the lasso is essentially a linear regression and is not even as flexible as regression splines; the linear mean function is very restrictive. We can do a lot better, and we will. The lasso can also be used as a model selection tool, but that is peripheral to our discussion.[20]

2.4 Penalized Regression Splines

Complexity penalties can be used to help solve the knot placement problem for regression splines. We proceed as before with regression splines but place a large number of equally spaced knots for different values of a single predictor X. For each knot, we compute a measure of roughness and then shrink the associated regression coefficients when the fitted values of Y are too rough. Recall that behind the scenes, X will be subject to a linear basis expansion using piecewise polynomials.

Figure 2.18 provides a simple visualization of how one can measure roughness when working with realized data. There is a numeric response variable Y and a single numeric predictor X. The blue line is an empirical estimate of the population approximation. There is a knot at $x = 11$ (in bold font) and at $x = 19$ (in bold font). Immediately above the blue approximation are the fitted values of Y for selected values of X. For example, when $x = 12$, $y = 4.1$.

Consider the knot at $x = 11$. The fitted values are changing slowly. The change from $x = 10$ to $x = 11$ is 0.03 (in red). The change from $x = 11$ to $x = 12$ is 0.08 (in red). The fitted values are changing more rapidly to the right of the knot. Each of those changes is an empirical approximation of a first derivative. For the knot at

Fig. 2.18 Changes in Y as measures of roughness where Δ stands for change and $\Delta\Delta$ stands for change in the change

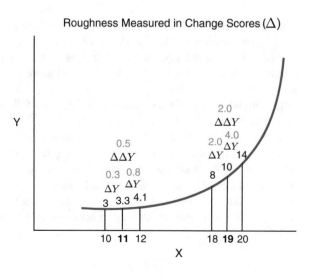

Roughness Measured in Change Scores (Δ)

$x = 19$, one can proceed in the same manner, which yields changes in the fitted values of 2.0 and 4.0 (in red). These too can be seen as empirical approximations of first derivatives.

In Fig. 2.18, first derivatives represent the changes in the fitted values, which do not directly measure roughness. Roughness is measured by the second derivatives, or the *change in change* of the fitted values. Two examples are shown. For the knot at $x = 11$ that value is 0.5 (in red). For the knot at $x = 19$ that value is 2.0 (in red). The second value is 4 times larger, and one can say that the change in the change is 4 times faster. Put another way, the fitted values are 4 times more rough at $x = 19$ than at $x = 11$. Change scores are commonly known as first differences, and changes in the change scores are commonly known as second differences.

Similar calculation can be undertaken at the x-value of each knot. One then has a set of empirical approximations of second derivatives. These are then squared and summed to become a measure of roughness for the full set of fitted values. One can use the sum as a measure of the complexity of the fitted values.

Suppose there are K equally spaced knots. We denote the roughness measure by $\sum_{k=2}^{K-1}(\hat{y}'')^2$. The summation of the penalty terms starts at $k = 2$ and ends at $k = K - 1$ because the second differences cannot be computed for first knot or the last knot (i.e., there are no knots to the left or to the right, respectively). As before, there is λ that determines how much weight should be given to the complexity measure as the fit of Y is undertaken. Conventional treatments usually represent the penalty in a more abstract manner as $\lambda \int [f''(t)]^2 dt$, where t is a placeholder for the fitted function. We adopt that shortly.

In practice, one minimizes

$$\hat{\beta} = \min_{\beta} \left[\sum_{i=1}^{n} [y_i - f(x_i)]^2 + \lambda \sum_{k=2}^{K-1} (\hat{y}'')^2 \right]. \tag{2.11}$$

The form of $f(x_i)$ is determined using a piecewise polynomial spline.[21] Just as for ridge regression and the lasso, the value of λ can be specified before the data analysis begins or determined empirically as part of the fitting process (e.g., using cross-validation). If the value of λ is known before the data analysis begins, one has a nonparametric approximation of the true response function but in the spirit of ridge regression or the lasso.[22] Statistical inference follows as before because there is no data snooping built into the procedure.

If the value of λ is determined as part of the estimation process, one can use training data and evaluation data to determine the value. Estimation is undertaken in test data. If there is interest in statistical inference, and one can make the case that the data are IID, conformal statistical inference can be used to obtain legitimate prediction intervals around fitted values. In short, once λ is determined, the formal data snooping is completed. One can proceed using the test data with a known value of λ.[23]

2.4.1 An Application

The data frame *Freedman* from the *car* library contains several variables potentially related to the crime rate per 100,000 in 1969 for 110 U.S. metropolitan areas with more 250,000 residents. One might seek to describe how the percent nonwhite is related to the crime rate. If a case can be made that the social process responsible for crime in larger U.S. cities were reasonably stable from the late 1960s to the early 1970s, one can postulate a joint probability distribution characterizing those process during that time period. The figures for 1969 can then be seen as IID realizations from that joint probability distribution. The crime rate in each metropolitan area is realized from the same joint probability distribution independently of the crime rate in any other metropolitan area. Level II may be a real option using training data and test data.

The results using a regression spline are shown in Fig. 2.19. Note that the data are split so that there are training data and test data, which reduces the number of observations available for training and testing. The procedure *gam* from the

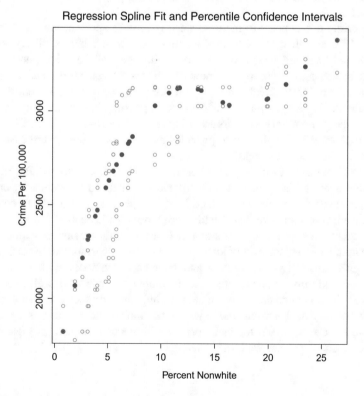

Fig. 2.19 A regression spline application (fitted values in blue, percentile confidence intervals in red. N = 110)

mgcv library was used. This software will be discussed in more depth later when regression splines for multiple predictors are considered.

The value of λ was determined automatically using tenfold cross-validation with the training data. A single "best" λ chosen using up a very large number of degrees of freedom as many different values of λ were tried. There are data snooping and overfitting issues. However, only the regression spline analysis of the training data is implicated, and its sole purpose was to arrive at a value for the penalty parameter λ.

With the value of the penalty parameter determined using the training data, the regression spline analysis can be run again with the test data and the estimated penalty parameter value fixed. There is now no data snooping. Nevertheless, blind fitting of the training data can be a risky way to determine λ because no subject-matter expertise can be brought to bear. We will revisit the issues shortly.

The blue filled circles in Fig. 2.19 are the test data fitted values. Using the nonparametric bootstrap, the test data were refit 1000 times. For each value of the predictor percentage nonwhite, the 95% confidence interval was computed and plotted as red open circles. The confidence interval behaves about as it should, although with just 55 test observations, we are a long way from from any asymptotic properties.

The crime rate appears to increase steadily until the percent nonwhite reaches around 15% and then starts to decline. Because the number of observations is modest, and there are several outliers, rerunning the analysis with a new split of the data can change this account somewhat. The confidence intervals are consistent with the pattern for the fitted values, which at the very least is a sanity check.[24]

Figure 2.19 provides an estimate of an approximation of the true response surface. Many important predictors are being ignored, and as a result, the description is incomplete. Whether the figure provides useful information nevertheless is for subject-matter experts to decide.

These ideas can be extended to the generalized linear model, so that, for example, one can smooth a binary response G. Instead of penalized least squares, one can apply penalized iteratively re-weighted least squares, which is a way to construct a penalized maximum likelihood estimator (Wood 2017: Section 3.4.1). One can further extend this approach to data that includes more than a single predictor.

The number and placement of knots still is not formally resolved. In particular, K can be set at 10 equally spaced knots, and the impact of unnecessary knots on the fit can be reduced through penalization. Such an approach can work well in practice. However, there is another, closed related formulation that seems to better capture the spirit of statistical learning and in which the number and locations of knots does not have to be specified. It too can work well in practice and can give results that are often much the same. We turn to that now.

2.5 Smoothing Splines

We now consider an alternative smoother that does not require a priori knots. A key feature of this approach is to saturate the predictor space with knots and then protect against overfitting by constraining the impact the knots can have on the fitted values. The influence that knots can have is diluted; the initial number of knots does not have to change but the impact of some can be shrunk towards zero.

We are still using a population approximation perspective in which the predictor and the response are random variables. For a single numeric predictor and a numeric response variable, there is a function for the population approximation $f(X)$ with two derivatives over its entire surface. This is a common assumption in the statistical learning literature and in practice does not seem to be particularly restrictive. The goal is to minimize a penalized residual sum of squares of the form

$$\text{RSS}(f, \lambda) = \sum_{i=1}^{N} [y_i - f(x_i)]^2 + \lambda \int [f''(t)]^2 dt, \tag{2.12}$$

where λ is, as before, a tuning parameter. The first term on the right-hand side captures how close the fitted values are to the actual values y_i. It is just the usual error sum of squares. The second imposes a cost for the complexity of the fit, much in the tradition of penalized regression splines, where t is a placeholder for the unknown function. The integral quantifies an overall roughness penalty, and λ once again determines the weight given to that penalty in the fitting process.[25]

At one extreme, as λ increases without limit, the fitted values approach the least squares line. Because no second derivatives are allowed, the fitted values are as smooth as they can be. At the other extreme, as λ decreases toward zero, the fitted values approach an interpolation of the values of the response variable.

For a Level I analysis, the larger the value of λ, the smoother the summary of the association between X and Y. For a Level II analysis, the estimation target is the smoothing splines function as a feature of the joint probability distribution with the empirically determined values of λ. If λ is larger, the smoother fitted values will likely lead to more bias and less variance. If λ is smaller, the rougher fitted values will likely lead to less bias and more variance. In short, the value of λ is used for tuning the bias–variance tradeoff. There is no need to think about the number and placement of knots.

Equation 2.12 can be minimized with respect to the $f(x)$, given a value for λ. Hastie et al. (2009: section 5.4) explain that a unique solution results, based on a natural cubic spline with N knots.[26] In particular,

$$f(x) = \sum_{j=1}^{N} N_j(x)\theta_j, \tag{2.13}$$

where θ_j is a set of weights, $N_j(x)$ is an N-dimensional set of basis functions for the natural cubic spline being used, and j stands for the knot index, of which there can be a maximum of N.

Consider the following toy example, in which x takes on values 0 to 1 in steps of 0.20. In this case, suppose $N = 6$, and one writes Eq. 2.13 in matrix form as $f(x) = \mathbf{N}\theta$, the result is

$$
f(x) = \begin{pmatrix}
-0.267 & 0 & 0 & -0.214 & 0.652 & -0.429 \\
0.591 & 0.167 & 0 & -0.061 & 0.182 & -0.121 \\
0.158 & 0.667 & 0.167 & -0.006 & 0.019 & -0.012 \\
0 & 0.167 & 0.667 & 0.155 & 0.036 & -0.024 \\
0 & 0 & 0.167 & 0.596 & 0.214 & 0.024 \\
0 & 0 & 0 & -0.143 & 0.429 & 0.714
\end{pmatrix}
\begin{pmatrix}
\theta_1 \\ \theta_2 \\ \theta_2 \\ \theta_4 \\ \theta_5 \\ \theta_6
\end{pmatrix}.
\tag{2.14}
$$

Equation 2.12 can be rewritten using a natural cubic spline basis and then the solution becomes

$$
\hat{\theta} = (\mathbf{N}^T\mathbf{N} + \lambda\mathbf{\Omega}_N)^{-1}\mathbf{N}^T\mathbf{y},
\tag{2.15}
$$

with $[\mathbf{\Omega}_N]_{ij} = \int N_j''(t)N_k''(t)dt$, where the second derivatives are for the function that transforms x into its natural cubic spline basis. One works with the product of these second derivatives because of the quadratic form of the penalty in Eq. 2.12. $\mathbf{\Omega}_N$ has larger values where the predictor is rougher, and given the linear estimator in Y, this is where the fitted values can be rougher as well. The penalty is the same as in Eq. 2.12.

To arrive at fitted values,

$$
\hat{\mathbf{y}} = \mathbf{N}(\mathbf{N}^T\mathbf{N} + \lambda\mathbf{\Omega}_N)^{-1}\mathbf{N}^T\mathbf{y} = \mathbf{S}_\lambda\mathbf{y},
\tag{2.16}
$$

where $\mathbf{S}_\lambda$ is a smoother matrix discussed in Chap. 1. For a given value of λ, we have a linear estimator for the fitted values. Equation 2.15 can be seen as a generalized form of ridge regression. With ridge regression, for instance, $\mathbf{\Omega}_N$ is an identity matrix.

The requirement of N knots may seem odd because it appears to imply that for a linear estimator all N degrees of freedom are used up. However, for values of λ greater than zero, the fitted values are shrunk toward a linear fit, and the fitted values are made more smooth. Fewer than N degrees of freedom are being used.

The value of λ can be determined a priori or through search procedures. One common approach is based on N-fold (drop-one) cross-validation, briefly discussed in the last chapter. The value of λ is chosen so that

$$
\text{CV}(\hat{f}_\lambda) = \sum_{i=1}^{N}[y_i - \hat{f}_i^{(-i)}(x_i)]^2
\tag{2.17}
$$

is as small as possible. In standard notation (Hastie et al. 2009: section 7.10), $\hat{f}_i^{(-i)}(x_i)$ is the fitted value for case i computed using a function fitted with all the data *but* the ith case, and y_i is the value of the response for the ith case. An in-sample estimate of CV, called the generalized cross-validation statistic (GCV), is computed as

$$
\text{GCV} = \frac{1}{N} \sum_{i=1}^{N} \left[\frac{y_i - \hat{f}(x_i)}{1 - \text{trace}(\mathbf{S})/N} \right]^2, \tag{2.18}
$$

where $\mathbf{S}$ is the smoother (or hat) matrix as before. Whether, the CV or GCV is used, all of the earlier caveats apply.

For a Level I analysis, there is no statistical inference and no formal adjustments for data snooping. For a Level II analysis and λ determined before the data analysis begins, one can proceed as before with asymptotically valid estimates, statistical tests, and confidence intervals for the approximation. As before, one is working in the spirit of ridge regression with a pre-determined value of λ. When λ is determined as part of the data analysis, data snooping complications are reintroduced, unless λ is determined using training data, and evaluation data, and statistical inference is undertaken with test data (although evaluation data are not mandatory). Examples will be provided later.

2.5.1 A Smoothing Splines Illustration

To help fix all these ideas, we turn to an application of smoothing splines. Figure 2.20 shows four smoothed scatterplots based on Eqs. 2.12 and 2.13. The R code can be found in Fig. 2.21. The procedure *gam* from the library *gam* is used.[27]

Each plot in Fig. 2.20 has the number of users of a particular server (centered) over time.[28] Time is measured in minutes. The penalty weight is *spar*, which can be thought of as a monotonic and standardized function of λ that is ordinarily set at a value from 0 to 1. The data, available in R—see Fig. 2.21—constitute a time series of 100 observations. Because the documentation in R does not explain how the data were collected, we proceed with a Level I analysis.

The number of users connected to the server varies dramatically over time in a highly nonlinear manner. Because details of the nonlinearity probably would have been unanticipated, an inductive approach available with smoothing splines is appropriate. For Fig. 2.20, there are four different plots with four different values of spar. The quality of the fitted values changes dramatically. But there is no right answer. For a Level I analysis, the goal is description. Choosing a value for spar depends heavily on subject-matter expertise and how the results might be used.

It could be very misleading to automatically choose the value of *spar* by some overall measure of in-sample fit. The fitted values are responding to both signal and

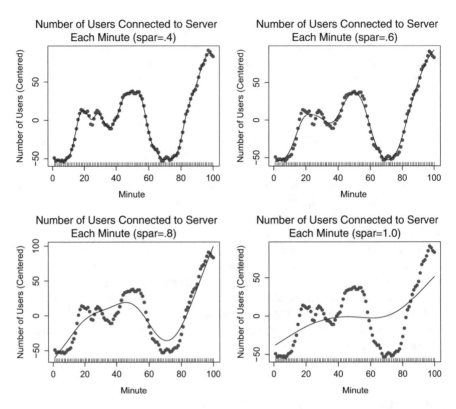

Fig. 2.20 Penalized smoothing spline fit for server use by minute with different penalty weights indexed by the tuning parameter *spar*

noise. For example, is the dip around minute 40 to be taken seriously? It would seem to be "real" when spar is 0.4 or 0.6, but not when spar is 0.8 or 1. Someone very familiar with the setting in which the data were collected and more generally knowledgeable about patterns of server use would need to make that call.

For a Level II analysis, one might want to consider the bias–variance tradeoff and in the absence of test data, set the value of spar using some approximation of out-of-sample performance. For these data, the default leave-one-out cross-validation selects a value of 8.5. But it is difficult to know what "out-of-sample" means. The data on hand are a sample of exactly what? To what does "out-of-sample" refer? Moreover, cross-validation is not a sensible procedure for time series data because cross-validation breaks up the temporal sequence of the data.[29]

More generally, the issues surrounding a Level II analysis are largely the same as those addressed for ridge regression and the lasso. If the value of λ (or the equivalent) is chosen before the data analysis begins, one can proceed as described in Chap. 1 with the response surface approximation perspective. If the value of λ is chosen as part of the data analysis, one is engaging in a form of model selection.

```
# Data
data(WWWusage)
Minute<-1:100
NumUsers<-WWWusage
internet<-data.frame(NumUsers,Minute)

# Smoothing Splines
library(gam)
par(mfrow=c(2,2))
out<-gam(NumUsers~s(Minute, spar=.4),data=internet)
plot(out,xlab="Minute",ylab="Number of Users (Centered)",
    main="Number of Users Connected to Server
    Each Minute (spar=.4)", col="blue", pch=19,
    residuals=T)

out<-gam(NumUsers~s(Minute, spar=.6),data=internet)
plot(out,xlab="Minute",ylab="Number of Users (Centered)",
    main="Number of Users Connected to Server
    Each Minute (spar=.6)",col="blue",pch=19,
    residuals=T)

out<-gam(NumUsers~s(Minute, spar=.8),data=internet)
plot(out,xlab="Minute",ylab="Number of Users (Centered)",
    main="Number of Users Connected to Server
    Each Minute (spar=.8)",col="blue",pch=19,
    residuals=T)

out<-gam(NumUsers~s(Minute, spar=1.0),data=internet)
plot(out,xlab="Minute",ylab="Number of Users (Centered)",
    main="Number of Users Connected to Server
    Each Minute (spar=1.0)",col="blue",pch=19,
    residuals=T)
```

Fig. 2.21 R code for penalized smoothing splines

With true test data or split samples, there may be a framework in which to proceed, but the longitudinal nature of the data would have to be maintained.[30]

2.6 Locally Weighted Regression as a Smoother

Thus far, the discussion of smoothing has been built upon a foundation of conventional linear regression. Another approach to smoothing also capitalizes on conventional regression, but through nearest neighbor methods. We turn to those.

2.6.1 Nearest Neighbor Methods

Consider Fig. 2.22 in which the ellipse represents a scatterplot of points for values of Y. For ease of exposition, there is a single target value of X, labeled x_0, for which a conditional mean $\bar{y}_0$ is to be computed. There may be only one such value of X or a relatively small number of such values. As a result, a conditional mean computed from those values alone risks being very unstable. One possible solution is to compute $\bar{y}_0$ from observations with values of X close to x_0. The rectangle overlaid on the scatterplot illustrates a region of "nearest neighbors" that might be used. Insofar as the conditional means for Y are not changing systematically within that region, a useful value for $\bar{y}_0$ can be obtained. For a Level I description, the conditional mean is a good summary for Y derived from the x-values in that neighborhood. If that conditional mean is to be used as an estimate in a Level II analysis of the true response surface, it will be unbiased and likely be more stable than the conditional mean estimated only for the observations with $X = x_0$. In practice, however, some bias is often introduced because Y actually does vary systematically in the neighborhood. As before, one hopes that the increase in the bias is small compared to the decrease in the variance.

A key issue is how the nearest neighbors are defined. One option is to take the k closest observations using the metric of X. For example, if X is age, x_0 is 24 years old, and k is 10, the ten closest x-values might range from 23 to 27 years of age. Another option is take some fixed fraction f of the observations that are closest to x_0. For example, if the closest 25% of the observations were taken, k might turn out to be 30, and the age-values might range between 21 and 29. Yet another option is to vary either k or f depending on the variability in Y within a neighborhood. For example, if there is more heterogeneity that is likely to be noise, larger values of k or f can be desirable to improve stability. For any of these approaches, the neighborhoods will likely overlap for different target values for X. For another target

Fig. 2.22 A conditional mean $\bar{Y}_0$ for X_0, a target value of X

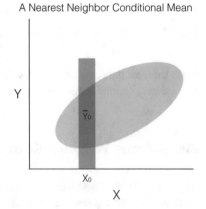

A Nearest Neighbor Conditional Mean

value near x_0, some near neighbors will likely be in both neighborhoods. There also is no requirement that the neighborhood be symmetric around x_0.

Suppose now that for each unique value of x, a nearest neighbor conditional mean for y is computed using one of the approaches just summarized. Figure 2.23 shows a set of such means connected by straight lines. The pattern provides a visualization of how the means of y vary with x. As such, the nearest neighbor methods can be seen as a smoother.

The values k or f are often referred to as the "bandwidth," "window," or "span" of a neighborhood. The larger the values of k or f, the larger the size of the neighborhood, and Fig. 2.23 will change. Larger neighborhoods will tend to make the smoothed values less variable. If the smoothed values are to be treated as Level II estimates of the true response surface, they will likely have more bias and less variance. Smaller neighborhoods will tend to make the smoothed values more variable. If the smoothed values are to be treated as Level II estimates of the true response surface, they will likely have less bias and more variance.

Where is the population approximation in all this? For an estimate of a single condition expectation, there is no population approximation of the true response surface. There is just a single conditional expectation whose value may be of interest. Figure 2.23 should make clear that there is likely to be concern for an approximation of the true response surface when lines are drawn between the empirical, conditional means. One has a visualization of how the condition mean of Y varies with X.

2.6.2 Locally Weighted Regression

Nearest neighbor methods can be effective in practice and have been elaborated in many ways (Ripley 1996; Shakhnarovich 2006). In particular, what if within each

Fig. 2.23 Interpolated conditional means

A Nearest Neighbor Interpolation of Conditional Mean

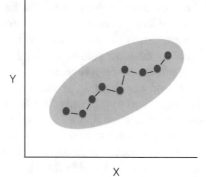

neighborhood the conditional means of Y vary systematically? At the very least, there is information being ignored that could improve the estimate of $\bar{y}_0$.

Just as in conventional linear regression, if Y is related to X in a systematic fashion, there can be less variation in the regression residuals than around the neighborhood mean of Y. More stable estimates can follow. The idea of applying linear regression within each neighborhood leads to a form of smoothing based on locally weighted regressions. The smoother commonly is known as "lowess."[31]

We stick with the one predictor case a bit longer. For any given value of the predictor x_0, a polynomial regression is constructed only from observations with x-values that are nearest neighbors of x_0. Among these, observations with x-values closer to x_0 are weighted more heavily. Then, $\hat{y}_0$ is computed from the fitted regression and used as the smoothed value of the response y at x_0. The process is repeated for all other values of x.

Although the lowess polynomial is often of degree one (linear), quadratic and cubic polynomials also are used. It is not clear that much is gained in practice using the quadratic or cubic form. In some implementations, one can also employ a degree zero polynomial, in which case no regression is computed, and the conditional mean of y in the neighborhood is used as $\hat{y}_0$. This is just the nearest neighbor approach except for the introduction of distance weighting. Perhaps surprisingly, the lowess estimator is linear for a given value of k or f (Hastie et al. 2009: section 6.1.1), although the smoothed relationship between X and Y may be highly nonlinear.

The precise weight given to each observation depends on the weighting function employed. The normal distribution is one option, although there is no formal statistical rationale. That is, the weights form a bell-shaped curve centered on x_0 that declines with distance from x_0.

The tricube is another option. Differences between x_0 and each value of x in the window are divided by the length of the window along x. This standardizes the differences. Then the differences are transformed as $(1 - |z|^3)^3$, where z is the standardized difference. Values of x outside the window are given weights of 0.0. As an empirical matter, most of the common weighting functions give about the same results, and there seems to be no formal justification for any particular weighting function.

As discussed for nearest neighbor methods, the amount of smoothing depends on the value of k or f. For f, proportions between 0.25 and 0.75 are common. The larger the proportion of observations included, the smoother are the fitted values. The span plays the same role as the number of knots in regression splines or λ in smoothing splines. Some software also permits the span to be chosen in the units of the regressor. For example, if the predictor is population size, the span might be defined as 10,000 people wide. Whatever the metric, one is assembling a set of linear basis expansions in X.

More formally, each local regression at each x_0 is constructed by minimizing the weighted sum of squared residuals with respect to the intercept and slope for the $M \leq N$ observations included in the window. Thus,

$$\text{RSS}^*(\boldsymbol{\beta}) = (\mathbf{y}^* - \mathbf{X}^*\boldsymbol{\beta})^T \mathbf{W}^*(\mathbf{y}^* - \mathbf{X}^*\boldsymbol{\beta}). \tag{2.19}$$

The asterisk indicates that only the observations in the window are included. The regressor matrix $\mathbf{X}^*$ can contain polynomial terms for the predictor, should that be desired. $\mathbf{W}^*$ is a diagonal matrix conforming to $\mathbf{X}^*$, with diagonal elements w_i^*, which are a function of distance from x_0. This is where the weighting-by-distance gets done.[32]

The overall algorithm then operates as follows.

1. Choose the smoothing parameter such as bandwidth, f, which is a proportion between 0 and 1.
2. Choose a point x_0 and from that the $(f \times N = M)$ nearest points on x.
3. For these M nearest neighbor points, compute a weighted least squares regression line for y on x.
4. Construct the fitted value $\hat{y}_0$ for that single x_0.
5. Repeat Steps 2 through 4 for each value of x. Near the boundary values of x, constraints are sometimes imposed much like those imposed on cubic splines and for the same reasons.
6. To enhance visualization, connect adjacent $\hat{y}$s with straight lines.

There also is a robust version of lowess. After the entire fitting process is completed, residuals are computed in the usual way. Weights are constructed from these residuals. Larger residuals are given smaller weights, and smaller residuals are given larger weights. Using these weights, the fitting process is repeated. This, in turn, can be iterated until the fitted values do not change much (Cleveland 1979) or until some pre-determined number of iterations is reached (e.g., 3). The basic idea is to make observations with very large residuals less important in the fitting.

Whether the "robustification" of lowess is useful will be application-specific and depend heavily on the window size chosen. Larger windows will tend to smooth the impact of outlier residuals. But because the scatterplot being smoothed is easily plotted and examined, it is usually easy to spot the possible impact of outlier residuals and, if necessary, remove them or take them into account when the results are reported. In short, there is no automatic need for the robust version of lowess when there seem to be a few values of the response that perhaps distort the fit.

Just as with penalized smoothing splines, a Level I analysis is descriptive and always an analysis option. For Level II, if the span is determined before the data analysis begins, one has an estimate of a population approximation of the true response surface for given span. But that approximation cannot be expressed as a single linear regression. There are many such regressions, one for each fitted value. Yet, on an intuitive basis, if each regression makes sense a feature of the joint probability distribution, all of them do. And if all of them do, so do the set of lowess fitted values. With IID data, we are back in business. The regression coefficients are of no interest, but one can use the nonparametric bootstrap to obtain confidence intervals around the fitted values, much as was done for Fig. 2.19. And one can resample the full dataset.

If the span is determined as part of the data analysis, one should have evaluation and test data. That is, the span is determined in the training (and evaluation data), and an approximation for that span is computed from the test data. The estimation target is still the lowess approximation of the true response surface, and one can proceed just as in Fig. 2.19.

2.6.2.1 A Lowess Illustration

Figure 2.24 repeats the earlier analysis of server use, but applies lowess rather than smoothing splines. The results are much the same over a set of different spans. The fraction for each reported span is the proportion of observations that define a given neighborhood. (See Fig. 2.25 for the R code.)

Figure 2.24 was produced in R by *scatter.smooth*.[33] One can also proceed with *loess*, which has more options and separates the plotting from the fitting. Both procedures require that the span (or an equivalent turning parameter) be hard coded although there have been proposals to automate the tuning, much as done for smoothing splines (Loader 2004: section 4).

In summary, lowess provides a good, practical alternative to smoothing splines except that the span is not determined automatically (at least in R). Otherwise, it has pretty much the same strengths and weaknesses, and performance will be similar. For example, the same issues arise about whether the dip in use at about minute 40 is "real." Or even if it is, whether the dip is substantively or practically important. The lower left-hand plot in Fig. 2.24 may be the most instructive rendering for these data.

2.7 Smoothers for Multiple Predictors

The last set of figures is only the most recent example in which the limitations of a single predictor are apparent. Many more things could be related to server use than time alone. We need to consider smoothers when there is more than one predictor.

In principle, it is a simple matter to include many predictors and then smooth a multidimensional space. However, there are three significant complications in practice. An initial problem is the curse of dimensionality addressed in the last chapter. As the number of predictors increases, the space the data need to populate increases as a power function. Consequently, the demand for data increases very rapidly, and one risks data that are far too sparse to produce a meaningful fit. There are too few observations, or those observations are not spread around sufficiently to provide the support needed. One must, in effect, extrapolate into regions where there is little or no information. To be sensible, such extrapolations would depend on knowing the approximation $f(X)$ quite well. But it is precisely because the approximation $f(X)$ is unknown that smoothing is undertaken to begin with.

The second problem is that there are often conceptual complications associated with multiple predictors. In the case of lowess, for example, how is the neigh-

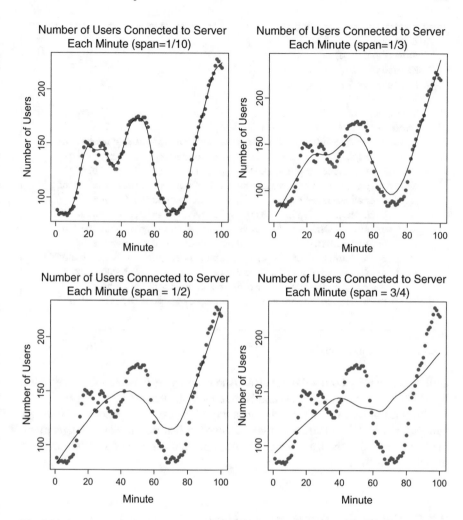

Fig. 2.24 Lowess conditional means for the number of server users per minute and different values for the tuning parameter span

borhood near x_0 to be defined (Fan and Gijbels 1996: 299–300)? One option is to use Euclidian distance. But then the neighborhood will depend on the units in which predictors happen to be measured. The common practice of transforming the variables into standard deviation units solves the units problem, but introduces new difficulties. When does it make substantive sense to claim that two observations that are close in standard deviations are close in subject-matter units? We considered very similar issues when ridge regression was discussed.

Another approach to neighborhood definition is to use the same span (e.g., 0.20) for both predictors, but apply it separately in each direction. Why this is a better

```
# Data
data(WWWusage)
Minute<-1:100
NumUsers<-WWWusage

# Lowess
par(mfrow=c(2,2))
scatter.smooth(Minute,NumUsers,xlab="Minute",ylab="Number of
     Users", main="Number of Users Connected to Server
     Each Minute (span=1/10)", span=1/10,pch=19,col="blue")
scatter.smooth(Minute,NumUsers,xlab="Minute",ylab="Number of
     Users", main="Number of Users Connected to Server
     Each Minute (span=1/3)", span=1/3, pch=19, col="blue")
scatter.smooth(Minute,NumUsers,xlab="Minute",ylab="Number of
     Users", main="Number of Users Connected to Server
     Each Minute (span = 1/2)", span=1/2, pch=19, col="blue")
scatter.smooth(Minute,NumUsers,xlab="Minute",ylab="Number of
     Users", main="Number of Users Connected to Server
     Each Minute (span = 3/4)", span=3/4, pch=19,col="blue")
```

Fig. 2.25 R code lowess smooth

definition of a neighborhood is not clear. And one must still define a distance metric by which the observation in the neighborhood will be weighted.

The third problem is that gaining meaningful access to the results is no longer straightforward. When there are more than two predictors, one can no longer graph the fitted surface in the usual way. How does one make sense of a surface in more than three dimensions?

2.7.1 Smoothing in Two Dimensions

Given the problems just summarized, the step from a single predictor to two predictors can be challenging. The step from a single predictor to many predictors will be addressed later. We will proceed drawing heavily on an empirical example.

A key issue in the study of climate is cyclical variation in rainfall for areas on the Pacific rim. An important driver is measured by the Southern Oscillation Index (SOI), which is the difference in sea level barometric pressure between Tahiti and Darwin, Australia. Negative values are associated with a phenomenon called "El Niño." Positive values are associated with phenomenon called "La Niña." Both are connected to patterns of rainfall in ways that are not well understood.

The illustrative data we will use has 101 observations. Predictors are years from 1900 to 2001 and the average yearly SOI. Average yearly rainfall in Australia is the response. The data are shown in Fig. 2.26, and the code is shown in Fig. 2.27.[34]

We begin by specifying an approximation of the true response surface. Rainfall is the response. Year and SOI are the predictors. A smoothing splines formulation for a single predictor is applied, but the single predictor is the product of year and SOI, just as one might represent an interaction effect between the two. The product variable is smoothed and then plotted in the 2-dimensional predictor space.[35]

Figure 2.28 shows the result for the Australian rainfall data from 1900 to 2001.[36] Values of the *spar* tuning parameter range from 0.2 to 1.0. Larger values of spar produce smoother surfaces. Any one of the values (or some other) could be preferred. (A spar-value of 1.0 was chosen using leave-one-out cross-validation.) The label on the vertical axis shows the expression by which the fitted values were computed.[37]

From a Level I analysis, there is a modest increase in rainfall over the time period with most of that increase occurring early. Rainfall increases when the SOI is larger, but the relationship is highly nonlinear. The association is especially pronounced for larger values of the SOI. For some smaller values of spar, the surface is "torqued." The relationship between SOI and rainfall is substantially stronger in some years

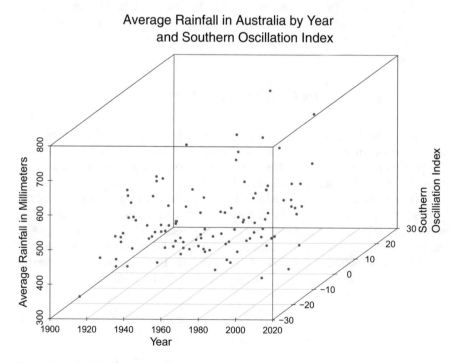

Fig. 2.26 A 3-Dimensional scatterplot of rainfall in Australia as a function year and the Southern Oscillation Index

```
library(DAAG)
data(bomsoi)
attach(bomsoi)
library(scatterplot3d)
scatterplot3d(Year,SOI,avrain,xlab="Year", ylab="Southern
             Oscilliation Index",zlab="Average Rainfall in
             Millimeters", main="Average Rainfall in Australia
             by Year and Southern Oscillation Index",pch=19,
             color="blue")
```

Fig. 2.27 R code for the 3-D scatterplot

than others. For example, with spar = 0.2, the strongest association is in the 1980s. However, with only 101 observations spread across the 2-dimensional predictor space, there are relatively few observations behind such interaction effects. That may be reason enough to prefer the fitted values with spar=1.0 and provides a small-scale object lesson about the curse of dimensionality.

Much as in several earlier analyses, thinking through a Level II analysis would be challenging. There data are longitudinal with year as one of the predictors. In the same fashion as the Tokyo water use data, the data were collected by year, but only summary statistics are reported. A lot more information is need to justify a Level II analysis.

2.7.2 The Generalized Additive Model

Moving beyond two predictors usually requires a different strategy. A more practical and accessible means needs to be found to approximate a response surface when the predictor space is greater than two. One approach is to resurrect an additive formulation that in practice can perform well.

The generalized additive model (GAM) is superficially an easy extension of the generalized linear model (GLM). Just as for GLMs, the response variables can be numeric, integer, or binary. Starting here with a numeric Y, GAM tries to circumvent the curse of dimensionality by assuming that the conditional mean of the response is a linear combination of functions of the predictors. Thus, the generalized additive model with a numeric Y (for now) and p predictors can be written as

$$Y = \alpha + \sum_{j=1}^{p} f_j(X_j) + \varepsilon, \tag{2.20}$$

where α is fixed at the mean of numeric Y. Using smoothing splines, we once again minimize the penalized regression sum of squares (PRSS) but with respect to all the p f_j's (Hastie et al. 2009: 297):

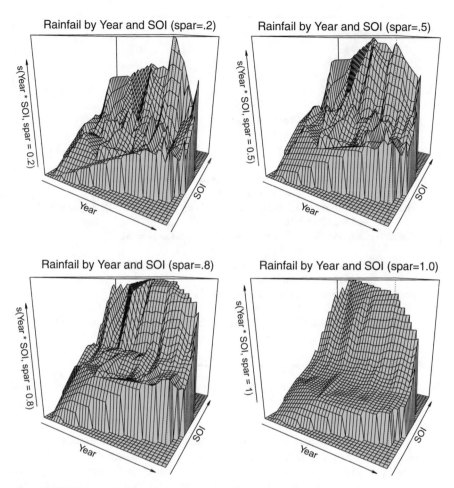

Fig. 2.28 GAM fitted values for rainfall in Australia plotted against year and the Southern Oscillation Index for different values of the tuning parameter spar

$$\mathrm{PRSS}(\alpha, f_1, f_2, \ldots, f_p) = \sum_{i=1}^{N} \left(y_i - \alpha - \sum_{j=1}^{p} f_j(x_{ij}) \right)^2 + \sum_{j=1}^{p} \lambda_j \int f_j''(t_j)^2 dt_j.$$

$$(2.21)$$

Equation 2.21 is a generalization of single-predictor smoothing splines that allows for a different value of λ_j for each function in the linear combination of functions; there are p values for λ that need to be specified in advance or more typically, determined as part of the data analysis. The pth second derivatives correspond to the pth function only.[38]

```
    library(DAAG)
    data(bomsoi)
    attach(bomsoi)
    llbrary(gam)
    library(akima)
    par(mfrow=c(2,2))
    out1<-gam(avrain~s(Year*SOI,spar=.2),data=bomsoi,
                    family=gaussian)
    plot(out1,theta=30, main="Rainfail by Year and SOI (spar=.2)",
          col="light blue")
    out2<-gam(avrain~s(Year*SOI,spar=.5),data=bomsoi,
                    family=gaussian)
    plot(out2, theta=30, main="Rainfail by Year and SOI (spar=.5)",
          col="light blue")
    out3<-gam(avrain~s(Year*SOI,spar=.8),data=bomsoi,
                    family=gaussian)
    plot(out3, theta=30, main="Rainfail by Year and SOI (spar=.8)",
          col="light blue")
    out4<-gam(avrain~s(Year*SOI,spar=1),data=bomsoi,
                    family=gaussian)
    plot(out4, theta=30, main="Rainfall by Year and SOI (spar=1.0)",
          col="light blue")
```

Fig. 2.29 R code for 3-Dimensional smooth of Australian rainfall data as a function of year and the Southern Oscillation Index

In the same manner as the generalized linear model, the generalized additive model permits several different link functions and disturbance distributions. For example, with a binary response, Y in our notation becomes G, and is assumed to have a conditional (on X) binomial distribution. The distribution of the conditional probabilities of G can be treated as logistic. When the conditional probabilities are transformed into the logarithm of the odds (called "logits") with an appropriate "link function," the right-hand side becomes a linear combination of the predictors. One now has the look and feel of a logistic regression (Hastie and Tibshirani 1990: Section 4.4).

There are no regression coefficients associated with the smoothed predictors. Regression coefficients would just scale up or scale down the functions of predictors. Whatever impact they would have is absorbed in the function itself. In other words, the role of the regression coefficients cannot be distinguished from the role of the transformation and, therefore, the regression coefficients are not identified. For the same reason, the usual regression intercept is also not identified and not included. Instead, the functions are centered on α, the mean of Y in the numeric response variable case. For binary G, the centering is on the mean logit. In either case, each function has a mean of 0.0 over the N observations in the data.

Each predictor can have its own functional relationship to the response. Because these functions are usually estimated using single-predictor smoothers of the sort addressed earlier, the term nonparametric is commonly applied despite the a priori commitment to an additive formulation. Alternatively, all of the functions may be specified in advance with the usual linear model as a special case.

All of the common predictor transformations are available, including the logs, polynomials, roots, product variables (for interaction effects), and indicator variables. As a result, GAM can be parametric as well and in this form, is really no different from the generalized linear model. The parametric and nonparametric specifications can be mixed so that some of the functions are derived empirically from the data, and some are specified in advance. Then the model is often called semiparametric.

One can use for GAM the same conception of "holding constant" that applies to conventional linear regression. Suppose that for a conventional regression analysis each of the predictors is transformed in a known manner. With least squares, each transformed predictor is covariance adjusted; the relationship between a given transformed predictor and the response is determined with the linear dependence between that transformed predictor and all other transformed predictors removed. One would like to do the same thing when each transformation is not known. But there can be no covariance adjustments until the transformations are determined, and there can be no transformations until each predictor is covariance adjusted. We have a chicken-egg problem. The backfitting algorithm provides a solution.

2.7.2.1 A GAM Fitting Algorithm

Proper estimation of generalized additive models can be undertaken with Eq. 2.21 generalized to penalized iteratively re-weighted least squares, in the spirit of GLMs. Backfitting, which for the generalized additive model is the Gauss–Seidel method (Breiman and Friedman 1985), can be a very effective way to proceed in practice. Backfitting has the following structure (Hastie et al. 2009: section 9.1.1).

1. Initialize with $\hat{\alpha} = \frac{1}{N} \sum_1^N y_i$, $\hat{f}_j \equiv 0, \forall i, j$. Each function is given initial values of 0.0, with α fixed at the mean of y.
2. Cycle: $j = 1, \ldots, p, 1, \ldots, p, \ldots,$

$$\hat{f}_j \leftarrow S_j \left[\{ y - \hat{\alpha} - \sum_{k \neq j} \hat{f}_k(x_{ik}) \}_1^N \right].$$

$$\hat{f}_j \leftarrow \hat{f}_j - \frac{1}{N} \sum_{i=1}^N \hat{f}_{ij}$$

Fitted values from all predictors but predictor j are linearly combined and subtracted from the response. A smoother S_j is applied to the resulting "residuals."

The result is a new set of fitted values for predictor j. These fitted values are then centered. All of the other predictors are cycled through one at a time in the same manner until each of the p predictors has a revised set of fitted values.
3. Repeat Step 2 until $\hat{f}_j$ changes less than some small, pre-determined amount. In the process, adjustments are made for linear dependence between the transformed predictors. For smoothed predictor, the other smoothed predictors are "held constant."

The backfitting algorithm is quite general and quite fast. A wide variety of smoothers can be introduced and in the past have been. For example, both lowess and penalized smoothing splines are available from *gam* procedure in the library *gam*. It can also include smooths of surfaces for two predictors at once, as illustrated earlier with the Australian rainfall data.

So what's not to like? The linear combination of smooths is not as general as a smooth of an entire surface, and sometimes that matters. Looking back at the El Niño example, the response surface was "torqued." The nonlinear function along one predictor dimension varied by the values of the other predictor dimension. This is a generalization of conventional interaction effects for linear regression in which the slope for one predictor varies over values of another predictor. The generalized additive model does not allow for interaction effects unless they are built into the mean function as product variables; interaction effects are not arrived at inductively. This is no different from conventional linear regression.

In addition, it apparently is difficult to introduce an automated search for good values of λ into the backfitting algorithm. Investigator-guided trial and error is required. Some may find this to be an inconvenience, but it forces a boots-on-the-ground examination of GAM performance. As before, subject-matter and policy implications can really matter, and there is no way to automate such considerations.

An excellent alternative implementation of the generalized additive model that provides for automated determination of λ values as well as trial-and-error methods is the *gam* implementation, discussed earlier, in the library *mgcv*. The procedure has many variants and options, but the underlying structure is penalized *regression* splines, with estimation undertaken by penalized maximum likelihood formulated as penalized iteratively re-weighted least squares. Extensions are provided for random effects models.

The number of knots can be specified by the user, which are spaced evenly over the range of each predictor to be smoothed. The number of knots determines an upper bound for complexity. The procedure can automatically search for satisfactory simpler approximations of the true response surface. One also can fix the weight given to the penalty function so that no search is undertaken.

A Bayesian approach to statistical inference is available, motivated by placing a prior distribution on λ. Readers who are intrigued should consult Wood's textbook (2017, section 4.2.4). Bayesian inference will not be pursued here. Bayesian inference begins with a perspective that is difficult to reconcile the population approximation approach on which we have built. There also are some very strict, and arguably fanciful, assumptions that need to be imposed.

The *gam* procedure in the library *gam* and the *gam* procedure in the library *mgcv* appear to have very similar performance. The implementation one prefers sensibly can be based on the form of the output. They can differ a bit, for example, in the details of the output information provided.

A Level II analysis can be viable if the data are IID, and there is no data snooping. Just as for smoothers of a single predictor, one requires that the values of any tuning parameters are determined before the data analysis begins. Alternatively, having valid test data can help, as illustrated later.

2.7.2.2 An Illustration Using the Regression Splines Implementation of the Generalized Additive Model

We turn to an application using the *gam* in the library *mgcv*. Although population counts from the U.S. census are highly accurate, they are certainly not perfect. In the absence of perfection, small differences between the actual number of residents in an area and the counted number of residents in that area can have very important consequences for the boundaries of voting districts, the number of elected representatives a county or state can have, and the allocation of federal funds. Beginning with the 1980 U.S. census, there were particular concerns about population undercounts in less affluent, minority-dominated voting districts.

The data we will now use come from a study by Ericksen et al. (1989) that sought correlates of census undercounts. Sixty-six geographical areas were included, 16 being large cities. The other geographical units were either the remainder of the state in which the city was located or other states entirely. Sampling was purposive.

We use the following variables:

1. Undercount—the undercount as a percentage of the total count;
2. Minority—the percentage of residents who are Black or Hispanic;
3. Language—the percentage of residents who have difficulty with English;
4. Housing—the percentage of residential buildings that is small and multi-unit;
5. Crime—reported crimes per 1000 residents; and
6. City—a major city as the geographical unit.

The first variable is the response. The others are predictors thought to be related to census undercounts. No doubt there are other predictors that subject-matter experts would claim should have been included. For example, we know nothing about the census enumeration procedures or the race and gender of enumerators. We also know nothing about any efforts by local authorities to encourage residents to cooperate. By conventional criteria, the mean function is misspecified. We proceed with an approximation of the true response surface.

Using the procedure *gam* in the library *mgcv*, the generalized additive model for a numeric response was applied to the data. For simplicity, all of the defaults were used. There was, as usual, information on the fit, much like provided for conventional linear regression, and for predictors that were not smoothed (e.g., factors), their regression coefficients were displayed along with standard errors and p-values. For each smoothed predictor, the effective degrees of freedom was

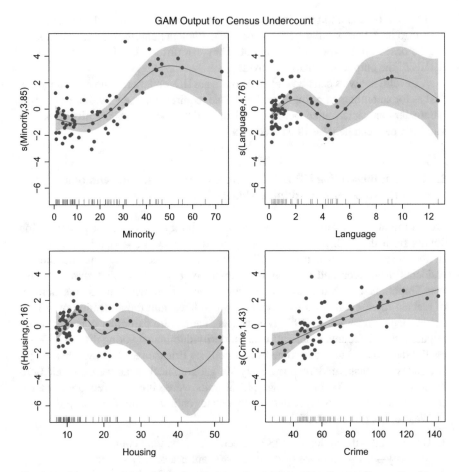

Fig. 2.30 Correlates of the estimated undercount for the U.S. 1980 Census (the predictor is on each horizontal axis, the centered fitted values are on each vertical axis, the shaded areas are error bands, rug plots are shown, and $N = 66$)

reported. Larger values for the effective degrees of freedom indicated that the corresponding fitted function was more complex. Because the effective degrees of freedom for each smoother was determined as part of the fitting process by GCV statistics, all of the results warrant scrutiny; they may not comport well with subject-matter expertise.

The model's predictors accounted for about 79% of the deviance. This is more than respectable, but there are 66 observations and the smoothers consume a substantial number of degrees of freedom. Were this a Level II analysis, generalization error could be quite large despite the good fit in the training data.

The regression coefficient for the city indicator of -0.28 is too small to matter in substantive terms. The reduction is about a quarter of a percent for city locations compared to all others. Figure 2.30 shows how the numeric predictors are related to

```
library(car)
data(Ericksen)
library(mgcv)

# make better variable names plotting
attach(Ericksen)
City<-as.numeric(ifelse(city=="city",1,0))
Minority<-minority
Language<-language
Housing<-housing
Crime<-crime
Undercount<-undercount
temp<-data.frame(Undercount,Crime,Housing,Language,Minority,City)

# GAM from mgcv
out<-gam(Undercount~s(Minority)+s(Language)+s(Housing)+
        s(Crime)+City ,data=temp, family=gaussian)
par(mfrow=c(2,2))
plot(out,residual=T,cex=1,pch=19,shade=T,
    shade.col="light blue",col="blue")
```

Fig. 2.31 R code for undercount analysis

the response after the backfitting algorithm removes any linear dependence between the transformed predictors. (See Fig. 2.31 for the R code.) For each graph, the response is centered around $\hat{\alpha}$, and there are rug plots just above the horizontal axes. Also shown are the response residuals. The vertical axis label includes the effective number of degrees of freedom used by the particular smoothed function, determined by the GCV statistic. For example, there are a little more than 6 degrees of freedom used by the housing variable and a little more than 1 degree of freedom used by the crime variable. The former is highly nonlinear. The latter is very nearly linear.

There are also shaded areas representing plus and minus two standard errors for the fitted values. Were one doing a Level II analysis, they are intended to convey the amount of uncertainty in the fitted values. But it is difficult to know what to make of this rendering of uncertainty. Although the error bands can be given a frequentist interpretation (Marra and Wood 2012), the estimation target apparently is the true response surface. We have already shown that under these circumstances, biased estimates are virtually certain, which means that the error bands confound the bias with the variance. As discussed above, one also needs to make the case that the observations were realized independently, conditional on the spatial areas chosen. But even if such a case could be made, model selection by the GCV statistic can make any Level II analysis problematic.

Perhaps the major take-away is that the "error bands" widen dramatically where the data are most sparse. Fitted values in those regions need very careful scrutiny and perhaps have no interpretive value. But one does not have anything like true confidence intervals to use as a guide.

If one had test data, error bands for the population approximation with far better statistical properties could be obtained conditional on the training data and the values of the penalty parameters selected through the GCV statistics computed in the training data. More discussion of this approach follows shortly; the key is to treat the estimated penalty parameters as fixed once they are estimated and then work with test data.[39]

In general, all four predictors show positive relationships with the size of the undercount in regions where the data are not sparse. For example, the relationship with the percentage of residents having problems with English is positive until the value exceeds about 2%. The relationship then becomes negative until a value of about 5% when the relationship turns positive again. But there is no apparent substantive explanation for the changes in the slope, which are based on very few observations. The twists and turns could be the result of noise or neglected predictors, but with so little data, very little can be concluded. The changing width of the shaded area makes the same point.

Do any of the estimated relationships matter much? The observed values for the undercount can serve as an effective benchmark. They range from a low of -2.3% to a high of 8.2%. Their mean is 1.9%, and their standard deviation is 2.5%. Where the data are not sparse, each predictor has fitted values that vary by at least 1% point. Whether changes variable by variable of a percentage point or two matter would need to be determined by individuals with subject-matter expertise.

Perhaps more telling is what happens when the four fitted relationships are combined in a linear fashion to arrive at overall fitted values. Fitted values range from little below -1% to about 7.5%, and as Fig. 2.32 shows, there is a substantial number of areas with fitted undercounts greater than 4%. Moreover, the distribution tends to decline over positive values up to about 4%, after which there is an curious increase. One might have expected continuing declines in the right tail. At least from a policy point of view, it might be instructive to know which geographical areas fall on the far right of the histogram. In short, insofar as the observed variability in the undercount matters, so does the variability in the fitted values.

2.8   Smoothers with Categorical Variables

Smoothers can be used effectively with categorical variables. When a predictor is categorical, there is really nothing to smooth. A binary predictor can have only two values. The "smoother" is then just a straight line connecting the two conditional means of the response variable. For a predictor with more than two categories, there is no way to order the categories along the predictor axis. Any imposed order would imply assigning numbers to the categories. How the numbers were assigned could make an enormous difference in the resulting fitting values, and the

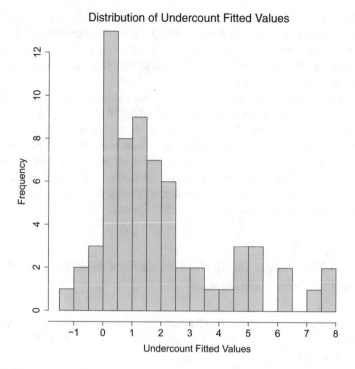

Fig. 2.32 Histogram of the undercount fitted values in percentages from the GAM procedure (N=66)

assigned numbers necessarily would be arbitrary. Consequently, the categories are reconfigured as indicator variables.

When the response is categorical and binary, smoothing can be a very useful procedure. All of the earlier benefits apply. In addition, because it is very difficult to see much in a scatterplot with a categorical response, a smoother may be the only way to gain some visual leverage on what may be going on. However, the earlier caveats apply too.

Within the generalized additive model, the analysis of binary response variables can be seen as an extension of binomial regression from the generalized linear model. The right-hand side is a linear combination of predictor functions. The left-hand side is the response transformed by a link function to logit units (i.e., the log of the odds of the outcome coded as 1). A key difference is that the functions for each predictor can be unknown before the analysis begins.[40]

Just as with logistic regression, the linear function of the predictors is in logit units. One usually can specify that those fitted values be transformed back into the units of the response, which are values between 0 and 1. Then, the fitted values for a Level I analysis can be treated as proportions, or for a Level II analysis, can be treated as probabilities. In either case, the deviance is a measure of fit although measures that take into account the degrees of freedom used are probably more instructive (e.g., AIC).

Usually, GAM with a binary outcome is meant to be a classifier. Just as in logistic regression, a threshold is imposed on the fitted values transformed to fall between 0.0 and 1.0. Commonly, that threshold is 0.50. Cases with fitted value larger than 0.50 are assigned the class usually coded 1. Cases with fitted values equal to or less than 0.50 are assigned the class usually coded 0.[41]

Classification error and functions thereof are, therefore, instructive. One can work with each observation's actual class and assigned class. Ideally, they are the same. When they are not, one has a classification error. The actual classes and fitted classes over observations can be tabulated in various ways to arrive at estimates of accuracy for binary outcomes. A rich story about accuracy also can be extracted from a confusion table, which is just a cross-tabulation over cases of each actual class against each fitted class. All such estimates should be obtained from test data. Confusion tables will be considered in depth in the next chapter.

2.8.1 An Illustration Using the Generalized Additive Model with a Binary Outcome

We consider again the low birthweight data, but now the response is binary: low birthweight or not. A birthweight is low when it is less than 2.5 kg. The following predictors are used:

1. Age—in years;
2. Mother's weight—in pounds;
3. Uterine—presence of uterine irritability; and
4. Smoke—whether the mother smokes.

We are proceeding with the approximation framework once again because there are no doubt important omitted variables (e.g., a mother's use of alcohol).

Using the defaults in *gam* (in the library *mgcv*), about 9% of the deviance can be attributed to the four predictors. Consider first the role of the two binary predictors. When the mother smokes, the odds of a low birthweight baby are multiplied by 2.05. When the mother has uterine irritability, the odds of a low birthweight baby are multiplied by 2.32. Both are exponentiated regression coefficients like those that can be obtained from a logistic multiple regression.[42] In practical terms, both associations are likely to be seen as substantial.

Figure 2.33 (code in Fig. 2.34) shows the smoothed plots for the mother's age and weight. The units on the vertical axis are logits centered on the mean of the response in logit units. Weight has a linear relationship with the logit of low birthweight. The relationship between age and the logit of birth weight is roughly negative overall, but positive between about the age of 20–25. Yet, to the eye, both relationships do not appear to be strong, and the impression of a negative relationship with age is driven in part by one observation for a woman who is 45 years old. However, looks can be deceiving. When the logit units are transformed into probability units,[43] the

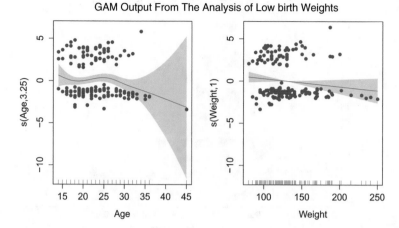

Fig. 2.33 A GAM analysis of newborn low birthweight as a function of background characteristics of mothers (the mother's age and weight are on the horizontal axes, the centered fitted logits are on the vertical axes, residuals are shown, and shaded area represents error bars. $N = 189$)

```
library(mgcv)
library(MASS)
data(birthwt)
attach(birthwt)

# Rename and Clean up variables
Low<-as.factor(low) # already coded low=1, not=0
Age<-age
Weight<-(lwt)
Uterine<-as.factor(ifelse(ui==1,"Yes","No"))
Smokes<-as.factor(ifelse(smoke==1,"Yes","No"))
temp<-data.frame(Low,Age,Weight,Uterine,Smokes)

# Apply GAM
out<-gam(Low~s(Age)+s(Weight)+Uterine+Smokes, family=binomial,
            data=temp)
par(mfrow=c(1,2))
plot(out, se=T, residuals=T, pch=19, col="blue", shade=T,
        shade.col="light blue")
```

Fig. 2.34 R code for low birthweight analysis

difference in the proportion of low birthweight babies can be about 0.30 greater when a mother of 35 is compared to a mother of 25. A similar difference in the proportion of low birthweight babies is found when women weighing around 100 pounds are compared to women weighing around 200 pounds.[44]

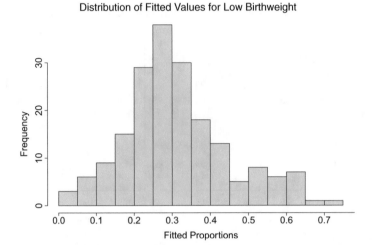

Fig. 2.35 Histogram of the fitted values in proportion units for low birthweight GAM analysis ($N = 189$)

As before, there is an effort to represent uncertainty in the fitted values, and as before, it is difficult to know exactly what to make of the shaded area. Where the shaded area is wider vertically, there is more uncertainty, but true confidence intervals are not represented. Perhaps the major conclusion is that the shape of the function for age is difficult to determine for values of age greater than about 35. We will return to how one can handle the uncertainty more properly in the next section.

GAM output automatically can include two kinds of fitted values for binary response variables: the linear combination of predictors in logit units and fitted proportions/probabilities. The former can be useful for diagnostic purposes because many of the conventional regression diagnostics apply. One has an additive model in logit units. The latter are useful for interpretation as approximate values of the response surface (i.e., probabilities).

Figure 2.35 is a histogram of the fitted values in proportion/probability units. One can see that substantial variation is found between different cases, which may imply that the cases differ in a consequential manner. Fitted values ranges from a little above 0.0 to nearly 0.80. At one extreme, virtually no women are at risk for having a low birthweight child, and at the other extreme, the risks are very substantial.

Some prefer to treat the fitted values as probability estimates, but that interpretation requires a clear and credible case that the realized observations are IID and that the fit was not tuned inductively. The latter we know to be false here. A Level II interpretation is not justified.

2.9   An Illustration of Statistical Inference After Model Selection

Significant parts of the discussion in this chapter have emphasized the risks in a Level II analysis when penalty weights are determined empirically as part of the data analysis. For readers who rely on "statistical significance" to extract subject-matter conclusions, the tone may be disappointing and even annoying. As a possible corrective, consider now a Level II analysis that perhaps can be properly be defended.

Assuming IID data, Fig. 2.36 in a refinement of the resampling strategy introduced in Chap. 1. Algorithmic tuning is done working back and forth between training data and evaluation data. Once the procedure is tuned, test data are used in conjunction with the tuned regression specification to get snooping free results. One estimates the population functionals of interest over B bootstrap samples of the test data. From these B bootstrap samples, there will likely be an empirical sampling distribution for each estimand of interest. Asymptotically valid statistical tests and confidence intervals can follow.

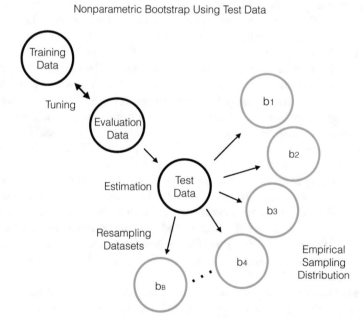

Fig. 2.36 A split sample approach for a Level II analysis that includes fitting with training data and evaluation data, assessment with test data, and honest uncertainty addressed with B bootstrap samples

For GAM in particular, once the values of the penalty parameters are determined, one essentially has a constrained least squares estimation procedure or more generally, constrained iteratively reweighted least squares estimation, which allows for the flexibility found in the generalized linear model (Dominici et al. 2004: Section 3). In Eq. 2.21, the values of λ_j are computed in a minuet between the training data and the evaluation data. Once the λ_j are determined, they are fixed. The fitting procedure is then applied to bootstrap samples of the test data from which empirical sampling distributions of interest can be constructed (e.g., the proportion of cases misclassified).[45] One has the requisite results from which to compute asymptotically valid statistical tests and confidence intervals.

Consider an empirical example. The data, available in R, are taken from the U.S. Panel Study of Income Dynamics (PSID). Funded by the National Science Foundation, the study began in 1968 and has been going for nearly 45 years. Households are followed over time and as the children of those households leave and form their own households, they are followed as well. New households are added when needed and feasible. Topics addressed in the survey have expanded over the years to include more than economic well-being: health, child development, time use, and others (McGonagle et al. 2012). The data available in R are on married women in 1975. (See the code in Fig. 2.37.)

Given the sampling design, it may be reasonable to treat each observation in the dataset as an IID realization from a joint probability distribution.[46] In this case, the population is real and finite, but very large. The response is whether a married woman is in the labor force (even if unemployed). Predictors include (1) the wife's age, (2) family income excluding the wife's income in thousands of dollars, (3) whether the wife attended college, (4) whether the husband attended college, and (5) the number of children in the household under 6 years of age. Clearly, there are other potentially important predictors such as the wife's health and the local availability of jobs. We are working within the wrong model perspective once again.

The R code used is shown in Fig. 2.37. With a sample of 753 cases, it is practical to construct a training sample, an evaluation sample, and a test sample. The code starts by providing more accessible names for the variables and recoding some stray observations — one cannot have negative family income. Then, three randomly chosen, disjoint, data subsets of equal size are constructed. The training data are analyzed using the generalized additive model as implemented in *gam* from the *mgcv* library. Several different values for the penalty parameters (i.e., *sp*) are tried beginning the smallest at 0.01. For each, performance is then assessed using the evaluation data.[47]

There is a wealth of information in the usual output, but it can be difficult to arrive at an overall assessment of what the *sp* value for each regressor function should be. For binary outcomes, a confusion table can be a very effective overall assessment tool. As noted earlier, a confusion table is nothing more than a cross-tabulation of the actual binary outcome and the fitted binary outcome. The smaller the proportion of cases misclassified, the better the fitted values perform.

```
library(car)
data(Mroz)
library(mgcv)
# Clean up labels and stray observations
Participates<-Mroz$lfp # in labor force
Age<-Mroz$age # age
FamIncome<-ifelse(Mroz$inc < 0,0,Mroz$inc) # family income
WifeColl<-Mroz$wc # Wife college degree
HusColl<-Mroz$hc # husband colleage degree
Kids5<-Mroz$k5 # Number of kinds under 6
temp1<-data.frame(Participates,Age,FamIncome,
                  WifeColl,HusColl,Kids5)

# Construct 3 random disjoint splits
index<-sample(1:753,753,replace=F) # shuffle row numbers
temp2<-temp1[index,] # put in random order
Train<-temp2[1:251,] # training data
Eval<-temp2[252:502,] # evaluation data
Test<-temp2[503:753,] # test data

# Bootstrap SEs for coefficients and Classification Error
Temp0<-rep(NA,2000)
Coefs<-matrix(Temp0,nrow=500)
Error<-as.vector(rep(NA,500))

for(i in 1:500) # 500 bootstrap samples
{
   index<-sample(1:251,251,replace=TRUE) # Random index
   NewTest<-Test[index,] # Select bootstrap sample
out3<-gam(Participates~s(Age,sp=1)+s(FamIncome,sp=1)+
             WifeColl+HusColl+Kids5,data=NewTest,family=binomial)
coefs<-out3$coefficients[1:4]
Coefs[i,]<-coefs
preds<-ifelse(out3$fitted.values>.5,"yes","no")
misclass<-(sum(preds != NewTest$Participates))/251
Error[i]<-misclass
}
SEs<-apply(Coefs,2,sd)
mean(Error)
bounds<-quantile(Error, probs=c(.025,.975))
hist(Error,col="lightblue",breaks=20,
     xlab="Proportion Misclassified",
     main="Histogram of Fitting Performance")
abline(v=.235, col="red",lwd=2)
abline(v=.346, col="red",lwd=2)
```

Fig. 2.37 R code for a Level II analysis of the PSID data

Confusion tables will play an important role in later chapters, and there are a number of complications and subtleties. For now, we simply will classify a case as in the labor force if the fitted value in the response metric is greater than 0.50 and not in the labor force if the fitted value in the response metric is equal to or less than 0.50. The marginal distribution of labor force participation provides a baseline for the GAM fitted values. Nearly 57% of the sample are in the labor force. Applying the Bayes classifier to the marginal distribution, classification error is minimized if all cases are classified as in the labor force. The proportion misclassified is then 0.43. How much better can be done using the predictors and good values for *sp*?

Regardless of the *sp* values tried, performance was modest. In the training data, about 22% of the deviance could be attributed to the five predictors with the misclassification proportion for those in the labor force of about 0.30. Improvement over the baseline is noticeable, but not dramatic.

For the *sp* values tried, out-of-sample performance using the evaluation data did not vary much. Confusion tables from the evaluation data were all rather similar. Because the functions for both smoothed predictors were essentially straight lines, smaller *sp* values did not improve the fit enough to overcome the loss of degrees of freedom. Therefore, the values of *sp* for both quantitative predictors were set to the relatively large value 1.0.[48]

The test data provide an antidote to data snooping. With the value of *sp* fixed at the "best" value, the generalized additive model was applied using the test data. About 33% of the cases in the labor force were misclassified, and a little more than 21% of the deviance could be attributed to the predictors. There is no evidence of meaningful overfitting earlier.

Among the three linear predictors, if a wife had attended college, the odds of labor force participation are multiplied by a factor of 2.5. A husband's college attendance hardly matter. For each additional child under six, the odds of labor force participation are multiplied by a factor of 0.40.[49]

Figure 2.38 shows in the test data the relationships between labor force participation and the two smoothed predictors. The near-linearity is apparent. Age has virtually no relationship with labor force participation, although there is a hint of decline for wives over 50. Family income (excluding the wife's income) has a very strong effect. The log odds decrease by about 3.9 logits when the lowest income households are compared to the highest. Higher income is associated with less labor force participation. So much for the Level I analysis.[50]

Thanks to the test data and how the full dataset was generated, it is relatively easy to move to Level II. All of the results just reported from the test data can be used as asymptotically unbiased estimates for the population's same generalized additive model with the same sp values. But, there is considerable uncertainty to address.

Although original sample had 753 observations, the test sample had only 251, and that is the relevant sample size. Using the nonparametric bootstrap to compute asymptotically valid standard errors, hypothesis tests for the parametric parameters rejected the usual null hypothesis for all but the husband's college variable and are probably sufficiently valid despite the formal requirement of large samples.

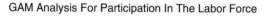

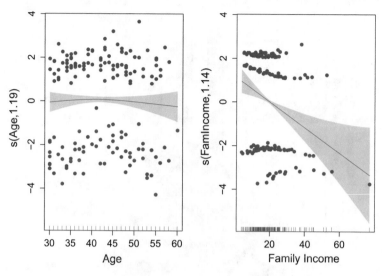

Fig. 2.38 Smoother estimates for age and family income in the test data (fitted values in the units of centered log odds are on the vertical axes, predictors age and family income are on the horizontal axes, the shaded areas show error bands, and $N = 251$)

In addition, we can properly represent uncertainty in overall estimate of classification error. Figure 2.39 shows the estimated sampling distribution for the proportion of cases misclassified. The code is shown near the bottom of Fig. 2.37. The bootstrap percentile method was used.

Even taking uncertainty into account, the GAM formulation still does better than simply using the more common category from the marginal distribution of the response variable. Again, the improvement is not dramatic, but now we know that the improvement is not easily explained by happenstance.[51]

2.9.1   Level I Versus Level II Summary

Decisions about when Level I is appropriate or when Level II is appropriate typically require extensive knowledge about how the data were generated. Subject-matter knowledge can also be essential. But, Level I is always a viable option. Getting to Level II often will be challenging, and sometimes one must proceed in a highly provisional manner. Inferential results then must include a user-beware label because the case for Level II is insufficiently compelling.

Figure 2.40 provides a decision guide to help structure thinking about a Level I versus Level II data analysis. The first challenge for Level II is to make a good case that each observation was at realized independently. The first I in IID is the key.

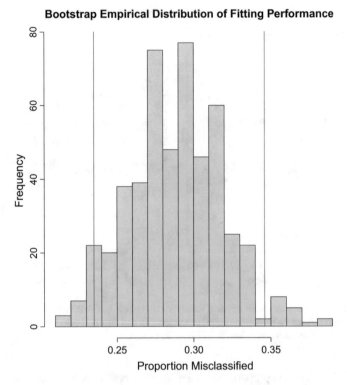

Fig. 2.39 Distribution of classification error estimates over 500 bootstrap samples with the 95% confidence interval displayed by the two vertical red lines (the 95% confidence interval is from 0.235 to 0.346)

Recent work, mentioned earlier, can allow for certain kinds of dependence. Look back at the discussion of the water use data for Tokyo.

Given IID data (or an acceptable approximation), the second Level II challenge is to consider the role of data snooping, whether automatic or informal. If there is no snooping, a Level II analysis can be justified for an acknowledged approximation of the true response surface estimated from the training data alone. If there is snooping, one is still estimating an acknowledged approximation of the true response surfaced but test data will likely be necessary. If there are no test data, one might well be limited to a Level I approach.

2.10 Kernelized Regression

In this chapter, much has been made of linear basis expansions as a way to make better use of the information a set of predictors contains. But each kind of expansion retained a matrix structure in which rows were observations and columns were variables. There is a very different and powerful way to transform the data from

Fig. 2.40 Decision guide for Level I and Level II data analyses

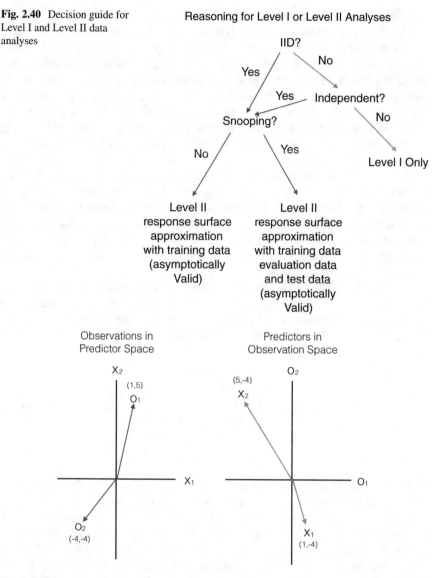

Reasoning for Level I or Level II Analyses

Fig. 2.41 Dimensional vector spaces that change the roles of variables and observations (the left figure has observations in predictor space, and the right figure has predictors in observation space)

observations located in predictor space to predictors located in observation space. The result can be a kernel matrix that with some regularization can form a new kind of predictor matrix for a wide range of regression applications.[52]

Figure 2.41 illustrates how one can represent observations in predictor space or predictors in observation space. O_1 and O_2 are observations, and X_1 and X_2 are predictors. The arrows represent vectors. Recall that vectors are lines with direction and length. We use them here primarily as a visualization tool.

The left plot shows observations in predictor space, and is the way one normally thinks about a scatterplot. There are two observations in a space defined by two predictors. The right plot shows predictors in observation space, and is one way to think about kernels. There are two predictors in a space defined by two observations. For example, in the plot on the left, O_1 has a value of 1 for X_1 and a value 5 for X_2. In the plot on the right, X_1 has a value of 1 for O_1 and a value of -4 for O_2. In practice, there would be many more predictors and many more observations. Plots would be totally impractical.

But why bother with predictors in observation space? Thinking back to the discussion of linear basis expansions in Chap. 1, kernels can alter the number of dimensions in which the values of a response variable are located. By increasing the number of dimensions, one may find good separation more easily. This is an important rationale for working with kernels. Kernels also have other desirable properties that can make them a very handy tool. These will be considered as the discussion of kernels proceeds.[53]

Consider Eq. 2.22, a very simple predictor matrix $\mathbf{X}$ with five rows and three columns. Rows and columns are labeled. The rows are people and the columns are predictors that are features of those people. Linear basis expansions of the sort we have considered so far could be applied to all three predictors or a subset.

$$
\mathbf{X} = \begin{pmatrix}
 & V1 & V2 & V3 \\
Ilene & 1 & 2 & 3 \\
Jim & 4 & 2 & 0 \\
Ken & 1 & 0 & 0 \\
Linda & 5 & 3 & 5 \\
Mary & 3 & 2 & 4
\end{pmatrix}. \tag{2.22}
$$

Figure 2.42 shows the $\mathbf{X}$ matrix, and the results from two different forms of matrix multiplication. The first is $\mathbf{X}^T\mathbf{X}$, which produces the usual sum of cross-products, a symmetric matrix that plays such an important role in the ordinary least squares estimator. Its main diagonal contains for each variable the sum of its squared values. For example, value of 21 in the second row and second column is the sum of the squared values of V2. The off-diagonal elements contain for each pair of variables their sum of element by element products, called inner products. The result is a scalar. For example, the value of 40 in the first row and third column and also in the third row and the first column results from $(1 \times 3) + (4 \times 0) + \cdots + (3 \times 4)$.

The second matrix is derived from $\mathbf{X}$ by computing $\mathbf{X}\mathbf{X}^T$. It too is symmetric. There are again sums of squared values or sums of cross-products, but the roles of predictors and observations are switched. The main diagonal now contains for each *person* the sum of that person's squared values over the three predictors. For example, Linda's diagonal value is 59: $5^2 + 3^2 + 5^2$. The off-diagonal elements are the sums of cross-products for *person* pairs over the three predictors. For example,

```
                    X # The predictor matrix

                        V1 V2 V3
                Ilene   1  2  3
                Jim     4  2  0
                Ken     1  0  0
                Linda   5  3  5
                Mary    3  2  4


            # Cross Product Matrix t(X)%*%X

                        V1 V2 V3
                    V1 52 31 40
                    V2 31 21 29
                    V3 40 29 50


            # Kernal Matrix X%*%t(X)

            Ilene Jim Ken Linda Mary
        Ilene   14   8   1    26   19
        Jim      8  20   4    26   16
        Ken      1   4   1     5    3
        Linda   26  26   5    59   41
        Mary    19  16   3    41   29
```

Fig. 2.42 R code inner products of **X**

the sum of cross products for Jim and Ilene is $(4 \times 1) + (2 \times 2) + (3 \times 0) = 8$. As before, these are sums of cross-products that result in a scalar.

Notice that this matrix has 5 columns rather than 3. Were one to use the matrix columns as a set of predictors, there would be 5 regressors. The response variable values would now reside in a 5-D predictor space, not a 3-D predictor space. The number of dimensions has been increased by 2.

$\mathbf{XX}^T$ is often called a "linear kernel" and can be viewed as a similarity matrix Murphy 2012: 479. The off-diagonal elements can be measures of the association between the different rows of **X**. One can learn which observations are more alike over the full set of variables. In this example, a close look at **X** indicates that Mary and Linda have the most similar values for V1, V2, and V3, and from the kernel matrix, the value of 41 is the largest off-diagonal element. A kernel matrix is conventionally denoted by **K**.

There are many kinds of kernels constructed with different kernel functions denoted in general by $\kappa(x, x')$. The notation x and x' means one row and another row, although it can also mean a row with itself in which case, each sum of cross-products is non-negative (i.e., $\kappa(x, x') \geq 0$). Any kernel matrix, **K**, is symmetric (i.e., $\kappa(x, x') = \kappa(x', x)$). For regression applications, it is common to work with Mercer kernels for which **K** is positive semi-definite.

The preference for Mercer kernel begins with **X**. Imagine linear basis expansions for the full set of predictors each represented by $h(x)$. For Mercer kernels, $\kappa(x, x') = \langle h(x), h(x') \rangle$, which means the inner products of the expansions are contained in Mercer kernels (Hastie et al. 2009: section 12.3.1).[54] There is no need the know the actual expansions because for regression applications one can proceed directly with the kernel. This is a very convenient computational shortcut, which means that in practice, model specification is usually a choice between different kinds of kernels without much regard for the implied basis expansions. More will be said about kernels in the chapter on support vector machines.[55]

However, there are several complications. Because the kernel function requires that all elements in **X** be numeric, categorical predictors are a problem. At best, they can be transformed into 1/0 indicator variables, but the gap between a 1 and a 0 is arbitrary. And actually, the problem is more general. **K** depends on the units in which each column of **X** is measured. With different units, there are different kernels even when the kernel function is the same. Standardization of each column of **X** is, therefore, a common practice. But the common units chosen are effectively arbitrary and make it difficult to understand what the similarities mean. Two rows that are the much alike in standard deviation units, may be very different in their original units, which is how one normally thinks about those rows. One should always ask, therefore, "similar with respect to what?"

A second complication is that a kernel matrix is necessarily $N \times N$. Therefore, some form of dimension reduction is required in a regression setting. Regularization is required. Options include using a subset of **K**'s principal components as regressors or a form penalized regression. For example, the latter can lead to a ridge regression approach. In the notation of Hastie et al. (2009: section 12.3.7),

$$\hat{f}(x) = h(x)^T \hat{\beta} = \sum_{i=1}^{N} \hat{\alpha}_i K(x, x_i), \qquad (2.23)$$

and

$$\hat{\alpha} = (K(x, x_i) + \lambda \mathbf{I})^{-1} \mathbf{y}. \qquad (2.24)$$

Equation 2.23 shows the fundamental equivalence between regressors as basis functions and regressors as columns of **K**. Equation 2.24 shows how the new regression coefficients $\hat{\alpha}$ for **K** are computed. Equation 2.24 is a close cousin of conventional ridge regression.

With $\hat{\alpha}$ in hand, the fitted values can follow as usual as long as one remembers to use **K** not **X**. For fitted values from *new* observations, the same reasoning carries over, but the new observations **Z** need to be "kernelized" (Exterkate et al. 2011: section 2.2). A prediction kernel is constructed as $\kappa(x, z') = \langle h(x), h(z') \rangle$ not as $\kappa(x, x') = \langle h(x), h(x') \rangle$. That is, the inner products are undertaken with respect to

X and **Z**, not with respect to **X** itself. For the linear kernel one computes $\mathbf{XZ}^T$ rather than $\mathbf{XX}^T$. That is,

$$\hat{f}(x, z) = \sum_{i=1}^{N} \hat{\alpha}_i K(x, z_i). \tag{2.25}$$

Also as before, λ in Eq. 2.24 is a tuning parameter whose value needs to be specified in advance or determined empirically. This leads to a third complication. Often it is desirable for λ to be large because, in effect, one starts with N predictors (much like for smoothing splines). But, empirically determining a sensible value for λ can be challenging, as we will soon see. There are usually additional tuning parameters.

A fourth complication is that kernel matrices produce a new kind of black box. In Eq. 2.23, for example, the regressors are columns of **K** not columns of **X**, and the estimated regression coefficients in Eq. 2.24 are $\hat{\alpha}$ not $\hat{\beta}$. It is a bit like trying to make sense of the regression coefficients associated with B-splines. Moreover, only in very special cases is it practical to work backwards from **K** to $h(x)$. The linear expansions of **X** typically are not accessible. As before, therefore, the story will be in the fitted values.

Finally, there are many different kinds of kernels, and several different kinds of Mercer kernels that can be used in practice (Murphy 2012: section 14.2; Duvenaud et al. 2013). Because of the black box, it is very difficult to know which kernel to use. The decision is usually based on experience with particular subject-matter applications and craft lore. We turn to two kernels that are popular for regression analysis.

2.10.1 Radial Basis Kernel

The bottom matrix in Fig. 2.42 is an example of a linear basis kernel. Formally, it is relatively easy to work with, but is not used much because there are other kernels that usually perform better. A good example is the radial basis kernel that is sometimes characterized as an "all-purpose" kernel. Perhaps its most important departure from the linear kernel is that row comparisons are made initially by subtraction not multiplication. With each variable standardized and $\|.\|$ denoting the Euclidian distance (i.e., the "norm"), the radial basis kernel is defined by

$$k(x, x') = exp(-\sigma \|x - x'\|^2), \tag{2.26}$$

where $\|x - x'\|^2$ is the squared Euclidian distance between two rows.

The first step is to compute the sum of squared *differences*. For the second and third row of our toy **X**, one has for the sum of squared differences: $(4 - 1)^2 + (2 - 0)^2 + (0 - 0)^2 = 13$. The sum of squared differences is multiplied by $-\sigma$ and then

```
library(kernlab)

# Radial Basis Kernel

tune<-rbfdot(sigma=.5)
kernelMatrix(tune,X)
An object of class "kernelMatrix"
          Ilene      Jim        Ken       Linda      Mary
Ilene 1.0000e+00 1.2341e-04 1.5034e-03 2.7536e-05 8.2085e-02
Jim   1.2341e-04 1.0000e+00 1.5034e-03 1.3710e-06 2.0347e-04
Ken   1.5034e-03 1.5034e-03 1.0000e+00 1.3888e-11 6.1442e-06
Linda 2.7536e-05 1.3710e-06 1.3888e-11 1.0000e+00 4.9787e-02
Mary  8.2085e-02 2.0347e-04 6.1442e-06 4.9787e-02 1.0000e+00

# ANOVA Basis Kernel

tune<-anovadot(sigma=2.0,degree=2)
kernelMatrix(tune,X)
An object of class "kernelMatrix"
          Ilene      Jim        Ken       Linda      Mary
Ilene 9.000000 1.000000 1.0007e+00 1.8407e-02 1.2898e+00
Jim   1.000000 9.000000 1.0007e+00 7.3263e-02 1.2810e+00
Ken   1.000671 1.000671 9.0000e+00 2.3195e-16 4.5014e-07
Linda 0.018407 0.073263 2.3195e-16 9.0000e+00 7.3444e-02
Mary  1.289748 1.288986 4.5014e-07 7.3444e-02 9.0000e+00
```

Fig. 2.43 R code for radial basis and ANOVA basis kernels

exponentiated. For the radial basis kernel, otherwise known as the Gaussian radial basis kernel (Murphy 2012: section 14.2.1), σ is a scale parameter specifying the spread in the kernel values. The kernel matrix $\mathbf{K}$ is always symmetric and $N \times N$. If the scale parameter σ happens to be 0.5, the value in $\mathbf{K}$ for the second and third row of $\mathbf{X}$ is $e^{(13 \times -0.5)} = 0.0015034$. The top matrix in Fig. 2.43 follows in the same manner.[56]

The diagonal entries of the radial basis kernel are always 1 ($e^0 = 1$), and the off-diagonal entries are between 0 and 1. Because radial kernels build on Euclidian distances, they can be viewed as similarity matrices. With a smaller distance between a pair of observations, there is a greater similarity. Thanks to the negative sign of σ, a larger kernel value conveys greater similarity.

When the value of σ is larger, the off-diagonal kernel values become smaller, so their measured similarities are reduced. The rows become more heterogeneous, which is consistent with a larger scale value. In language we used earlier, the bandwidth, span, or window have gotten smaller. A more complex set of fitted values can be accommodated. Consequently, σ typically is treated as a tuning parameter.

Radial basis kernels have proved to be useful in a wide variety of applications but for regression, there can be a better choice (Katatzoglou et al. 2004: section 2.4).

2.10.2 ANOVA Radial Basis Kernel

The ANOVA radial basis kernel builds on the radial basis kernel. Using common notation for the ANOVA kernel,

$$k(x, x') = \left(\sum_{k=1}^{p} exp(-\sigma(x^k - x'^k)^2) \right)^d, \qquad (2.27)$$

where x^k and x'^k are the two values for predictor k, p is the number of predictors in $\mathbf{X}$, and σ is again a scale parameter typically used for tuning. As before, larger values of σ allow for a more complex fit.[57] The values for d are usually 1, 2, or 3. Because the computations begin with differences that after being transformed are added together, the calculations are linear when $d = 1$, and one has a linear, additive effects expression. When $d = 2$, one has an expression with products that can be seen as two-way interaction variables. By the same reasoning, when $d = 3$, one has three-way interaction variables. In practice, d is treated as a tuning parameter along with σ.[58] Larger values for d allow for a more complex set of fitted values.

The lower matrix in Fig. 2.43 shows the results for the same predictor matrix $\mathbf{X}$ when σ is set to 2.0 and d is set to 2. Because there are 3 predictors in $\mathbf{X}$, the main diagonal elements are all equal to 9 (i.e., $(1 + 1 + 1)^2$). Off-diagonal elements no longer have an upper bound of 1.0.

2.10.3 A Kernel Regression Application

In a regression context, the radial kernel and the ANOVA kernel can be used as predictor matrices that replace $\mathbf{X}$ in a regression analysis. Both kernels provide a very rich menu of complicated transformations that are directly given to the fitting machinery. One hopes that $\mathbf{K}$ can find relationships with the response that $\mathbf{X}$ cannot. Complicated nonlinear relationships are in play through what is effectively a nonparametric formulation.

As usual, "nonparametric" can be used in different ways. What one means for kernelized regression is that the regression structure is not meant to be a model of anything. The regression structure is just part of an algorithm linking input to outputs. There are regression coefficients for the columns in $\mathbf{K}$, but they have no subject-matter interpretation. Just as for smoothing splines, the goal is to interpret and use the relationship between inputs and outputs.

The heavy emphasis on fitted values has meant that for kernel regression ways to visualize how inputs are related to outputs are not yet as well developed. Some of the visualization procedures discussed in later chapters could be applied, but at least in R, they apparently have not been applied yet. Where kernel regression method can shine is in forecasting.

A natural question, therefore, is what kernel methods estimate. In principle, kernel regression methods can be used to estimate an approximation of the true response surface as a feature of nature's joint probability distribution. That approximation has the same structure, and same values for the tuning parameters used when the fitted values estimated. The fitted values from the data are biased (even asymptotically) estimates of the true response surface. In short, a Level II analysis has the same features as a Level II analysis for smoothing splines. And as before, one has to make a credible case that a Level II analysis is justified. But, what about data snooping? Even if the choice of kernel is made before looking at the data, in practice the kernel's parameters will be tuned, and the regularization parameter will be tuned as well. So, here too data snooping issues have to be addressed. As before, access to training data, evaluation data, and test data can really help.

Consider Eqs. 2.23 and 2.24. What may look to be a simple application of ridge regression is not so simple. There are three tuning parameters, two for the ANOVA kernel and one for the regularization, that typically need to be determined empirically. A first impulse might be to use some in-sample fit measure such as the GCV statistic. A search is undertaken over values of the tuning parameters. Their values are determined by the best fit value. However, any credible in-sample fit statistics should take the effective degrees of freedom (EDF) into account because the effective degrees of freedom is changing as the values of the tuning parameters are varied. If the effective degrees of freedom is ignored, a better fit may result simply from more degrees of freedom being used in the fitting process. This matters even for a Level I analysis because the data analyst could be faced with unnecessarily complicated fitted values that will be challenging to interpret.

Yet, as discussed in Chap. 1, even the idea of an effective degrees of freedom (or effective number of parameters) in such a setting is being questioned. What does the effective degrees of freedom mean when there is tuning? In practice, therefore, a sensible Level I analysis requires a careful examination of plots showing the fitted values against actual response values. Subject-matter knowledge can be critical for determining which sets of fitted values are most instructive. In short, the Level I concerns for conventional ridge regression carry over but now with more tuning parameters to specify.

For a Level II analysis, we are again faced with data snooping that can introduce challenging problems for statistical inference. Rather than using some in-sample fit statistics, why not employ cross-validation? The issues are tricky. A kernel matrix is $N \times N$, and the tuning is done with respect to the full kernel matrix. Yet, cross-validation necessarily fits subsets of the data, each with fewer than N observations. Tuning could be quite different, and with respect to the full kernel matrix, misleading. Probably the best cross-validation approach is N-fold because for each pass through the data only one observation is lost.[59]

Alternatively, one might employ a split sample strategy. As before, the training and evaluation samples are exploited to determine the values for the tuning parameters. The kernel regression coefficients $\hat{\alpha}$ from the training sample are used to obtain fitted values in the evaluation data, from which one or more performance measures are computed. With the values of the tuning parameters determined, the test data can be employed to obtain honest performance assessments. But one is still faced with a smaller N than had the data not be split. If one is prepared to settle for working with and tuning for a kernel fit based on a substantially smaller sample, a split sample approach can work well. The new estimation target is test sample version.

There are apparently no fully satisfactory procedures currently in R that implement the kind of penalized kernel regression shown in Eqs. 2.23 and 2.24.[60] But with split samples and the *kernelMatrix* procedure from the library *kernlab* to construct the requisite kernels, it is relatively easy to write a "one-off" R-script that implements a version of Eqs. 2.24 and 2.25 cycling through the training data many times using different sets of values for σ, d, and λ.[61] Each set of $\hat{\alpha}$ is then used to produce fitted values in the evaluation data. Once acceptable tuning parameter values are determined, they are used to compute a penalized kernel ridge regression in the test data.

To see how this plays out, suppose one wanted to analyze variation in the gross domestic earnings for movies made in the USA immediately after the movie opens. There are data on 471 movies for which one has the following regressors: (1) the budget for making each movie, (2) the number of theaters in which it opened, and (3) opening day's earnings. The response is gross domestic earnings over the next 24 months. These data were randomly split into a training sample, an evaluation sample, and a test sample of equal sizes. The performance criterion was mean squared error.

From the search over the movie training data and evaluation data, σ was a chosen to be 10, d was chosen to be 2.0, and λ was chosen to be 3. There were several sets of tuning parameters that performed approximately as well, and the among those, the set with the smallest tuning parameter values for the kernel and the largest value for penalty parameter was selected. There seemed to be no reason to unnecessarily use up degrees of freedom.

A kernel regression with the same number of observations and tuning parameters values was used with the test data. In the same spirit as expected prediction error, a plot of the observed response values against the fitted response values for the test data is shown in Fig. 2.44. Overlaid is the least squares line from which the R^2 of 0.92 was computed. Overall, the scatterplot has a sensible pattern although the fitted values do not track some of the highest or lowest gross sales as well. This means that if the goal is to represent very soon after a movie is released its gross domestic sales over the next 2 years, the results look promising except for the few "flops" and "blockbusters." It is easy to capture those response values too with a more complex

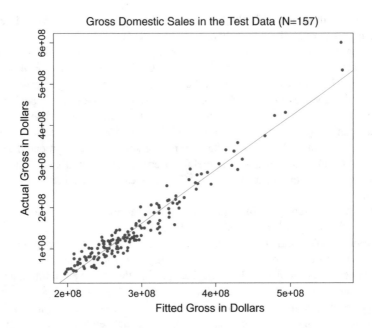

Fig. 2.44 Domestic gross sales in millions of dollars by the fitted values from a penalized kernel regression using the test data (N = 157)

set of fitted values (e.g., with a σ of 20, a d of 3, and a λ of 1), but that leads to unrealistic measures of fit (e.g., an R^2 of 0.99). The likely problem is that far too many degrees of freedom are being used.

For a Level II analysis, the estimation target is the kernel regression approximation of the true response surface with the same values for the tuning parameters. If one can define a substantively relevant joint probability distribution or finite population from which each observation was independently realized, the test data results can provide an asymptotically unbiased estimates. And much as in the previous example, one can then apply a nonparametric bootstrap to the test data and obtain information on the uncertainty built into the R^2 of 0.92.

2.11 Summary and Conclusions

Regression splines and smoothing splines, sometimes as features of generalized additive models, can be very useful Level I tools for describing relationships between a response variable and one or more predictors. As long as one is content to "merely" describe, these methods are consistent with the goals of an exploratory data analysis. Moving to a Level II analysis can be challenging because there needs to be a credible data generation backstory consistent with the formal requirements of statistical inference. One also must be satisfied working with approximations of the true response surface, and when data snooping is part of the data analysis, there are significant obstacles that in practice can be difficult to overcome. Level III analyses are generally not an option in part because one is estimating an approximation whose relationship to proper causal inference is unclear.

Experience suggests that for most datasets, it does not make a great difference which brand of smoother one uses. The dominant factor is usually the values of λ or other tuning parameters that determine smoothness and the bias–variance tradeoff. Less clear is how their values are best determined. Most methods emphasize some measure of generalization error. This is certainly sensible given the empirical focus on fitted values. But fitted values with low generalization error do not necessarily make scientific or policy sense. Moreover, any overall measure of out-of-sample performance can neglect that performance will usually be better for some predictors than others. Often a subset of predictors is of special interest, and it is on their performance that a useful evaluation should rest. These complications and others suggest that it can be a mistake to automatically defer to default tuning values or default tuning procedures. There is no substitute for subject-matter expertise and a careful examination of a wide range of data analysis output. Judgment matters. It is very important to avoid what a number of philosophers and social scientists call "statisticism" (Finch 1976; Lamiell 2013).

Finally, there are other smoothers that have not been discussed either because they perform best in a relatively narrow set of applications or because they are not yet ready for widespread use. An example of the former is wavelet smoothing (Hastie et al. 2009: section 5.9). "Wavelet bases are very popular in signal processing and compression, since they are able to represent both smooth and/or locally bumpy functions in an efficient way—a phenomenon dubbed time and frequency localization" (Hastie et al. 2009: 175). An example of the latter is very recent work that applies trend filtering to nonparametric regression (Tibshirani 2015). The key idea is to define the fitting penalty in a novel way, not using second derivatives, by a discrete differencing operator on the regression coefficients. The result is a smoother that adapts locally. It will fit a rougher function where the data are more rough and a smoother function where the data are more smooth.[62] In short, the book is not closed on smoothers, and readers interested in such procedure should at least skim the relevant journals from time to time.

For a wide range of problems, there are statistical learning techniques that arguably perform better than the procedures discussed in this chapter. They can fit the data better, are less subject to overfitting, and permit a wider range of information to be brought to bear. One price, however, is that the links to conventional regression analysis become even more tenuous. In the next chapter, we continue down this path.

Demonstrations and Exercises

Just as for the first chapter, these demonstrations and exercises emphasize the analysis of data. What substantive insights can be properly extracted? You may need to install some packages depending on what you have already installed. (Have you updated R and the procedures you will be using lately?)

Set 1: Smoothers with a Single Predictor

1. Load the dataset called airquality using the command *data(airquality)*. Attach the data with the command *attach(airquality)*. Use *gam* from the *gam* library with Ozone as the response and Temp as the sole predictor. Estimate the following three specifications assigning the output of each to its own name (e.g., output1 for the first model).

   ```
   gam(Ozone ~ Temp)
   gam(Ozone ~ as.factor(Temp))
   gam(Ozone ~ s(Temp))
   ```

   The first model is the smoothest model possible. Why is that? The second model is the roughest model possible. Why is that? The third model is a compromise between the two in which the degree of smoothing is determined by the GCV statistic. (See the textitgam documentation followed by the smoothing spline documentation.)

   For each model, examine the numerical output and plot the fitted values against the predictor. For example, if the results of the first model are assigned to the name "output1," use *plot.gam (output1, residuals=TRUE)*. Also, take a look at the output object for the variety of gam features and output that can be accessed. Extractor functions are available.

   Which model has the best fit judging by the residual deviance? Which model has the best fit judging by the AIC? Why might the choice of the best model differ depending on which measure of fit is used? Which model seems to be most useful judging by the plots? Why is that?

2. Using *scatter.smooth*, overlay a lowess smooth on a scatterplot with the variable Ozone on the vertical axis and the variable Temp on the horizontal axis. Vary three tuning parameters: span: 0.25, 0.50, 0.75; degree: 0, 1, 2; family as Gaussian or symmetric. How do the fitted values change as each tuning parameter is varied? Which tuning parameter seems to matter most? (You can get the same job done with *loess*, but a few more steps are involved.)

3. The relationship between temperature and ozone concentrations should be positive and monotonic. From the question above, select a single set of tuning parameter values that produces a fit you like best. Why do you like that fit best? If there are several sets of fitted values you like about equally, what it is about these fitted values that you like also?

4. For the overlay of the fitted values you like best (or select a set from among those you like best) describe how temperature is related to ozone concentrations.

Set 2: Smoothers with Two Predictors

1. From the library *assist* load the dataset TXtemp. Load the library *gam*. With mmtemp as the response and longitude and latitude as the predictors, apply *gam*. Construct the fitted values using the sum of a 1-D smoothing spline of longitude and a 1-D smoothing spline of latitude. Try several different values for the degrees of freedom of each. You can learn how to vary these tuning parameters with *help(gam)* and *help(s)*. Use the *summary* command to examine the output, and *plot.gam* to plot the two partial response functions. To get both plots on the same page use *par(mfrow=c(2,1))*. How are longitude and latitude related to temperature? (If you want to do this in *gam* in the *mgcv* library, that works too. But the tuning parameters are a little different.)

2. Repeat the analysis in 1, but now construct the fitted values using a single 2-D smoother of longitude and latitude together. Again, try several different values for the degrees of freedom. Examine the tabular output with *summary* and the plot using *plot.gam*. You probably will need to load the library *akima* for the plotting. How do these results compare to those using two 1-D predictor smooths? (For 2-D smoothing, the plotting at the moment is a little better using *gam* in the *mgcv* library.)

Set 3: Smoothers with More Than Two Predictors

1. Still working in *gam*, build an additive model for mmtemp with the predictors longitude, latitude, year, and month. Use a lowess smooth for each. Try different spans and polynomial degrees. Again use the *summary* and *plot.gam* command. To get all four graphs on the same page use *par(mfrow=c(2,2))*. How is temperature related to each of the four predictors?

2. Repeat the analysis just done using smoothing splines in *gam*. See if you can tune the model so that you get very close to same graphs. Does it matter which kind of smoother you use? Why or why not? (Keep in mind that you tune *s* differently from *lo*.)

Set 4: Smoothers with a Binary Response Variable

1. From the *car* library, load the dataset *Mroz*. Using *glm*, regress labor force participation on age, income, and the log of wages. From the library *gam*, use *gam* to repeat the analysis, smoothing each of the predictors with the smoother of your choice. Note that labor force participation is a binary variable. Compare and contrast your conclusions from the two sets of results. Which procedure seems more appropriate here? Why?

Endnotes

[1] Loosely speaking, a plug-in estimator uses as an estimator the computations in the data that correspond to the function responsible for the population parameter to be estimated (Efron and Tibshirani 1993: section 4.3). A common illustration is when the mean of a sample is used to estimate a population mean.

[2] Using conventional multiple regression, Zelterman (2014: 40–41) finds more internet references to zombies in states with fewer Miss America winners and fewer shopping centers per capita. Who knew?

[3] It is best for this particular linear piecewise mean function. There may be many other reasonable linear piecewise mean functions. Each would also be best by the least squares criterion for its linear piecewise mean function.

[4] The data were provided by the Tokyo Municipal Water Works as part of a project funded by The Asian-Pacific Network for Global Change Research.

[5] For these data, there is only one value of Y for each unique value of X. The y-values may be treated as if they were means. "Binning" entails ordering the values of a variable and then organizing those values into ranges. For example, instead of $1, 2, \ldots, 30$, one might have categories $1–5, 6–10, \ldots, 26–30$.

[6] The issues are too technical for this venue, but the paper by Chernozhukov et al. (2018) is an instructive illustration of the challenges that can arise with temporal (and spatial) data.

[7] Also notice that with so few observations, asymptotic performance is not a realistic option.

[8] More generally, how one can formulate the boundary constraints is discussed in Hastie et al. (2009: section 5.2.1).

[9] There can be lots of other options, depending on the application. For example, there are special issues when the intent is to smooth a 2-dimensional surface. An excellent discussion can be found in Wood(2017: Chapter 5).

[10] Some accounts use the term B-spline for a certain kind of linear basis expansion. Some use the term B-spline for the result when that linear basis expansion is used as the x-values on which a variable Y is conditioned. We will adopt the former.

[11] Suppose the error sum of squares for a given amount of fitted value complexity is 1000. Ordinarily, an increase in the complexity of the fitted values that reduces the error sum of squares to less than 1000 would be accepted. But suppose there is a penalty of 100. Now the penalized error sum of squares is 1100. Still, the error sum of squares threshold remains at 1000. Improvement in the fit has to overcome the penalty of 100. Unless the penalty value of 100 is overcome by the increase in complexity, the increase is not implemented.

[12] For both expressions, the regression intercept β_0 is irrelevant. It does not influence the roughness of the fitted values.

[13] The true units often matter a great deal when the regression coefficients are interpreted. It can be difficult to determine, for example, if a given regression coefficients is large enough to matter. One standard deviation may represent substantively trivial variation for one predictor and substantively important variation for another.

[14] There is a good reason to be uneasy proceeding exactly in this manner because the uncertainty in the λ estimated from training data is ignored when the test data are analyzed. Moreover, the meaning of degrees of freedom used in this two-step process is unclear (Dijkstra 2011). A valid characterization is that the value of λ is given for whatever statistical inference one undertakes for the test data. But that framing does not take into account all sources of uncertainty. In some sense, part of the problem has been defined away. One has at best a formally valid but incomplete assessment. As before, one risks falsely optimistic assessments of precision.

[15] The data, named *socsupport*, can be obtained as part of the *DAAG* library in R.

[16] Several different forms of sandwich standard errors can be estimated with *hccm()* in the *car* library. There is little formal guidance on which to use. One might as well work with the default.

[17] In the output object from *glmnet*, the 3s are labeled "df," presumably for degrees of freedom. But the documentation makes clear that df is actually the number of predictors. In conventional

linear regression, the degrees of freedom used is usually taken to be the number of predictors plus 1 for the intercept. As already mentioned, when the value of λ is determined empirically, many more degrees of freedom are used than the number of parameters to be estimated in the regression mean function. There is a regression estimated for each of the folds. In short, the number of predictors should not be confused with the degrees of freedom used.

[18]Lasso is sometimes written as "lasso," Lasso," or "LASSO.'

[19]Should one be interested in model selection per se, there are at least two other visible players within the penalized regression perspective: The Danzig Selector (Candes and Tao 2007; Gareth and Radchenko 2007; Liu et al. 2012) and the Regularization and Derivative Expectation Operator—RODEO—(Lafferty and Wasserman 2008). As mentioned earlier, model selection is sometimes called variable selection or feature selection.

[20]Lasso regularization is an example of "soft thresholding" because the regression coefficients gradually arrive at 0. Backward stepwise regression selects predictors by "hard thresholding" because regression coefficients, or functions of regression coefficients, smaller than some value are abruptly dropped from the analysis.

[21]Some software will allow for different polynomial orders, but a variant on cubic functions seems most common.

[22]This is a good example why terms like nonparametric can be a little slippery. Regression coefficients are in play in the piecewise natural cubic spline engine under the hood. But they are means to the end of obtaining a good approximation of the true response surface. They are not inherent features of the true response surface nor of its approximation.

[23]One has a penalized least squares estimator very much like the estimator used in ridge regression. The details depend substantially on how the knots are coded (Wood 2017: Section 4.2.2). Different expositions can appear to be quite different.

[24]Getting the bootstrap work to properly with the data was easily hand coded and straightforward. But the sampling with replacement necessarily scrambled the order of the observations. Getting the confidence intervals for each value of the predictor took a bit of data wrangling.

[25]In practice, the integral of the second derivatives would need to be estimated empirically in the same spirit as for penalized regression splines.

[26]There will be fewer knots if there are fewer than N distinct values of x.

[27]This implementation of the generalized additive model is discussed in some detail shortly. The estimation procedure for the multiple-predictor extension of Eq. 2.15 is a local scoring algorithm implemented as backfitting, which for generalized additive models is essentially the Gauss–Seidel method (Breiman and Friedman 1985).

[28]The plotted fitted values vary around the mean of the response. More will be said about this later when the generalized additive model is introduced.

[29]When there is an empirical determination of spar, the *gam* procedure reports the degrees of freedom used, not spar. With a little trial and error, however, one can figure out what the value of spar is.

[30]For example, one might have another dataset for the same 100 min at the same time the next day. If day-to-day variation is essentially noise, one might well have valid test data.

[31]Lowess is sometimes said to stand for locally weighted scatter plot smoothing. But Cleveland, who invented the procedure (Cleveland 1979), seems to prefer the term "local regression" known as "loess" (Cleveland 1993: 94).

[32]Because the weights are known within each window, the weighted least squares solution has a closed form. No iteration is required.

[33]The plots produced by *scatter.smooth* are not centered around the mean of the response, but whether the plot is centered or not should have no effect on an interpretation of the relationship between Y and X unless variation relative to the mean of Y matters. It also might if the actual values of the approximate response surface were important (e.g., in forecasting).

[34]The data can be obtained from the *DAAG* library under the name *bomsoi*.

[35]Recall, there is no need to specify neighborhoods for smoothing splines. The predictor space is saturated with knots whose impacts are penalized as needed. But the curse of dimensionality can still be an issue.

[36]The procedure used was again *gam* in the *gam* library. Documentation on plotting in 3-Dimensions was very skimpy. Be prepared for lots of trial and error.

[37]The use of the ∗ operator means multiplication. (See Fig. 2.29.) Year is multiplied by SOI. Currently, the plotting procedure "knows" when it sees ∗ that the plotting the surface should be in 2-D predictor space. If one does the multiplication in advance and uses the product as a predictor, *gam* produces the same fit and summary statistics. But the plot treats the product as the vector it is. The procedure does not know that the vector is the product of two predictors. Figure 2.28 shows the results as perspective plots. Contour plots would convey much the same information with more numerical detail but in a less easily understood visual format.

[38]The notation t_j is a placeholder for the unknown jth function.

[39]Each function's effective degrees of freedom is stored in the *gam* object as "edf." Based on the *mgcv* documentation in *choose.k*, one can impose some control over the penalty values chosen by a GCV statistic. For any smoothing function to be estimated, the tuning parameter "k" sets an upper bound to the number of equally spaced knots and, therefore, an upper bound on the effective degrees of freedom that is used. There is also the capacity to force the value of k on the fit for a given function by setting *fx=FALSE*. If the value of k is fixed before the analysis is undertaken, the prospect of asymptotically valid error bands for the fitted approximation would be improved. Another way to fix smoothness is with the *sp* tuning parameter, where *sp* stands for "smoothing parameter." This can be a very flexible approach, but for our purposes is just an alternative to using a fixed value of k, and the issues are very similar. Its main problem in practice is that the units of *sp* are not intuitive and can in practice range at least between 0.001 and 10. A larger value forces a smoother fit. An example will be provided shortly.

[40]Equation 1.11 shows the functional form for logistic regression before the link function is applied and corresponds to the discussion of logistic regression in Chap. 1.

[41]This can get a little tricky in R if the binary response is a factor such as graduated high school or not. If the researcher does not code these classes as 1 or 0 in advance, it may not be clear how R is representing each outcome. It is important to check with the documentation for the version of gam being used and then do some experimentation. This will be an ongoing issue with most classifiers discussed in later chapters.

[42]The regression coefficients are usually reported with the response in logit units. They are part of the routine tabular output from *gam*.

[43]How to transform logits into probabilities and interpret them properly will be discussed in later chapters. There can be subtle issues. Because such transformations are nonlinear, although monotonic, shapes of relationships shown will change, but the overall visual impressions are usually very similar.

[44]The relationship reported in Chap. 1 was rather different. In Fig. 1.2, the relationship between birthweights and mothers' weights was generally positive. But for that analysis, the mother's weight was the only predictor. Conditioning on other predictors makes a difference. One has the relationship between a mother's weight and her baby's birthweight with all other included predictors "held constant" (in the manner described earlier).

[45]Keep in mind that in practice the penalty parameters associated with each smoothed function can have different names and be computed somewhat differently. Recall the earlier discussion of edf, k, and sp. Make sure you precisely know what has been fixed when the software is applied.

[46]In practice, one would have to know a lot more about the sampling design. There may be some stratification and/or clustering sampling in play. But recall that the key requirement is that each case is sampled independently. Constant variance is a secondary concern.

[47]The evaluation data provide out-of-sample performance measures, but with each new *sp* value, the out-of-sample benefits decline a bit. The model is being tuned to the evaluation data so that the fitting responds to both its random and systematic variation. Nevertheless, the evaluation data are very instructive here. It was easy to see that with small values of *sp*, the overfitting in the training is substantial. More generally, the issue of hold-out data reuse gets very messy when the *test* data are used many times, and some interesting, partial solutions have been proposed (Dwork et al. 2015, 2017). But here, it is the *evaluation* data that are being reused. The test data remain pristine.

[48]Effectively the same results were obtained when the default of fitting by the GCV statistic was used.

[49]The number of children under 6 ranged from 0 to 2. With only 3 predictor values, smoothing was not an option.

[50]In the later chapters, methods to transform logits into more interpretable units will be provided. But one must not forget that the fitted values are centered.

[51]Because, the number of observations in the test data is modest, one cannot count on the ideal asymptotic properties. That helps explain the lumpy nature of the histogram, which in the limit will be normal. But the weight of the evidence still favors the estimated improvement in classification accuracy.

[52]In statistics, there are other meanings of "kernel" such as when the term is used for localized estimators (Hastie et al. 2009: section 6.6.1). In computer science, "variables" are sometimes called "feature vectors" that are located in "input space."

[53]Adam Kapelner and Justin Bleich helped extensively with the exposition of kernels. They deserve much of the credit for what clarity there is. Lack of clarity is my doing.

[54]Imagine a predictor $\mathbf{X}$ expanded so that each original column can now be many columns defined by some linear basis expansion (e.g., polynomials or indicator variables). In this context, the inner product means multiplying two rows (i.e., vectors) of the expanded predictor so that a scalar is produced. As before, it is just the sum of cross products. More generally, if there are two (column) vectors v_1 and v_2, the inner product is $v_1^T v_2$. The outer product is $v_1 v_2^T$, which results in a matrix. The same reasoning applies when a vector is multiplied by itself.

[55]There is a lot of very nice math involved that is actually quite accessible if it is approached step by step. For readers who want to pursue this, there are many lectures taught by excellent instructors that can be viewed for free on the internet. These are generally more helpful than formal textbook treatments because the intuitions behind the math are often well explained. A good example is the lecture by MIT professor Patrick Winston "Lecture 16—Learning: Support Vector Machines."

[56]For consistency, the kernel expressions and notation are the same as in the documentation for *kernlab* in R (Katatzoglou et al. 2004), the excellent library containing the kernel procedures used. In some expositions, λ is used instead of σ and then $\lambda = \frac{1}{2\sigma^2}$, where σ is another constant. In that form, the radial basis kernel commonly is called the Gaussian radial basis kernel. Note that this λ is not the same λ as in Eq. 2.24.

[57]The computational translation is a little tricky. These are the steps for any given entry i, j in $\mathbf{K}$. (1) As before, one does an element by element subtraction of observations i and j over each of the predictors. These are rows in $\mathbf{X}$. (2) Square each of the differences. (3) Multiply each of these squared differences by minus σ. (4) Exponentiate each of these products. (5) Sum each of the exponentiated products. (6) Raise the sum to the power of d.

[58]To illustrate, consider $\mathbf{X}$ with three predictors. For the pair of observations from, say, the first and second row of $\mathbf{X}$ and $d = 1$, the sum of differences is $(x_{11} - x_{21})^2 + (x_{12} - x_{22})^2 + (x_{13} - x_{23})^2$. This is linear and additive in the squared differences. For $d = 2$, the result is $[(x_{11} - x_{21})^2 + (x_{12} - x_{22})^2 + (x_{13} - x_{23})^2]^2$. All of the terms are now products of two squared differences, which are two-way interaction effects. For $d = 3$, the result is $[(x_{11} - x_{21})^2 + (x_{12} - x_{22})^2 + (x_{13} - x_{23})^2]^3$. All of the terms are now products of three squared differences, which are three-way interaction effects. Hence the name ANOVA kernel.

[59]The folds will need to be "kernelized." The same applies to a split sample strategy.

[60]There is in the *CVST* library a procedure with which to do penalized kernel ridge regression. However, the documentation is very spare, and the references cited often do not seem germane. It is, therefore, very difficult to know what the underlying code is really doing, and some of the output is problematic.

[61]The library *kernlab* was written by Alexandros Karatzoglou, Alex Smola, and Kurt Hornik. It has an excellent collection of functions for working with kernels in a wide variety of ways.

[62]The idea of allowing for locally varying complexity in fitted values is an old one. Fan and Gijbels (1992, 1996), who have made important contributions to the topic, attribute the idea to Breiman et al. (1977).

References

Beck, A. T., Ward, C. H., Mendelson, M., Mock, J., & Erbaugh, J. (1961). An inventory for measuring depression. *Archives of General Psychiatry, 4*(6), 561–571.

Berk, R. A., Buja, A., Brown, L., George, E., Kuchibhotla, A. K., Su, W., et al. (2019a). Assumption lean regression. *The American Statistician*, published online, April 12, 2019.

Breiman, L., & Friedman, J. H. (1985). Estimating optimal transformations for multiple regression and correlations (with discussion). *Journal of the American Statistical Association, 80*(391), 580–619.

Breiman, L., Meisel, W., & Purcell, E. (1977). Variable kernel estimates of multivariate densities. *Technometrics, 19*, 135–144.

Bring, J. (1994). How to standardize regression coefficients. *The American Statistician, 48*(3), 209–213.

Bühlmann, P., & van de Geer, S. (2011). *Statistics for high dimensional data*. New York: Springer.

Candes, E., & Tao, T. (2007). The Dantzig selector: Statistical estimation when p is much larger than n (with discussion). *Annals of Statistics, 35*(6), 2313–2351.

Cleveland, W. (1979). Robust locally weighted regression and smoothing scatterplots. *Journal of the American Statistical Association, 78*, 829–836.

Cleveland, W. (1993). *Visualizing data*. Summit: Hobart Press.

Chernozhukov, V., Wuthrich, K., & Zhu, Y. (2018). *Exact and robust conformal inference methods for predictive machine learning with dependent data*. arXiv:1802.06300 [stat.ML].

de Boors, C. (2001). *A practical guide to splines* (Revised edition). New York: Springer.

Dijkstra, T.K. (2011). *Ridge regression and its degrees of freedom*. Working paper, Department Economics & Business, University of Gronigen, The Netherlands.

Dominici, F., McDermott, A., & Hastie, T. J. (2004). Improved semi-parametric times series models of air pollution and mortality. *Journal of the American Statistical Association, 9*(468), 938–948.

Duvenaud, D., Lloyd, J. R., Grosse, R., Tenenbaum, J. B., & Z. Ghahramani (2013). Structure discovery in nonparametric regression through compositional kernel search. *Journal of Machine Learning Research W&CP, 28*(3), 1166–1174

Dwork, C., Feldman, V., Hardt, M., Pitassi, T., Reingold, O., & Roth, A. (2015). The reusable holdout: Preserving validity in adaptive data analysis. *Science, 349*(6248), 636–638.

Dwork, C., Feldman, V., Hardt, M., Pitassi, T., Reingold, O., & Roth, A. (2017). Guilt-free data reuse. *Communications of the ACM, 60*(4), 86–93.

Efron, B., & Tibshirani, R. (1993). *Introduction to the bootstrap*. New York: Chapman & Hall.

Ericksen, E. P., Kadane, J. B., & Tukey, J. W. (1989). Adjusting the 1980 census of population and housing. *Journal of the American Statistical Association, 84*, 927–944.

Exterkate, P., Groenen, P. J. K., Heij, C., & Van Dijk, D. J. C. (2011). *Nonlinear forecasting with many predictors using kernel ridge regression*. Tinbergen institute discussion paper 11-007/4.

Fan, J., & Gijbels, I. (1992). Variable bandwidth and local linear regression smoothers. *The Annals of Statistics, 20*(4), 2008–2036.

Fan, J., & Gijbels, I. (1996). *Local polynomial modeling and its applications*. New York: Chapman & Hall.

Fan, J., & Li, R. (2006). Statistical challenges with dimensionality: Feature selection in knowledge discovery. In M. Sanz-Sole, J. Soria, J. L. Varona, & J. Verdera (Eds.), *Proceedings of the International Congress of Mathematicians* (Vol. III, pp. 595–622).

Finch, P. D. (1976). The poverty of statisticism. *Foundations of Probability Theory, Statistical Inference, and Statistical Theories of Science, 6b*, 1–46.

Gareth, M., & Radchenko, P. (2007). Sparse generalized linear models. Working Paper, Department of Statistics, Marshall School of Business, University of California.

Gifi, A. (1990) *Nonlinear multivariate analysis*. New York: Wiley.

Green, P. J., & Silverman, B. W. (1994). *Nonparametric regression and generalized linear models.* New York: Chapman & Hall.

Hastie, T. J., & Tibshirani, R. J. (1990). *Generalized additive models.* New York: Chapman & Hall.

Hastie, T., Tibshirani, R., Friedman, J. (2009). *The elements of statistical learning* (2nd ed.). New York: Springer.

Katatzoglou, A., Smola, A., Hornik, K., & Zeileis, A. (2004). kernlab: An S4 package for kernel methods in R. *Journal of Statistical Software, 11*(9), 1–20. http://www.jstatsoft.org

Kuchibhotla, A. K., Brown, L. D., & Buja, A. (2018). Model-free study of ordinary least squares linear regression. arXiv: 1809.10538v1 [math.ST].

Lafferty, J., & Wasserman, L. (2008). Rodeo: Sparse greedy nonparametric regression. *Annals of statistics, 36*(1), 28–63.

Lamiell, J. T. (2013). Statisticism in personality psychologists' use of trait constructs: What is it? How was it contracted? Is there a cure? *New Ideas in Psychology, 31*(1), 65–71.

Leeb, H., Pötscher, B. M. (2005). Model selection and inference: Facts and fiction. *Econometric Theory, 21,* 21–59.

Leeb, H., & Pötscher, B. M. (2006). Can one estimate the conditional distribution of post-model-selection estimators? *The Annals of Statistics, 34*(5), 2554–2591.

Leeb, H., Pötscher, B. M. (2008). Model selection. In T. G. Anderson, R. A. Davis, J.-P. Kreib, & T. Mikosch (Eds.), *The handbook of financial time series* (pp. 785–821). New York: Springer.

Liu, J., Wonka, P. & Ye, J. (2012). Multi-stage Dantzig selector. *Journal of Machine Learning Research, 13,* 1189–1219.

Loader, C. (2004). Smoothing: Local regression techniques. In J. Gentle, W. Hardle, & Y. Mori (Eds.), *Handbook of computational statistics.* New York: Springer.

Lockhart, R., Taylor, J., Tibshirani, R. J., & Tibshirani, R. (2014). A significance test for the lasso. (with discussion). *Annals of Statistics, 42*(2), 413–468.

Marra, G., & Wood, S. N. (2012). Coverage properties of confidence intervals for generalized additive model components. *Scandinavian Journal of Statistics, 39*(1), 53–74.

McGonagle, K. A., Schoeni, R. F., Sastry, N., & Freedman, V. A. (2012). The panel study of income dynamics: Overview, recent innovations, and potential for life course research. *Longitudinal and Life Course Studies, 3*(2), 268–284.

Meinshausen, N., & Bühlmann, P. (2006). High dimensional graphs and variable selection with the lasso. *The Annals of Statistics, 34*(3), 1436–1462.

Murphy, K. P. (2012). *Machine learning: A probabilistic perspective.* Cambridge: MIT Press.

Ran, J., & Lv, J. (2008). Sure independence screening for ultrahigh dimensional feature space. *Journal of the Royal Statistical Society, Series B, 70*(5), 849–911.

Ripley, B. D., (1996). *Pattern recognition and neural networks.* Cambridge: Cambridge University Press.

Rosset, S., & Zhu, J. (2007). Piecewise linear regularized solution paths. *The Annals of Statistics, 35*(3), 1012–1030.

Ruppert, D., Wand, M. P., & Carroll, R. J. (2003). *Semiparametric regression.* Cambridge: Cambridge University Press.

Shakhnarovich, G. (Ed.) (2006). *Nearest-neighbor methods in learning and vision: Theory and practice.* Cambridge: MIT Press.

Sill, M., Heilschher, T., Becker, N., & Zucknick, M. (2014). c060: Extended inference with lasso and elastic-net regularized Cox and generalized linear models. *Journal of Statistical Software, 62*(5), 1–22.

Tibshirani, R. J. (1996). Regression shrinkage and selection via the lasso. *Journal of the Royal Statistical Society, Series B, 25,* 267–288.

Tibshirani, R. J. (2015). Adaptive piecewise polynomial estimation via trend filtering. *Annals of Statistics, 42*(1), 285–323.

Wang, H., Li, G., & Jiang, F. (2007). Robust regression shrinkage and consistent variable selection through the LAD-lasso. *Journal of Business and Economic Statistics, 25*(3), 347–355.

Wood, S. N. (2017). *Generalized additive models* (2nd ed.) New York: Chapman & Hall.

Zelterman, D. (2014). A groaning demographic. *Significance, 11*(5): 38–43.

Zou, H. (2006). The adaptive lasso and its oracle properties. *The Journal of the American Statistical Association, 101*(467) 1418–1429.

Zou, H., & Hastie, T. (2005). Regularization and variable selection via elastic net. *Journal of the Royal Statistical Association, Series B, 67* Part 2, 301–320.

Chapter 3
Classification and Regression Trees (CART)

Summary In this chapter, we turn to recursive partitioning, which comes in various forms including decision trees and classification and regression trees (CART). We will see that the algorithmic machinery successively subsets the data. Trees are just a visualization of the data subsetting processes. We will also see that although recursive partitioning has too many problems to be an effective, stand-alone data analysis procedure, it is a crucial component of more powerful algorithms discussed in later chapters. It is important, therefore, to get into the details.

3.1 Introduction

In stagewise regression, the results of a stage are fixed no matter what happens in subsequent stages. Earlier stages are not re-visited. Forward stepwise regression is not a stagewise procedure because all of the included regression coefficients are re-estimated as each new regressor is added to the model. In a similar fashion for backwards stepwise regression, all of the remaining regression coefficients are re-estimated as each additional regressor is dropped from the model.

If you look under the hood, conventional classification and regression trees (CART), also called decision trees in computer science, has important parallels to stagewise regression with predictors that are indicator variables. The CART algorithm determines which predictors are to be included and how each is to be transformed into a binary variable. In the end, one has a specification for a linear model from the GLM family. The discussion of linear approximations from Chap. 1 applies.[1]

In CART, the stagewise steps are typically displayed in a tree-like structure, which accounts for how the technique is named. Some data analysts use that structure as if it were a model from which substantive insights can be drawn. As

© Springer Nature Switzerland AG 2020   157
R. A. Berk, *Statistical Learning from a Regression Perspective*,
Springer Texts in Statistics, https://doi.org/10.1007/978-3-030-40189-4_3

will be more clear as we proceed, this is usually a bad idea. The tree structure more properly is viewed as a visualization of what the CART algorithm is doing. Let's begin there.

3.2 An Introduction to Recursive Partitioning in CART

Suppose one has a single quantitative response variable and several predictors. There is interest, as before, in $Y|X$, but the predictors are just inputs to CART algorithm. An essential task of the algorithm, repeated at each stage in the stagewise process, is to find the single "best" binary split of the data using information obtained from the full set of predictors.

Consider the first stage in which one works with all of the training data. Two kinds of searches are undertaken. First, for each predictor, all possible binary splits of the predictor values are considered. For example, if the predictor is age in years, and there are age-values of 21 through 24, all possible splits maintaining order would be 21 versus 22–24, 21–22 versus 23–24, and 21–23 versus 24.

Ordinal predictors can be handled in the same fashion. For example, the possible answers to a questionnaire item might be "strongly agree," "agree," "can't say," "disagree," and "strongly disagree." Then, all possible binary splits of the data are considered with the order maintained (i.e., in strength of agreement). Unlike conventional regression, ordinal predictors pose no special problems. Order is maintained for each possible split, which is all that really matters for CART.

Closely related reasoning can be applied when a predictor is categorical. For instance, if the predictor is marital status with categories never married, married, and divorced, all possible splits would be never married versus married and divorced, married versus never married and divorced, and divorced versus never married and married. For categorical variables, there is no order to maintain.

How is the "best" split for each predictor defined? For quantitative response variables, the metric usually is the response variable error sum of squares or its mean squared error. For count data, the metric can be the deviance or some function of the deviance, just as in Poisson regression. For binary response variables, there are several options including the deviance.

Each possible binary split of each predictor implies a different two-way partitioning of the data. For example, one partition might include all individuals under 25 years of age, and the other partition would then include all individuals 25 years of age or older. For a numeric response variable, an error sum of squares is computed separately within each partition and then added together. That sum will be equal to or less than the error sum of squares for the response variable before the partitioning. The best split for each predictor is defined as the split that reduces the error sum of squares the most. Analogous reasoning can be applied for binary response variables or count response variables, but using a different fitting metric.

With the best split for each predictor determined, the best split *overall* is determined as the second step. That is, the best split for each predictor is compared by the reduction in the error sum of squares. The predictor with the largest reduction wins the competition. It is the predictor that when properly split leads to the greatest reduction in the error sum of squares compared to the error sum of squares before that partitioning is undertaken. Again, similar reasoning applies to binary or count response variables.

With the two-step search completed, the winning split is used to *subset the data.* In other words, the best split for the best predictor defines two subsets. For example, if the best split were to be 21–22 versus 23–24 years of age, all individuals 21–22 would form one subset, and all individuals 23–24 would form the other subset.

There are now two partitions of the original data, defined by best split within and between the predictors. Next, the same two-step procedure is applied to each partition separately; the best split within and between predictors for each subset is found. This leads to four partitions of the data. Once again, the two-step search procedure is repeated, but now separately for each of the four data partitions. The recursive process can continue until there is no meaningful reduction in the response variable measure of fit. Then, the results are conventionally displayed as an inverted tree: roots at the top and canopy at the bottom. One nice feature of the partitioning process is that one can have more predictors than observations. This is not true of the other procedures discussed so far.

As addressed in more detail shortly, the recursive partitioning results can be represented within a linear basis expansion framework. The basis functions are indicator variables defined by the best splits. With these determined, one has a regression of the response on the basis functions yielding regression coefficients and fit statistics as usual. Because the partitions are determined empirically from the data, there are complications for any Level II analysis.

There is a remarkably large number of tree-based statistical methods (Loh 2014). In this chapter, we consider classification and regression trees (CART) introduced by Breiman, Friedman, Olshen, and Stone in 1984, which has been in use for about 30 years and remains a popular data analysis tool. We will focus on CART as it has traditionally been implemented. There are some interesting refinements and extensions (Chaudhuri et al. 1995; Lee 2005; Chipman et al. 1998; Loh 2014; Xiaogang et al. 2008; Choi et al. 2005; Hothorn et al. 2006; Zeileis et al. 2008), and even some major reformulations (Grubinger et al. 2014). There are also CART-like procedures such as CHAID (Kass 1980) and C5.0 (Quinlan 1993), which has a computer science lineage. A discussion of these variants would take us some distance from the approach emphasized in here in part because they treat CART primarily as a stand-alone data analysis tool. CART on occasion can be an effective stand-alone procedure as well, but more important for our purposes, it has become an integral component of several statistical learning algorithms discussed in subsequent chapters. A discussion of CART provides an essential foundation for understanding those algorithms.

Chapter 2 was devoted almost entirely to quantitative response variables. Equal time and more is now given to categorical, and especially binary, response variables. As noted earlier, procedures that assign observations to classes are often called "classifiers." When CART is used with categorical response variables, it is an example of a classifier. One grows a classification tree.

Categorical response variables introduce a number of issues that either do not apply to quantitative response variables or apply only at a high level of abstraction. We now need to get this material on the table in part because it applies to classifiers in addition to CART. We also emphasize again the differences between Level I, Level II, and Level III regression analyses and remind readers of the critical difference between explanation and forecasting.

This is a somewhat plodding, tedious chapter. An effort has been made to include only the material that is really needed. But that's a lot, and it is probably useful to slog through it all.

3.3   The Basic Ideas in More Depth

We begin with conceptual overview of the CART computational machinery. Mathematical details are provided later. They are at this point a detail.

For a binary response variable coded "A" or "B," and predictors X and Z, Fig. 3.1 is the three-dimensional scatterplot illustrating a simple classification problem as it might be attacked by CART. CART's algorithm is called "greedy" because it searches in a stagewise fashion for the best outcome without looking back to past splits or forward to future splits. The algorithm lives only in the present.

The vertical red line at, say, $Z = 3$ produces the first partition. It represents the best split in a competition between all possible splits of X or Z. The A-values tend to be concentrated on the left, and the B-values tend to be concentrated on the right. The green horizontal line at $X = 5$ produces the subsequent partition of the left subset. It represents the best split of the left partition. The upper left corner is now homogeneous in A. This is an ideal outcome. The yellow horizontal line at $X = -2$ produces the best subsequent split of the right partition. The lower right corner is

Fig. 3.1 A recursive partitioning for a binary response variable and predictors X and Z (the response is coded A or B. The red line shows the first partition. The green and yellow lines show the next two partitions)

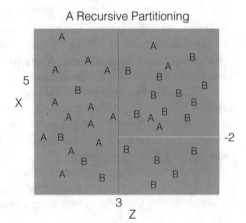

now homogeneous in B. This too is an ideal outcome. In principle, the lower left partition and the upper right partition would be further subdivided.

Figure 3.1 makes clear that CART constructs partitions with a series of straight-line boundaries perpendicular to the axis of the predictor being used. These may seem like serious constraints on performance. Why linear? Why perpendicular? These constraints are simple to work with and can perform very well in practice.

The values at which the partitioning is done matter. For example, Fig. 3.1 reveals that cases with $Z \leq 3$ and $X > 5$ are always A. Likewise, cases with $Z > 3$ and $X \leq -2$ are always B. Indeed, we are able to describe all four conditional distributions of the binary response variable conditioning on the four partitions of X and Z. Within each partition, the proportion of A-values (or B-values) might be a useful summary statistic for the binary outcome. How do these proportions vary over the different partitions? We are doing a regression analysis of $G|X$ summarized in a Level I analysis as conditional proportions.

3.3.1 Tree Diagrams for Showing What the Greedy Algorithm Determined

CART partitioning is often shown as an inverted tree. A tree visualization allows the data analyst to see how the data partitions were constructed and to consider the conditional relationships implied. Explanation can be in play within a Level I regression analysis, although one has an algorithm's machinations, not a model.

Figure 3.2 is a simple, schematic illustration of an inverted tree. The full dataset is contained in the root node. The data are then broken into two mutually exclusive pieces. Cases with $X > C_1$ go to the right, and cases with $X \leq C_1$ go to the left. The latter are then in terminal node 1, which is not subject to any more subsetting; no meaningful improvements in fit can be made. The former are in an internal node that can be usefully subdivided further, and the internal node is partitioned again. Observations with $Z > C_2$ go to the right and into terminal node 3. Observations with $Z \leq C_2$ go to the left and into terminal node 2. Further subsetting is not productive.

In this case, all splits beyond the initial split of the root node imply, in regression language, interaction effects. The right partition imposed at the internal node only includes observations with X-values that are greater than C_1. Consequently, the impact of Z on the fit depends on observations with $X > C_1$. The conditional relationship is itself conditional.

When there is no natural order to a predictor's values, the partitioning criterion selected is usually represented by the name of the variable along with the values that go to the right (or left, depending on the software) side. For example, if ethnicity is a predictor and there are five ethnicities represented by the letters a through e, the software might represent the partitioning criterion for a given split as *ethnicity = ade*. All cases belonging to ethnic groups a, d, and e are being placed in the right-hand partition.

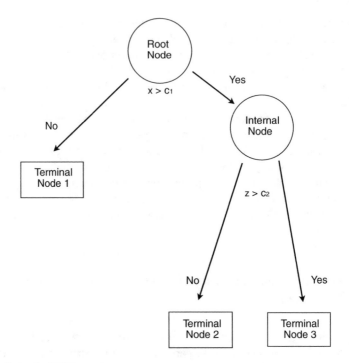

Fig. 3.2 A simple CART tree structure

Splits after the initial split do not have to represent interaction relationships. If an immediately subsequent partitioning of the data uses the same predictor (with a different breakpoint), the result is an additional step in the step function for that predictor. A more complicated nonlinear function results.

One can represent the terminal nodes in Fig. 3.2 as sets of linear basis expansions within a conventional regression mean function that can reproduce the tree fitted values. One just defines all of the terminal nodes with indicator variables, each of which is a function of one or more predictors (including the constant term). Thus,

$$f(X, Z) = \beta_0 + \beta_1[(I(x \leq c_1)]$$
$$+ \beta_2[I(x > c_1 \,\&\, z \leq c_2)] + \beta_3[I(x > c_1 \,\&\, z > c_2)]. \quad (3.1)$$

Equations like Eq. (3.1) can depict when a terminal node is composed of different binary splits of a single predictor, when a terminal node is composed of interactions between binary splits across predictors, and when both apply. However, representation of the terminal nodes within a conventional regression mean function—in practice, usually as part of a linear regression, binomial regression, or multinomial logistic regression[2]—disregards for each terminal node the *order* in which the predictors were selected. For any terminal node, the regression specification does not capture whether, say, income was chosen before age or whether age was chosen before income.[3] If a researcher wishes to make claims about predictor importance from that order, the regression equation cannot help. In practice, this is not an important loss, because there is no compelling rationale for treating selection order as a measure of predictor importance, especially because CART outputs are derived from an algorithm, not a model. Moreover, as considered below, tree structures can be very fragile.

The conventional regression representation can be more than a curiosity for Level II analyses. The lengthy discussion in Chap. 1 about statistical inference for regression functionals immediately becomes relevant. If asymptotically valid statistical inference can be undertaken for GLM approximations, why not for CART output represented as a GLM? The answer, in brief, is that sometimes this formulation works, but there are complications to think through, which are discussed later.[4]

The application of CART is always an opportunity for a Level I analysis. For a Level II analysis, we once again must treat the data as random, independent realizations from a nature's joint probability distribution. But what is the estimand? For a variety of technical reasons, the tree structure itself is not a useful estimation target.[5] Alternatively, the estimation target can be the regression formulation derived from the tree structure as a feature of the joint probability distribution, much as shown in Eq. (3.1). One has, once again, an approximation of the true response surface. In principle, proper statistical inference can be undertaken for the regression coefficients, but interest usually centers on the fitted values. The regression coefficients are a means to that end. Unfortunately, because CART has built-in data snooping, we are returned to the inferential complications discussed in the last chapter. Test data can be essential. More details will be provided as we proceed.

3.3.2   An Initial Application

To illustrate some of these initial ideas, consider passenger data from the sinking of the Titanic.[6] What predictors are associated with those who perished compared to those who survived? Figure 3.3 shows the CART results as an inverted tree. Survived is coded as a 1, and perished is coded as a 0. In each terminal node, the left number is the count of those who perished, and the right number is the count of those who survived. If the majority perished, the node is colored red. If the majority survived, the node is colored blue. Figure 3.4 contains the code.[7]

For this analysis, predictors used include:

1. sex—the gender of the passenger;
2. age—age of the passenger in years;
3. pclass—the passenger's class of passage;
4. sibsp—the number of siblings/spouses aboard; and
5. parch—the number of parents/children aboard.

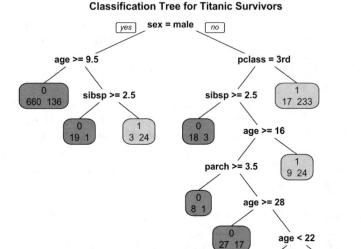

Fig. 3.3 A classification tree for the Titanic data: 1 = Survived, 0 = Perished (in each terminal node, the number who perished and the number who survived are shown to the left and right, respectively. In red nodes, the majority perished. In blue nodes, the majority survived. N=1309)

```
### CART Code
library(PASWR) # To get the data
data(titanic3) # Load the data

library(rpart) # Load the CART library
library(rpart.plot) # Load the fancy plotting library

# Partition the data
out<-rpart(survived~sex+age+pclass+sibsp+parch, data=titanic3,
method="class")
#Plot the tree
prp(out,extra=1,faclen=10,varlen=15,cex=1.2,
    main="Classification Tree for Titanic Survivors",
    box.col=c("red","lightblue")[out$frame$yval])
```

Fig. 3.4 R code for the CART Analysis of the Titanic data

The first split is on sex. Males are sent down the left branch. Females are sent down the right branch. The two subsequent splits for males are at an ages of 9.5 years and the number of siblings or spouses aboard at 2.5. For males, there are three terminal nodes. For the older males, 136 survived and 600 did not. Because the majority did not survive, the node is labeled with a 0 for not surviving. For males, only those younger than 9.5 with less than 2.5 siblings or spouses aboard were likely to survive (i.e., 24 to 3). For females, the splits are much more complicated but can be considered with the same sort of reasoning. For example, most of the females traveling in first or second class survived, and the terminal node is given a label of 1 accordingly (i.e., 233 to 17). If one takes the cinematic account seriously, some of the association broadly make sense, and a Level I analysis of the data has been undertaken. But many of the associations represent high level interaction relationships whose meanings are somewhat mysterious.

It is challenging to make a credible case for a Level II analysis. What is the joint probability distribution responsible for the data? It could perhaps be the joint probability distribution for passengers on ocean liners using as a response of whether or not each survived the passage. But much more specificity would be needed. For example, it is likely that such a distribution would change with new ship technology and better training of captains, crews, and navigators. The sinking of the Titanic itself led to revisions of marine safety regulations governing such things as the number of lifeboats required on board. And even if a reasonable joint probability distribution could be defined, one would still need to argue that each passenger's data were realized independently of all others even though some were traveling in families. Indeed, it is in part because of the many families that the Titanic sinking is such a compelling tragedy.

In addition, the partitioning algorithm is clearly an example of concerted data snooping. Therefore, in-sample performance is formally unjustified and potentially very misleading. Test data are required. What would be proper test data for the passengers on the Titanic? Unless there is a good answer, the fallback of cross-validation is also badly compromised. What exactly does an out-of-sample estimate mean?

3.3.3   Classification and Forecasting with CART

There is far more to the output from CART than a tree diagram. Indeed, probably the most important output is found in the terminal nodes. Suppose the response variable is binary, and the task is classification. Within each of the terminal nodes, the proportion of "successes" and proportion of "failures" can be calculated. These conditional proportions are often of significant descriptive interest as one kind of fitted value. For example, in Fig. 3.2 if the proportion of successes in terminal node 3 is 0.70, one can say for cases with $x > c_1$ and $z > c_2$ that the proportion of successes is 0.70. Analogous statements can be made about the other terminal nodes. For example, the proportion of success for cases with $x \leq c_1$ (terminal node 1) might be 0.25. Ideally, terminal node proportions will vary substantially, implying that the partitioning is making important distinctions between different kinds of cases. If one knows for any given case the value of x and the value of z, it really matters for the proportion of successes.

In addition, the conditional proportions can be used to attach class labels to terminal nodes that, in turn, can be assigned to observations. Technically, these class labels are not fitted values because, as will be more clear shortly, they are not a direct product of the CART minimization process. Nevertheless, there is no harm in thinking about the assigned classes as a second kind of fitted value. If the majority of observations in a terminal node are As, all of the observations in that partition are assigned to class A. If the majority of observations in a terminal node are Bs, all of the observations in that partition are assigned to class B. These labels convey what is most typical in a terminal node and, therefore, is most typical for cases with that particular configuration of indicator variables. If all of the observations in a terminal node need to be placed into a single response category, the terminal node class label provides the means. When CART is used in this manner, it is Bayes classifier, applied individually to each terminal node.

Think back to the discussion of logistic regression in Chap. 1. Recall that there were fitted proportions and assigned classes. Cases with fitted proportions that exceeded some threshold were assigned to one of the two classes. Cases with fitted proportions that did not exceed that threshold were assigned to the other class. Much the same is going on within each of the terminal nodes of classification trees, where by the Bayes classifier, the threshold is 0.50.

But why would anyone care about the class labels? The class labels can be critical for a Level II analysis if new data are provided that contain the same predictors but with the binary outcome unknown ("unlabeled"). The labels are a good guess for the unknown binary outcome for each case. Often, this plays out as forecasting. Suppose one knows that observations with certain values for predictors fall in a particular terminal node, and that the majority of observations in that partition have, say, the outcome category A. Then, new observations that fall in that terminal node, but for which the response is unknown, sensibly might be predicted to be A as well. If a Level II analysis is credible, the class label can be thought of as a predicted value to be used for forecasting.

3.3.4   Confusion Tables

If CART assigns classes to observations, it is sensible to ask how accurate those assigned classes actually are. Instructive assessments can be obtained from "confusion tables," briefly introduced earlier, which here cross-tabulate the observed classes against the classes that CART assigns. Ideally, the two will correspond much of the time. But that will be a matter of degree, and confusion tables can provide useful measures of fit. We will consider confusion tables many times in the pages ahead, but a few details are important to introduce now. For ease of exposition at this point, the categorical outcome variable is binary.

Table 3.1 shows an idealized confusion table. There are two classes for the response variable: success and failure. The letters in the cells of the table are cell counts. For example, the letter "a" is the number of observations falling in the upper-

Table 3.1 Confusion table structure

	Failure fitted	Success fitted	Classification error
Failure observed	a	b	$b/(a+b)$
Success observed	c	d	$c/(c+d)$
Prediction error	$c/(a+c)$	$b/(b+d)$	Overall error $= \frac{(b+c)}{(a+b+c+d)}$

left cell. All of the observations in that cell are characterized by an observed class of failure and a fitted class of failure. It follows that these are all correct classifications. When the observations are from training data, "fitted" means "assigned." They are a product of the CART fitting process. If the observations are from test data, "fitted" often means "forecasted." The difference between fitting and forecasting is critical in the next several chapters.

In many situations, having training data, evaluation data, and test data can help enormously. Also, a split-sample strategy can be employed so that the values of tuning parameters are determined by fitting performance in the evaluation data. Once a satisfactory tree has been grown and honestly assessed with the test data, it is ready for use when the outcome class is not known, but the predictor values are.

There are generally four kinds of performance assessments that are made from confusion tables.

1. The overall proportion of cases incorrectly classified is an initial way to assess performance quality. It is simply the number of observations in the off-diagonal cells divided by the total number of observations. If all of the observations fall in the main diagonal, CART has, by this measure, performed perfectly. None of the observations has an observed class that does not correspond to its fitted class. When no cases fall in the main diagonal, CART is a total failure. All of the observations have an observed class that does not correspond to its fitted class.

   Clearly, a low proportion for this "overall error" is desirable, but how good is good depends on the baseline for fitting skill when no predictors are used. The real issue is how much better one does once the information in the predictors is exploited. A lot more is said about this shortly.

2. The overall error neglects that it will often be more important to be accurate for one of the response variable classes than for another. For example, it may be more important to correctly diagnose a fatal illness than to correctly diagnose excellent perfect health. This is where the row proportions shown in the far right-hand column become critical. One conditions on the observed class outcome. For each observed class, the row proportion is the number of observations incorrectly classified divided by the total of observations of that class. Each row proportion characterizes errors made by the fitting procedure. When the true outcome class is known, how common is it for the procedure to miss it?

   The two kinds of classification failures are often called "false positives" or "false negatives." Successes incorrectly called failures are false negatives. Failures incorrectly called successes are false positives.[8] The row proportions representing the relative frequency of false negatives and false positives should, ideally, be small. Just as for overall error, the goal is to do better using information contained in the predictors than can be done ignoring that information. But, the exercise now is undertaken for each row separately. It is common for the fitting procedure to perform better for one outcome class than the other.

3. The column proportions address a somewhat different question. One conditions on the fitted class and computes the proportion of times a fitted class is wrong. Whereas the row proportions help evaluate how well the CART algorithm has performed, the column proportions help evaluate how useful the CART results are likely to be if put to work. They convey what would happen if a practitioner used the CART results to impute or forecast. One conditions on either a fitted success or on fitted failure from which two different estimates of errors in use can be obtained. Just as for classification error, it is common for prediction error to differ depending on the outcome class. The goal is much the same as for classification error: for each column, to be wrong a smaller fraction of the time than if the predictors are ignored.

4. The ratio of the number of false negatives to the number of false positives shows how the algorithm is trading one kind of error for the other. For example, if b is five times larger than c, there are five false positives for every false negative. This means that the CART procedure produces results in which *false negatives* are five times more important than false positives; one false negative is "worth" five false positives. Ratios such as this play a key role in our discussion later about how to place relative costs on false negatives and false positives.

In summary, confusion tables are an essential diagnostic tool. We rely on them in this chapter and all subsequent ones when a classifier is discussed. They also raise some important issues that are very salient in the pages ahead.

3.3.5 CART as an Adaptive Nearest Neighbor Method

The earlier discussion of lowess introduced in some detail the concepts of a statistical neighborhood and of nearest neighbors. Recall that there were several different ways to operationalize "nearest" and that the size of a neighborhood was determined by the span tuning parameter. The tuning led to data snooping, but if the value for the span was determined before the data analysis began (or using training data followed by test data), one could have a Level II linear estimator with desirable properties of a population approximation.

The data partitions represented in Fig. 3.1 can be viewed as neighborhoods defined by its nearest neighbors. But CART arrives at those neighborhoods adaptively. Like all stagewise (and stepwise) procedures, CART data snoops.

Consider, for example, terminal node 3 in Fig. 3.2. Within that node, are all observations whose values of x are greater than c_1, and whose values of z are greater than c_2. For these observations, a conditional mean or proportion can be computed. In other words, the nearest neighbors for either of these summary statistics are defined as all cases for which $x > c_1$ and $z > c_2$. All of the observations for which this condition holds can be used to arrive at a single numerical summary for the response variable.

Thinking in adaptive nearest neighbor terms provides another perspective on the bias-variance tradeoff. Suppose for a Level II analysis the true response surface is the estimation target, and for a given terminal node, a goal is to estimate the proportion of 1s over all observations in the terminal node whose neighborhood is defined by a particular set of x-values. For example, the binary response could be whether a high school student graduates; graduation is coded as 1 and dropout is coded as 0. The terminal node neighborhood in question contains high school students, self-identified as Asian, who have family incomes in excess of $75,000.

But suppose there are omitted predictor variables; there are other predictors associated with family income, say, and graduating that are not used to define this terminal node neighborhood. Even if these predictors happened to be in the dataset, they were not selected (e.g., the labor market for white- collar jobs). A more subtle specification error occurs when the correct predictor is chosen, but at the wrong breakpoint (e.g., family incomes > $6000 rather than > $75,000). One also has to wonder whether the relationship between graduating and family income is really a step function. Because the neighborhood is not defined correctly, there is a good chance that the estimated proportion graduating will be biased with respect to the true response surface.

A potential remedy is to further refine the terminal nodes by *growing a larger tree*. There is an opportunity for more predictors to determine the terminal node neighborhoods leading to a more homogeneous sets of cases. But for a given sample size, a larger tree implies that on the average, there will be fewer cases in each terminal node. Although bias may be reduced, variance may be increased.

If the estimation target is the population approximation of the true response surface, the issues differ. Any terminal node having a misspecified neighborhood with respect to the true response surface can define a neighborhood that is part of a population approximation. For a Level II analysis, the estimand is that approximation, which as shown earlier can be represented as regression equation. It is important to remember that this regression is not a model. It is a convenient summary of algorithmic results.

Because all terminal node neighborhoods are assembled adaptively, the handy asymptotic properties emphasized in Chap. 1 can be elusive. We will see later that using test data in concert with the regression formulation can help, but the challenges are greater than for smoothers. To prepare for this material, we need to examine CART in more formal detail.

3.4 The Formalities of Splitting a Node

A crucial matter the CART algorithm needs to address is exactly how to split each node using information contained in the set of predictors. For a quantitative predictor with m distinct values, there are $m - 1$ splits that maintain the existing ordering of values. So, $m - 1$ splits on that variable need to be evaluated. For example, if there are 50 distinct high school GPA scores possible, there are 49 possible splits that maintain the existing order. However, there are often algorithmic shortcuts that can capitalize, for instance, on ordering the splits by the size of the conditional mean or proportion. The same logic holds for ordinal predictors.

Order does not matter for categorical predictors. Consequently, a categorical variable with k categories has $(2^{k-1} - 1)$ possible splits. For example, if there are five ethnic group categories, there are 15 possible splits. Hence, although there are sometimes shortcuts here too, the computational burdens are generally much heavier for categorical variables.

How at each splitting opportunity is "best" partitioning to be formally defined? Traditional expositions focus on the "impurity" of a node. Impurity is essentially heterogeneity. The goal is to have as little impurity (heterogeneity) overall as possible. Consequently, the best split is the one that reduces impurity the most. To help simplify the details follow, assume a binary response variable G coded 1 or 0. The term "success" is used to refer to outcomes coded 1, and the term "failure" to refer to outcomes coded 0.

A discussion of impurity can work well using the proportions of successes and failures in a node or the probabilities of a success or a failure in a node. Most expositions favor probabilities and assume that they are known. There is really no didactic cost to this assumption for now. We too will for now abandon proportions for probabilities.

Suppose that the observations in a dataset are realized independently from a joint probability distribution; the concept of a probability can apply. Consider a given node, designated as node A. The impurity of node A is taken to be a nonnegative function of the probability that $G = 1$, written as $P(G = 1|A)$.

Any node A ideally should be composed of cases that are all equal to 1 or all equal to 0. Then $P(G = 1|A)$ would be 1.0 or 0.0. Intuitively, impurity is the smallest it can be. If half the cases are equal to 1 and half the cases are equal to 0, the probability of either is 0.50. A is the most impure it can be because a given case is as likely to be a 1 as a 0.

One can more formally build on these intuitions. Let the impurity of node A be:

$$I(A) = \phi[P(G = 1|A)], \tag{3.2}$$

with $\phi \geq 0$, $\phi(P) = \phi(1 - P)$, and $\phi(0) = \phi(1) < \phi(P)$. In other words, impurity is nonnegative, and symmetrical with a minimum when A contains all 0s or all 1s, and a maximum when A contains half of each.[9]

There remains a need to define the function ϕ. For classification, three definitions have been used in the past: Bayes error, the cross-entropy function,[10] and the Gini loss. In order, they are:

$$\phi(P) = \min(P, 1 - P); \tag{3.3}$$

$$\phi(P) = -P \log(P) - (1 - p) \log(1 - P); \tag{3.4}$$

and

$$\phi(P) = P (1 - P). \tag{3.5}$$

All three functions for impurity are concave, having minimums at $P = 0$ and $P = 1$ and a maximum at $P = 0.5$. Entropy and the Gini loss are the most commonly used, and in CART generally give very similar results except when there are more than two response categories. Then, there is some reason to favor the Gini loss (Breiman et al. 1984: 111). The Gini loss is more likely to partition the data so that there is one relatively homogeneous node having relatively few cases. The other nodes are then relatively heterogeneous and have relatively more cases. For most data analyses, this is a desirable result. Cross-entropy tends to partition the data so that all of the nodes for a given split are about equal in size and homogeneity. This is generally less desirable.[11]

One might legitimately wonder why CART does not directly minimize classification error. Direct minimization of classification error is discussed in some detail by Breiman and his colleagues (1984: section 4.1). A key problem is that there can be several splits for a given stage minimizing classification error. Recall that the assigned class is a product of a vote. A terminal node having a winning vote of 60% for a given class will assign the same class had the winning vote been 90% for that class. Yet, the node with the winning vote of 90% is far more homogeneous. Important information has been lost undermining the ability to find a single best split. In addition, minimizing classification error at each stage has a tendency, like cross-entropy, of producing a tree structure that is more difficult to interpret. For now, we focus on node impurity as just defined. Direct minimization of classification error resurfaces as an instructive consideration when boosting is introduced in Chap. 6.

For real applications, the probabilities are not likely to be known. Suppose one uses data to estimate the requisite probabilities. It should be apparent by now that obtaining good estimates involves conceptual and technical complications, but for didactic purposes, assume that the complications have been effectually addressed.

Building on Zhang and Singer (1999; chapters 2 and 4), for any internal node, consider a potential left "daughter" node A_L, and a right "daughter" node A_R, whose impurities need to be computed. Table 3.2 provides the information required. The entries in each cell are counts, with rows as the first subscript and columns as the second subscript.

As before, we let $G = 1$ if there is a success and 0 otherwise. The estimate of $P(G = 1|A_L)$ is given by $n_{12}/n_{1.}$. Similarly, the estimate $P(G = 1|A_R)$ is given by $n_{22}/n_{2.}$.

Consider calculations for entropy as an example. Cross-entropy impurity for the left daughter is

Table 3.2 Counts used to determine the usefulness of a potential split

	Failure	Success	Total
Left node: $x \leq c$	n_{11}	n_{12}	$n_{1.}$
Right node: $x > c$	n_{21}	n_{22}	$n_{2.}$
	$n_{.1}$	$n_{.2}$	$n_{..}$

The cell entries are counts, with the first subscript for rows and the second subscript for columns

$$I(A_L) = -\frac{n_{11}}{n_{1.}}\log(\frac{n_{11}}{n_{1.}}) - \frac{n_{12}}{n_{1.}}\log(\frac{n_{12}}{n_{1.}}). \qquad (3.6)$$

Cross-entropy impurity for the right daughter is

$$I(A_R) = -\frac{n_{21}}{n_{2.}}\log(\frac{n_{21}}{n_{2.}}) - \frac{n_{22}}{n_{2.}}\log(\frac{n_{22}}{n_{2.}}). \qquad (3.7)$$

Imagine that for the left daughter there are 300 observations with 100 successes and 200 failures. The impurity is $-0.67(-0.40) - 0.33(-1.11) = 0.27 + 0.37 = 0.64$. Imagine now that for the right daughter there are 100 observations with 45 successes and 55 failures. The impurity is $-0.55(-0.60) - 0.45(-0.80) = 0.33 + 0.36 = 0.69$.

To put these numbers in context, it helps to consider the smallest and largest possible values for the impurity. The greatest impurity one could obtain would be for 50% successes and 50% for failures. The computed value for that level of impurity would be 0.693. For proportions of 1.0 or 0.0, the value of cross-entropy impurity is necessarily 0. In short, the minimum value is 0, and the maximum is a little more than 0.69. The closer one gets to 50–50, where the impurity is the greatest, the closer one gets to 0.693. The impurity numbers computed are rather close to this upper bound and reflect, therefore, substantial heterogeneity found in both daughter nodes. It is likely that this split would not be considered to be very good, and if there are better options, would not be implemented.

Once all possible splits across all possible variables are evaluated in this manner, a decision is made about which split to use. The impact of a split is not just a function of the impurity of a node. The importance of each node must also be taken into account. A node in which few cases are likely to fall is less important than a node in which many cases are likely to fall. The former probably will not matter much, but the latter probably will matter a lot.

We define the improvement resulting from a split as the impurity of the parent node minus the weighted left and weighted right daughter impurities. If this is a large number, impurity is reduced substantially. More formally, the benefits of the split s for node A,

$$\Delta I(s, A) = I(A) - P(A_L)I(A_L) - P(A_R)I(A_R), \qquad (3.8)$$

where $I(A)$ is the value of the parent impurity, $P(A_R)$ is the probability of a case falling in the right daughter node, $P(A_L)$ is the probability of a case falling in the left daughter node, and the rest is defined as before. Impurity can be measured by cross-entropy or the Gini loss. The two probabilities can be estimated from information such as provided in Table 3.2; they are just the marginal proportions $n_{1.}/n_{..}$ and $n_{2.}/n_{..}$. They serve as weights.

In short, CART finds the best $\Delta I(s, A)$ for each variable. The variable and split with the largest value are then chosen to define the new partition. The same approach is applied to all subsequent nodes.

3.5   An Illustrative Prison Inmate Risk Assessment Using CART

A key issue for prison administrators is understanding which inmates are likely to place themselves and others in harm's way. Use of narcotics, assaults on prison guards, and homicides are examples. Although such events are relatively rare, they have very serious consequences. Consequently, it would be very useful if such conduct could be anticipated. Then, for the high-risk inmates, preventive measures might be taken. For example, inmates from rival street gangs might be housed in different prisons. Low-risk inmates might be given far greater freedom to participate in job training and educational programs. A prerequisite, however, is a way to find effective predictors of misconduct in prison.

Using data from the administrative records of a large state prison system, Fig. 3.5 shows a classification tree suggesting which kinds of inmates are reported for some form of misconduct within 18 months of intake.[12] From Fig. 3.6, one can see that there are two tuning parameters. A relatively large minimum node sample size of 100 was imposed to stabilize the results and to keep the diagram very simple. More will be said soon about the complexity parameter cp, but a small value allows splits that do not reduce node impurity very much. According to the documentation of *rpart*, cp is a threshold on the proportional improvement in fit. Only splits improving the fit by at least the value of cp will be permitted. A large value for the threshold means that acceptable splits must improve the fit a lot.[13]

The three predictors in Fig. 3.5 were selected by the CART procedure from a larger set of 12 predictors.

1. Term: Nominal sentence length in years. (A nominal sentence is the sentence given by the trial judge. Inmates are often released before their nominal sentence is fully served.)
2. AgeArr: Age at arrival at the prison reception center in years using 16–20, 21–26, 27–35, and 36 or older.
3. Gang: gang membership with Y for "yes" and N for "no."

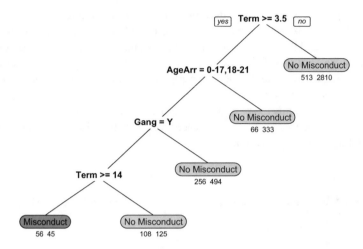

Fig. 3.5 CART recursive partitioning of the prison data (the value on the left below each terminal node is the number of inmates who engaged in misconduct. The value on the right is the number of inmates who did not engage in misconduct. A red node means that the majority in that node engaged in misconduct. A blue node means that the majority in that node did not engage in misconduct. N=4806)

```
library(rpart) # Load the CART library
library(rpart.plot) # Load the fancy plotting library

# Partition the data
out<-rpart(Fail~AgeArr+Gang+CDC+Jail+Psych+Term,
           data=temp, method="class",
           minbucket=100,cp=.001)
# Plot a tree
prp(out,extra=1,faclen=10,varlen=15,
box.col=c("red","lightblue")[out$frame$yval])
```

Fig. 3.6 R code for CART analysis of prison misconduct

Terminal nodes are labeled "No Misconduct" if the majority in that node do not engage in misconduct and "Misconduct" if the majority do. The numbers within each terminal node show left to right the counts of misconduct cases and no-misconduct cases, respectively.[14] There are 4806 observations in the root node. Among these, observations are sent left if the nominal prison term is equal to or greater than 3.5 years and to the right if the nominal prison term is less than 3.5 years. Likewise, at each subsequent split, the observations meeting the condition specified are sent left.

The story is simple. Inmates with nominal prison terms over 14 years, who are under 22 years of age, and who are gang members are more likely than not to be reported for misconduct (i.e., 56 cases v. 45 cases). Inmates with nominal terms of less than 3.5 years are relatively unlikely to be reported for prison misconduct regardless of age, gang membership, or any other nine predictors in the data (i.e., 513 cases v. 2810 cases). In the other three terminal nodes, no-misconduct cases are the majority. One might say that a very long nominal terms puts an observation over the top but by itself is not associated with a preponderance of reported misconduct. Each of the five terminal nodes but the one on the far right is defined by interaction relationships.

There are readily available (post hoc) explanations for these results. Judges impose far longer prison terms on individuals who have committed very serious, usually violent, crimes. The data suggest that the judges are on to something. And it is well known that young gang members can be atypically difficult, especially when housed with members of rival gangs.

At the same time, a classification tree is not a model. It summarizes the results of a greedy algorithm. But if one insists in treating Fig. 3.5 as a model, the implied regression equation is no doubt badly misspecified. For example, there is no information on the security level in which the inmate is placed, and higher security levels are thought to reduce incidents of serious misconduct.[15] Finally, because the data partitions were arrived at inductively as part of an extensive search, there can be both data snooping and substantial overfitting affecting Fig. 3.5. There is data snooping because a single "best" split is chosen for each partitioning; one has an exemplar of a problematic approach to data analysis in Level II settings. There is overfitting because unsystematic as well as systematic patterns in the data are being aggressively exploited.[16]

Nevertheless, suppose at intake, prison administrators wanted to intervene in a manner that could reduce prison misconduct. Absent other information, it might make sense to distinguish young gang members with very long sentences from other inmates. In effect, the prison administrators would be using the classification tree to make forecasts to help inform placement and supervision decisions.

Although such thinking can have real merit, there are complications. We will have shifted into a Level II analysis if the results are to be used for forecasting. One would need to consider how the data were realized, the impact the CART's extensive data snooping, and out-of-sample performance. These problems have now been raised several times. Near the end of the chapter, the issues and potential solutions will be squarely faced.

In addition, the consequences of failing to identify a very dangerous inmate at intake can be enormously different from the consequences of incorrectly labeling a low-risk inmate as dangerous. The different consequences can have very different costs. In the first instance, a homicide could result. In the second instance, an inmate might be precluded from participating in prison programs that could be beneficial. It stands to reason, therefore, that the differential costs of forecasting errors should be introduced into the CART algorithm. We turn to that now.

3.6   Classification Errors and Costs

Looking back at the earlier details on how splits are determined, there was little explicit concern about costs of classification errors, but it can be shown that all three impurity functions treat classification errors symmetrically. Incorrectly classifying an A as a B is treated the same as incorrectly classifying a B as an A.

Consider, for example, the second terminal node from the left in Fig. 3.5. The vote is close, but the 125 no-misconduct cases win. It follows that the 108 inmates who in fact had reported misconduct are misclassified. But suppose the 125 cases counted half as much. The misconduct vote would carry the day, and the terminal node would be assigned to the misconduct class. There would then be 125 classification errors, but each would count half as much as before. Whereas the original cost ratio was 1 to 1, it is now 2 to 1. In concrete terms, a misclassified misconduct case is taken to be twice as costly as a misclassified no-misconduct case.

As we examine in depth shortly, introducing "asymmetric" costs for classification errors can be a game changer that actually begins with the criteria by which splits are determined and involves far more than re-weighting the votes in terminal nodes. We will see that by altering the prior, the two impurities in Eq. (3.8) are weighted differently when a split is determined. That changes the relative improvement in the fit so that different splits may be selected.[17] Whether there actually are asymmetric costs resulting from classification errors depends on what is to be done with the classification tree results. If the CART results are just archived in some academic journal, there are probably no costs one way or the other. If the results are used to guide future research, costs can be a real issue. In genomic research, for example, follow-up research would be wasted if a genomic snip is incorrectly identified as important. Conversely, a significant research lead might be missed if an important genomic snip is incorrectly overlooked. These two costs are probably not the same. In applied research, costs can be very important, as the prison example should make clear. A way is needed to build in the differential costs classification errors.

3.6.1   Default Costs in CART

Without any apparent consideration of costs, the CART algorithm can make classification decisions about the misconduct of inmates. But in fact, costs are built in. To see how, we need to examine Table 3.3, which is constructed from the earlier prison misconduct analysis.

As noted earlier, tables of the form of Table 3.3 are often called confusion tables. They can summarize the classification performance (or as we see later, forecasting performance) of a particular classifier. Here, that classifier is CART. There is a row for each actual outcome. There is a column for each classified outcome. Correct classifications are in the main diagonal. Misclassifications are the off-diagonal

Table 3.3 CART confusion table for classifying inmate misconduct using the empirical prior distribution of the outcome variable (N=4816)

	Fitted as no misconduct	Fitted as misconduct	Classification error
No misconduct	3762	45	0.01
Misconduct	953	56	0.95
Predicting error	0.20	0.45	Overall error = 0.21

elements. Thus, we learn that 998 out of 4816 cases were incorrectly classified. But, how good this is depends on the baseline.

Had no predictors been used, classification could have been done from the misconduct marginal distribution alone. Applying the Bayes classifier, all cases would have been classified as having no reported misconduct. Then, 1009 (i.e., 953+56) out of 4816 of the cases would have been incorrectly classified. The CART classifier in this case is of little help (i.e., 998 errors compared to 1009 errors).

But, there is lots more going on in the table that is relevant to the costs of classification errors. The overall fit ignores how well CART does when the two response variable categories separated. Consider first what happens when one conditions on the actual outcome class. In this case, the absence of misconduct can be classified very well; 99% of the cases are classified correctly. In contrast, instances of misconduct are misclassified about 95% of the time. The overall error rate masks these important differences. CART performs very well when there is no misconduct and very poorly when there is misconduct.

The columns in Table 3.3 are also instructive. Now the conditioning is with respect to the fitted class, not the actual class. If the no-misconduct class is assigned, it is wrong for about 20% of the observations. If the misconduct class is assigned, it is wrong for about 45% of the observations. So, mistakes are relatively more common when misconduct is assigned, but we do better with the misconduct class that one might expect. If one is thinking ahead to possible forecasting applications, there may be some hope.

Where are costs in all this? Key information about empirical costs is contained in the two off-diagonal cells. There are 45 no-misconduct cases incorrectly classified and 953 misconduct cases incorrectly classified. The former one might call false positives, and the latter one might call false negatives. The ratio of the cell counts is $953/45 = 21.2$. There are about 21 false negatives for each false positive. Stated a little differently, one false positive is "worth" about 21 false negatives, and its cost is, therefore, about 21 times greater. According to the confusion table, it is 21 times more costly to misclassify a case of no misconduct (i.e., a false positive) than to misclassify a case of misconduct (i.e., a false negative).

The performance results in the table depend on the 21 to 1 cost ratio produced by default, and one has to wonder if corrections administrators and other stakeholders think that the 21 to 1 cost ratio makes sense. The analysis is shaped de facto by treating false positives as far more costly than false negatives. In practice, prison misconduct, false negatives are usually thought to be more costly (Berk 2018), so this analysis looks to have it upside down. And if that's right, all of the various measures of classification performance are highly suspect and potentially very misleading.

Important lessons follow. First, the CART algorithm (and every other classification procedure for that matter) *necessarily* introduces the costs of classification errors at least implicitly when classes are assigned. There is no way to circumvent this. Even if the data analyst never considers such costs, they are built in. To not consider the relative costs of misclassifications is to leave the relative cost determinations to the data and the classification algorithm. Second, the way cases are classified will vary depending on the cost ratios. As a result, the entire confusion table can change dramatically depending on the cost ratio. Finally, the outcome class assigned can serve as a forecast when the predictor values are known but the outcome class is not. If the assigned classes depend on the false negative to false positive cost ratio, so do the forecasts.

If costs are so important, there is a need to understand how they are incorporated into the CART algorithm. This will set the stage for a data analyst to introduce costs explicitly. In other words, it is desirable — some might say essential — to treat the relative costs of classification/forecasting errors as an *input* to the algorithm. Unless this is done, the results risk being unresponsive to the empirical questions being asked.

3.6.2 Prior Probabilities and Relative Misclassification Costs

Priors and relative costs are intimately related and address the need to take asymmetric costs of classification errors into account. To make the links, some preparation is needed. There are lots of details.

The marginal distribution of any categorical response variable will have a proportion of the observations in each response category. In the prison example, 0.21 of the inmates had a reported incident of misconduct, and 0.89 of the inmates had not. For a Level II analysis, such proportions can be conceptualized as the "prior probabilities" associated with the response variable. The word "prior" comes from Bayesian statistical traditions in which the "prior" refers to the beliefs of the data analyst, before the data are examined, about the probability density or distribution of some parameter.

There has been some work within Bayesian traditions capitalizing on several different kinds of CART priors (Chipman et al. 1998, 1999), including a "pinball prior" for tree size and some features of tree shape (Wu et al. 2007). That is, key features of the tree itself are given a prior probability distribution. The ideas advanced are truly interesting, and have led to some important statistical learning spinoffs (Chipman et al. 2010). But in practice, the technical complications are considerable, and it is not even clear that there will commonly be credible information available to make such priors more than tuning parameters. Tuning parameters are important and useful, but they are not a feature of probability distributions specified before the data analysis begins. Consequently, for present purposes, we will use the term "prior" only with reference to the empirical, marginal distribution of the response variable in the data.

Consistent with most expositions of CART, we will proceed as if a Level II analysis is appropriate, but in broad brush strokes the lessons learned apply as well to Level I approaches. Assume that a credible Level II analysis can be undertaken with CART. Drawing heavily on Therneau and Atkinson (2015), suppose the training data has N observations and C classes for the response variable. The CART algorithm produces K terminal nodes. Define π_i for $i = 1, 2, \ldots, C$ as the prior probability of a case being in class i. Often, $C = 2$. For the binary outcomes, i is often represented by 1 or 0 or by 1 or -1.

$L(i, j)$ is the binary outcome loss matrix, i for rows and j for columns. The elements in the main diagonal (i.e., $i = j$) are the costs of a correct classification, assumed to be 0.0. The off-diagonal elements (i.e., $i \neq j$) are the costs of classification errors, taken to be positive. We will not make direct use of the full loss matrix in the exposition to follow, but will employ certain elements of it. We present the loss matrix in part because *rpart* provides an option to work directly with the loss matrix.

A is any node and, therefore, a subset of the data derived from recursive partitioning. $\tau(x)$ is the true class for an observation, where x represents the vector of predictor variable values for that observation. We let $\tau(A)$ be the class assigned to the observations in node A. N_i and N_A are the number of observations for the full sample that are in class i and for node A, respectively, with N_{iA} the number of observations of class i for node A.

Table 3.4 provides the numbers needed for a simple illustration of why the prior matters and how changing it affects relative costs. There are 10,000 high school students. According to the marginal distribution, 20% of the students drop out. This translates into 2000 students (i.e., $0.2 \times 10,000$). 80% of the students graduate, which translates 8000 students (i.e., $0.8 \times 10,000$). Table 3.4 shows the composition of some partition A_L.

Consider again the expression for determining whether a given split will be made. As before, for node A, s stands for the split to be evaluated, L and R stand for left and right respectively, $I(.)$ is impurity, for which we will use the Gini measure, and $P(.)$ stands for probability. Then,

$$\Delta I(s, A) = I(A) - P(A_L)I(A_L) - P(A_R)I(A_R). \qquad (3.9)$$

We can now examine how the prior affects $\Delta I(s, A)$.

Table 3.4 Hypothetical partition A_L with a prior of (.20, .80) for dropping out of high school and graduating high school respectively and a total of 10,000 high school students

	Dropout	Graduate	Total
Number of cases	250	650	900

1. Consider $P(A_L)$. The issues are exactly the same for $P(A_R)$. For the left partition, $P(A_L)$ is the probability of cases appearing in node A_L, which is equivalent to $\sum_{i=1}^{C} \pi_i P[x \in A_L | \tau(x) = i]$, where π_i is a prior probability. For each class i, the prior probability of a case being in class i is multiplied by the probability that class i cases will be in node A_L. This product is summed over classes. $P(A_L)$ can be estimated by $\sum_{i=1}^{C} \pi_i (N_{A_L,i}/N_i)$. From Table 3.4 we have, rounded to two decimal places, $(0.20 \times 250/2000) + (0.80 \times 650/8000) = 0.09$. The prior probabilities affect the probability of landing in A_L. If the prior distribution were different, the probability of landing in A_L would be different as well, other things equal.

2. Then, $P(i|A)$ is the conditional probability of class i given that a case is in node A, or $P[\tau(x) = i | x \in A]$. The value of $P(i|A)$ can be estimated by the number of cases of class i in node A, divided by the total number of cases in that node and equals $\pi_i P[x \in A | \tau(x) = i]/P[x \in A]$, which can be estimated by $\pi_i (N_{iA}/N_i)/\sum_{i=1}^{C} \pi_i (N_{iA}/N_i)$. The conditional probability of a case with true class i landing in A depends in part on the prior probability that a case is class i to begin with. From Table 3.4, the two probabilities, rounded to two decimal places, are $(0.20 \times (250/2000))/(900/10,000) = 0.28$ and $(0.80 \times (650/8000))/(900/10,000) = 0.72$. The Gini value is the product of these two probabilities, which here is about 0.20. A key point is that the prior affects the Gini value too, and if the prior is altered, the Gini value is altered as well, other things equal. From Eq. (3.9), the contribution of the left partition to the reduction in impurity, rounded to two decimal places, is $0.20 \times 0.09 = 0.02$. The value of 0.02 probably would be different with a different prior.

3. At this point, we make a transition to terminal nodes only; the recursive partitioning has been completed. Each terminal node has an outcome class assigned by majority vote. Cases that fall in the minority represent errors. $R(A)$ is the "risk" associated with node A, such that $\sum_{i=1}^{C} P(i|A)L(i, \tau(A))$. It is conventional to attach a loss of 0 to members of the majority and a loss greater than 0 (e.g., 3) to members of the minority. One can allow for a different losses depending on which cases are being misclassified. For example, classifying a high school dropout as a high school graduate can have different costs from classifying a high school graduate as a high school dropout. Risk is a product of probability of a given outcome class falling in terminal node A and the loss associated with that landing node. Looking back point #2, the probability of a given outcome class falling in terminal node A is determined in part by the prior. Other things equal, if one changes the prior, that probability changes and, therefore, so does the risk. The risk can also be altered by changing the losses attached to misclassifications. Finally, because risk is a product of $P(i|A)$ and $L(i, \tau(A))$, one can alter the risk by altering the prior *or* by altering the loss (or both).

4. $R(T)$ is the risk for the entire tree T, which equals $\sum_{j=1}^{K} P(A_j)R(A_j)$, where A_j is for each of the K terminal nodes of the tree. (There is no left or right). We are now just adding the risk associated with each terminal node, weighted

by the probability of cases falling in that node. It follows that $R(T)$ is just cost weighted overall classification error that one could compute directly from a confusion table.

How does all this correspond to our earlier material on costs? First, there is a close correspondence once some translations are provided. One key translation is that the loss attached to a misclassification effectively is the same as the cost attached to a misclassification. Here, the terms here mean the same thing.

Second, what matters is the relative costs, just as before. If one multiplies the costs by any constant, all that changes is the units of risk. (e.g., like going from feet to inches). This helps to explain why the cost ratio is so easy to interpret; the units don't matter.

Third, the information responsible for $R(T)$ can be displayed in a confusion table as a summary of performance aggregated across all of the terminal nodes. This does not work for any single node because there is for a single node only one assigned class. For a binary outcome, one of the columns of a confusion table would be missing. For categorical outcomes with more than two classes, $C - 1$ of the columns would be missing.

Fourth, working backward from point #4 to point #3 to point #2 to point #1 — and here is the punch line — *changing the prior can change the confusion table.* The impact of any altered prior cascades in a complicated manner through all of the calculations is just summarized and is also necessarily shaped by properties of the data. Using the prior to alter particular features of a confusion table in specified ways will usually require some trial and error, although *rpart* in R provides an argument with which to directly alter the prior.[18]

Fifth, although one can alter a confusion table by changing the prior or by changing the costs of misclassifications, changing the prior has some conceptual advantages. One important advantage is that in many applications, a prior can be understood as a base rate. Base rates play a central role in discussion of algorithmic fairness, which is addressed toward the end of the book. Also, because one can change a base rate by re-weighting the data, re-weighting can be used to alter the confusion table as well. The option to use weighting can be very important when the software one might prefer does not provide for direct changes in the prior. We will see this play out in later chapters.

3.7 Varying the Prior and the Complexity Parameter

Figure 3.7 shows again the tree diagram for the CART analysis of inmate misconduct. Recall that the empirical distribution of the response variable was used as the prior distribution, the role of asymmetric costs was not considered, and the number of terminal nodes was constrained by setting the minimum terminal node sample size.

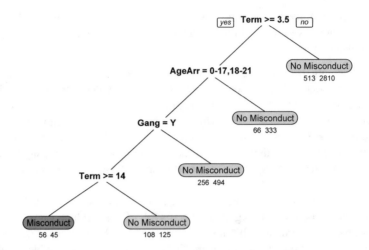

Fig. 3.7 CART recursive partitioning of the prison data with default costs (the red nodes represent misconduct, the blue nodes represent no misconduct, N=4806)

Table 3.5 CART confusion table for classifying inmate misconduct with default cost ratio (as discussed above, even with the same data, N's can vary over different analyses because of missing data patterns, $N = 4816$)

	Classify as no misconduct	Classify as misconduct	Classification error
No misconduct	3762	45	0.01
Misconduct	953	56	0.95
Prediction error	0.20	0.45	Overall error = 0.21

Recall also the confusion table. It is reproduced here as Table 3.5. One questionable feature of the table was that there were about 21 false negatives for each false positive, implying that false positives were far more costly than false negatives.

Conversations with prison officials indicated that from their point of view, false negatives were worse than false positives. Failing to anticipate inmate misconduct, which could involve fatal violence, was of far greater concern than incorrectly labeling an inmate as high risk. When pushed, a prison official said that the cost of a false negative was at least twice the cost of a false positive. Hence, the earlier analysis got things upside down.

Figure 3.8 shows the tree diagram that results when the target cost ratio of false negatives to false positives in the confusion table is 2 to 1. The changes are dramatic. The code is shown in Fig. 3.9.

Setting appropriate values for *prior* and *cp* is explicit tuning.[19] The process can involve some trial and error and in this illustration, the task was complicated by a tree with relatively few terminal nodes. When there are few terminal nodes, the distribution of fitted classes can be lumpy so that getting the empirical cost ratio exactly right — or even close — in the confusion table may not be possible.

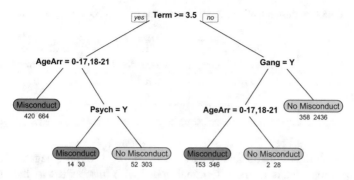

Fig. 3.8 CART recursive partitioning of the prison data with 2 to 1 target cost ratio (N=4797)

```
# Partition the data
out<-rpart(Fail~AgeArr+Gang+CDC+Jail+Psych+Term,
          data=temp, method="class",
          parms = list(prior = c(.52,.48)),cp=.004)
# Plot a Tree
prp(out,extra=1,faclen=10,varlen=15,under=T
    box.col=c("red","lightblue")[out$frame$yval])
```

Fig. 3.9 R code for CART analysis of prison misconduct with a 2 to 1 target cost ratio

With a specified prior of 52% misconducts and 48% no misconducts, the confusion table cost ratio was approximately 2.5 false positives for every false negative. False negatives are about 2.5 times more costly. The results do not change materially with cost ratios between approximately 1.5 and 3.5.

At first, the terminal nodes in Fig. 3.8 may seem a little odd. There is not a single terminal node in which there are more misconduct cases than no-misconduct cases and yet, there are three terminal models with misconduct as the fitted class. The reason is that the counts shown in each terminal node are weighted by the new prior. Misconduct cases constitute about 21% of the observations but are now treated as if they constitute a little over half. The number of misconduct cases in each terminal node is multiplied by about 2.5 when the fitted class is determined. The ratio of the new prior for misconduct of 0.52 to the old prior misconduct of 0.21 is about 2.5.

The partitioning in Fig. 3.8 returns a somewhat different story from the partitioning in Fig. 3.7. Misconduct is the fitted class for young inmates with long nominal terms. Gang membership is not required. For older inmates with long nominal terms, a diagnosed psychological problem leads to a misconduct fitted class. Inmates with shorter nominal terms who are young and gang members are also classified as misconduct cases. All of these results are produced by interaction effects. There are no terminal nodes defined by main effects.

Table 3.6 CART confusion table for classifying inmate misconduct with 2 to 1 target cost ratio (N=4797)

	Fitted as no misconduct	Fitted as misconduct	Classification error
No misconduct	2767	1040	0.27
Misconduct	412	578	0.42
Prediction error	0.13	0.64	Overall error = 0.30

Table 3.6 shows dramatic changes. Increasing the costs of false negatives relative to false positives leads to more terminal nodes with misconduct as the assigned class. This is precisely what was intended. As a result, there is a dramatic increase in CART's ability to accurately classify misconduct and in trade, a dramatic reduction in CART's ability to accurately classify no-misconduct cases.

Overall error for Table 3.6 is increases a bit, but as already explained, the overall error rate is misleading when the costs of classification errors are asymmetric. The overall error rate incorrectly treats all classification errors the same. With asymmetric costs, this is no longer valid.

Finally, prediction errors have changed as well. When no misconduct is the fitted class, it is incorrect 13% of the time rather than 20% of the time. In trade, the prediction error when misconduct is the fitted class increases from 45% to 64%. The increase results from the decision to make false positives less costly. It follows that there are now many more of them.

The confusion table is constructed from training data only and is no doubt subject to overfitting. For a Level I analysis, that comes with the territory. Nevertheless, the changes in prediction error could have important implications for Level II forecasting because the fitted class becomes the forecasted class for new cases when that outcome is not known; generalization error is now a key measure of forecasting success. By making false negatives more costly, the CART algorithm is, in effect, accepting weaker statistical evidence when misconduct is the fitted class or when misconduct is forecasted; the algorithm is trying harder not to overlook potential misconduct cases. The flip side is that for no misconduct to be the fitted or forecasted class, the algorithm requires stronger statistical evidence. As a result, classification and forecasting accuracy (i.e., conditioning on the fitted class) will decline for misconduct outcomes and improve for no-misconduct outcomes. Ideally, one would see this all play out in test data.

There is nothing mandatory about these results. One might think that there is some sensible way to define an optimal result and a way to produce it. But, even when one has training data, evaluation data, and test data, optimality is usually a pipe dream. As a technical matter, several different configurations of tuning parameters values often can lead to very similar results. As already explained, for example, the minimum node size argument and the cp tuning parameter can accomplish much the same thing.

The preferred cost ratio complicates matters further. It should be determined by stakeholders, not the data analyst, and depends on decisions that will be informed by the CART tree and confusion table. Such decision-making responsibilities usually are not included in the job description of a data analyst.

But even with a given cost ratio, how well CART performs is not easily reduced to a single number. For example, some observers might want the tree structure to make subject matter sense. There is no single number by which that can be measured. Other observers may just want a tree structure that is easily interpreted. Again, there is no single number. Still other observers may care little about the tree structure and focus instead on classification accuracy. However, there can be several measures of classification accuracy extracted from a confusion table. In short, there will often be a substantial disconnect between the goals of explanation, classification, and forecasting. Even when one dominates, there may well be no single evaluation yardstick to optimize. This is a very important lesson to carry forward into subsequent chapters. Typically, a statistical learning data analysis cannot be boiled down solely to an optimization problem.

There also can be pragmatic complications. In this illustration, prison officials might want to place all inmates forecasted to be problematic in high security settings. But high security incarceration is very expensive (about like Ivy League tuition), and if too many misconduct cases are forecasted, the requisite resources will not be available. In effect, there is some threshold above which the number of false positives and true positives breaks the bank. There can be, as well, legal and political complications if too many false positives are forecasted. Prison officials can be criticized for "over-incarceration."

In short, a reasonable stance is that CART will sometimes provide useful information but rarely definitive guidance. How helpful the information turns out to be will depend on the information with which it competes. When decision-makers are operating in an information vacuum, very weak CART results can be valuable. When a lot is already known, strong CART results can be irrelevant. Fortunately, there are much more powerful statistical learning procedures coming.

3.8 An Example with Three Response Categories

In broad brush strokes, there is no formal problem extending CART to three or more response variable categories. But the bookkeeping is much more demanding and getting the cost ratios right is sometimes quite difficult. To see how this happens, the prison data are reanalyzed with the three-category response variable: serious and substantial misconduct, some minor form of misconduct, and no misconduct. About 78% of the cases have no reported misconduct, about 20% have some minor reported misconduct, and about 2% have serious and substantial reported misconduct. The 2% represents very rare cases that ordinarily present a difficult classification challenge. The available predictors are the same as before.

The first hurdle is arriving at sensible cost ratios for classification errors. Prison administrators were concerned about even minor misconduct because it can be a challenge to staff authority and lead to more serious problems. Still, reported cases

Table 3.7 CART confusion table for classifying inmate misconduct with three outcome classes and target cost ratios ($N = 4736$)

	Fitted as none	Fitted as some	Fitted as substantial	Classification error
None	2438	1181	188	0.36
Some	301	443	117	0.49
Substantial	31	70	37	0.73
Prediction error	0.11	0.74	0.89	Overall error = 0.39

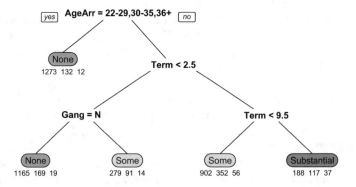

Fig. 3.10 CART recursive partitioning of the prison data with three outcome classes (red terminal nodes represent serious and substantial misconduct, yellow terminal nodes represent some minor misconduct, and green terminal nodes represent no misconduct. The order of the numbers below each terminal node is alphabetical: none, some, substantial. $N = 4806$)

of serious and substantial misconduct were of somewhat greater concern. After some back and forth, the following cost ratios were provisionally agreed upon, which can be compared to the results in Table 3.7. The agreement is about as good as one can get without a large number of terminal nodes.

- Misclassifying a "substantial" as a "none" was taken to be about five times worse than misclassifying a "none" as a "substantial." In fact, cell 31/cell 13 = 188/31 = 6.1.
- Misclassifying a "substantial" as a "some" was taken to be about about two times worse than misclassifying a "some" as a "substantial." In fact, cell 23/cell 32 = 117/70 = 1.7.
- Misclassifying a "some" as a "none" was taken to be about two times worse than misclassifying a "none" as a "some." In fact, cell 12/cell 21 = 1181/301 = 3.9.

Given cost ratios in the confusion table, Fig. 3.10 shows the associated classification tree. The R code is provided in Fig. 3.11. With three outcome classes, one reads the classification tree much like before. The main difference is that in each terminal node there is one count for each class arranged in alphabetical order from left to right. As before, the outcome with the largest prior-weighted count determines the

```
library(rpart) # Load the CART library
library(rpart.plot) # Load the fancy plotting library
# Partition the data
out<-rpart(Fail3Way~AgeArr+Gang+CDC+Jail+Psych+Term,
            data=temp, method="class",
            parms = list(prior = c(.35,.35,.30)),cp=.01)
#Plot a tree
prp(out,extra=1,faclen=10,varlen=15,under=T
    box.col=c("green","yellow","red")[out$frame$yval])
```

Fig. 3.11 R code analysis of prison misconduct

class assigned to a terminal node. But here is where the bookkeeping starts to matter. Because the prior has three classes, the weighting is more complicated. Tuning is more intricate. For example, 2% of the cases in the empirical priors are reported for serious and substantial misconduct, but cost-sensitive prior arrived at assigns a value of 30%. Such cases are upweighted by a factor of about 15. At the other extreme, the no-misconduct cases account for 78% of the cases in the empirical prior but only 35% of the tuned cost-sensitive prior. These cases are down weighted by a factor of about 0.45. In short, all of the votes in each terminal node are given more or less weight than their raw counts indicate.

With the weighting, Fig. 3.10 has no substantive surprises. Young inmates (i.e., < 22) with longer nominal sentences (i.e., > 9.5 years) land in the only terminal node assigned the class of serious misconduct. Older inmates and younger inmates with shorter terms and no gang associations land in the two terminal nodes that have no misconduct as the assigned class. But if the latter are gang members, they placed in the node assigned some, less consequential misconduct. There is also an apparent break point for nominal sentences less than 9.5. years. Inmates with terms of more than 2.5 years but less than 9.5 years land in a terminal node with the "some" assigned class.

The performance measures in the confusion table are interpreted as before with one important exception. With three outcome categories, there are always two ways to misclassify. For example, when there is no misconduct, the classification is wrong about a third of the time. But the vast majority of those errors are not for cases of serious and substantial misconduct. Perhaps, the performance is better than it first seems. When the class assigned is no misconduct, it is correct nearly 90% of the time. As before, the cost ratios require that there be strong statistical evidence before a case is classified as a no misconduct. Related reasoning can be applied to the other two outcomes.

Outcomes with more than two classes are common and often very desirable. For example, forecasting how an inmate will do on parole has historically been done such that any form of recidivism counts as a failure. The absence of recidivism is a success. Of late, and in response to expressed needs to criminal justice stakeholders, more than two outcome classes are increasingly being used (Berk 2018). One might want to distinguish, for example, between new arrests for crimes of violence and new arrests for crimes in which there is no violence. There are then three outcome classes: no arrest, an arrest for a crime that is not violent, and an arrest for a violent crime.

Just as with the earlier, two-outcome analysis of prison misconduct, the results are derived solely from training data. Ideally, one would work with training data, evaluation data, and test data. In a forecasting setting, the three data sets can be essential because before forecasting with real consequences is undertaken, one must have a classification tree that is tuned well and provides an honest assessment of out-of-sample performance.

3.9 Regression Trees

The emphasis in this chapter has been on categorical response variables. By concentrating on categorical response variables, the full range of fundamental issues surrounding CART are raised. But CART is certainly not limited to categorical response variables; quantitative response variables are also fair game. And with the discussion of categorical response variables largely behind us, a transition to quantitative response variables is relatively straightforward. It is possible to be brief.

Perhaps, the major operational complication is the kind of regression method to be applied. For example, there are three options in *rpart* labeled as "anova," "poisson," and "exp." The first is for conventional quantitative response variables such as income. The second is for count response variables such as the number of hurricanes in a given hurricane season. The third is for survival response variables such as the time from prison release until a new arrest. The code to be written, options available, and output differ a bit over the three. Beneath the hood, the algorithmic details differ a bit too. The splitting criterion is now some variant on the deviance.

Consider a conventional regression application as an illustration. Node impurity is represented by the response within-node sum of squares:

$$I(\tau) = \sum (y_i - \bar{y}(\tau))^2, \tag{3.10}$$

where the summation is over all cases in node τ, and $\bar{y}(\tau)$ is the mean of those cases. Then, much as before, the split s is chosen to maximize

$$\Delta(s, \tau) = I(\tau) - I(\tau_L) - I(\tau_R). \tag{3.11}$$

Recall that for the split decision when the response is categorical, the Gini or deviance impurities are weighted by the proportion of cases in each potential daughter node. For the sum of squares impurities, there is no weighting. Because the sum of squares is a sum over observations, the number of cases in each daughter node automatically matters; there is implicit weighting. One can be more direct by reformulating the problem in units of variances. Impurity for the parent node is represented by the variance of its y-values. Likewise, impurity in the derived nodes is represented by each of their variances. Before they are added, the two variances are weighted by the proportion of cases in their respective node. The proportion weights provide the opportunity to employ different weights. Ishwaran (2015) examined three kinds: no weighting, weighting by the node proportions, and weighting by the node proportions squared (called "heavy" weighting). Conventional weighting is said to work best for regression trees when predictors are very noisy.[20]

No asymmetric cost weights can be used because there is no reasonable way to consider false positives and false negatives without a categorical response variable. Ideally, one would alter the way impurity is computed. This is easily done for quantile regression applications, but not for least squares applications. There is interesting work on quantile regression trees (Chaudhuri and Loh 2002; Meinshausen 2006; Bhat et al. 2011), but the most recent efforts have moved on to more useful forms of machine discussed in later chapters.

To get the impurity for the entire tree, one sums over all terminal nodes to arrive at $R(T)$. In *rpart*, regression trees can be pruned using the *cp* tuning parameter. Just as with categorical response variables, one can also "pre-prune" using the *cp*.

The summary statistic for each terminal node is usually the node's mean. In principle, a wide variety of summary statistics could be computed (e.g., the median). And just like for conventional regression, one can compute overall measures of fit. Unfortunately, with all of the searching over possible splits and predictors, it is not clear how to adjust for the degrees of freedom used up. There is no summary measure of fit that can account for this form of overfitting. As usual, the best course of action is to use test data to get an honest assessment of fit.

Just as in parametric regression, the fitted values can be used for forecasting. Each new observation for which the outcome is unknown is dropped down the tree. The fitted value for the terminal node in which an observation lands become the forecast. Typically, that is the conditional mean. And as before, a linear regression equation can be used to summarize how the terminal nodes are related to the response variable.

All of the earlier concerns about CART still apply, save for those linked to the classes assigned. Potential bias and instability remain serious problems. Possible remedies, insofar as they exist, are also effectively the same.

3.9.1 A CART Application for the Correlates of a Student's GPA in High School

Figure 3.12 shows a regression tree for applicants to a large public university. Figure 3.13 shows the code. The response variable is a student's GPA in high school.

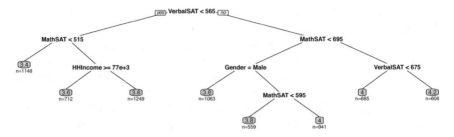

Fig. 3.12 CART recursive partitioning high school GPA data (the number in each terminal node is the conditional mean. $N = 6965$)

```
# Construct CART Partitions
out<-rpart(GPA~VerbalSAT+MathSAT+HHIncome+Gender,
           data=temp, method="anova", cp=.005)
# Construct a CART tree
prp(out,extra=1,faclen=10,varlen=15,under=T)
# Get Fit Plots
par(mfrow=c(1,1))
rsq.rpart(out)
```

Fig. 3.13 R code analysis of high school GPA

Predictors include the verbal SAT score, the mathematics SAT score, gender, and household income. Grade point average can be as high as 5.0 because the scoring gives performance in advanced placement classes extra weight. The mean GPA in each node is shown along with the number of cases in that node.[21]

Students with Math SAT scores above 695 and verbal SAT scores above 675 have the highest mean grade point average. Their mean is 4.2. Students with verbal SAT scores less than 565 and math SAT scores below 515 have the lowest mean grade point average. Their mean is 3.4. The two terminal nodes are characterized by interaction effects between the verbal and math SATs. All of the other branches suggest rather complicated and not easily explained relationships. For example, students with verbal SAT scores below 565 and math SAT scores above 515 get an extra boost if they are from families with income over $77,000. That students from higher income household do a bit better is no surprise. But why that boost only materializes within a certain set of SAT score values is not apparent. The role of gender is even more obscure. Claims are sometimes made that one of CART's assets is the ease with which a classification or regression tree can be interpreted. In practice, splits based on reductions in impurity often do not lead to results with credible subject-matter interpretations.

There are no confusion tables for quantitative response variables. But one can get a sense of fit performance from Fig. 3.14 produced by *rsq.rpart*.[22] Both plots

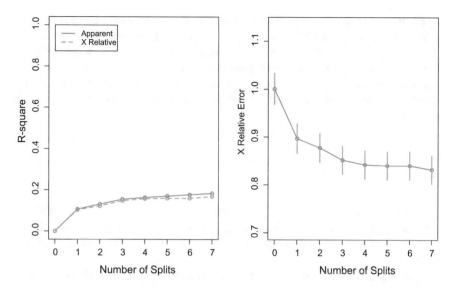

Fig. 3.14 Plots of GPA regression fit (the left figure shows the increase in R^2 with increases in the number of splits. The solid line is computed in-sample. The dashed line is computed through cross-validation. The left figure shows the reduction in relative fitting error with increases in the number of splits. The vertical lines are error bars)

show the number of splits on the horizontal axis. On the vertical axis for the plot on the left is the usual R^2. The "Apparent" R^2 (in blue) is computed from the data used to grow the regression tree. The "X relative R^2" (in green) is computed using cross-validation in an effort to get a more honest measure of fit. In this case, the two are almost identical and approach .20 as the number of splits increases. The cross-validation R^2 levels out a bit sooner. There is little improvement in the quality of the fit when the number is greater than 3. It is also apparent from the similarity of the two lines that the CART search procedures do not seem to have produced problematic overfitting in this instance. This follows from the large number of observations and small number of predictors. Relative to the number of observations, the amount of data snooping is modest. Relatively few degrees have been spent.

The plot on the right side shows the relative improvement in fit. On the vertical axis is the proportional reduction in mean squared error. The vertical lines show plus and minus one standard error estimated by cross-validation. For this plot, we see that there is little evidence of systematic improvement after the first split, and no evidence of systematic improvement after the third split. The first two error bars do not overlap at all. Subsequent error bars overlap to varying degrees. The availability of these error bars is helpful, but given all of the problems with CART Level II analyses, they should not be taken literally. Moreover, there seems to be no formal justification for using "the 1-SE rule" rather some other rule (e.g., a 2-SE rule).

For this application, one could probably make a good case for a Level II analysis. A relevant joint probability distribution could probably be defined as representing all recent applicants to this university with each applicant realized independently.[23] Figure 3.14 suggests that the consequences of data overfitting may not be serious. However, the inherent data snooping cannot be so easily dismissed. Any Level II analysis should be done with test data. We return again to the issues shortly and in more depth.

3.10 Pruning

The size of a decision tree, CART or otherwise, is usually defined by the number of splits or by the number of terminal nodes. They measure somewhat different things, but for our purposes are interchangeable. The larger the values of either, the larger the tree.

The bias-variance tradeoff with respect to the true response surface is usually affected by the size of tree. For a fixed number of observations, large trees can reduce the bias but increase the variance. The reverse holds for small trees. In *rpart*, one especially relevant tuning parameter is *minbucket*. The user can specify the minimum number of observations allowed in any data partition. The larger the value imposed, the smaller the tree tends to be. Even for a Level I analysis *minbucket* can be of help. Larger trees lead to greater complexity to digest.

Another way to tune depends on some minimum reduction in impurity before a new partitioning of the data is undertaken. In *rpart*, the relevant tuning parameter is *cp*. As mentioned earlier, the value of *cp* is the minimum proportion reduction in impurity that is acceptable for a split of the data to be made. If *cp* is larger, an acceptable split must produce a larger reduction in impurity.

Tuning by *minbucket* or *cp* is done while growing the tree. It is common for data analysts to try several values of either and then evaluate how the tree looks and performs. Having evaluation data as well as training data can help.

Alternatively, tree size can be addressed by "pruning" after a tree is grown. The pruning process removes undesirable branches by combining nodes that do not reduce heterogeneity sufficiently in trade for the extra complexity introduced. The process starts at the terminal nodes and works back up the tree until all of the remaining nodes are satisfactory. One can think of the tuning parameters *minbucket* and *cp* as serving to "pre-prune" the tree. The material on pruning that follows draws heavily on Therneau and Atkinson (2015, section 4).

Of late, pruning has not gotten a lot of attention. The problems that pruning addresses are very real. But, as CART has been superseded as stand-alone procedure, pruning has become less salient. Consequently, the discussion of pruning here is relatively short. The main objectives are acquaint readers with the topic should it ever arise and to highlight some issues that figure significantly in subsequent chapters. Tree size can be an important matter for some more advanced statistical learning procedures.

For a tree T, recall that the overall risk over K terminal nodes is

$$R(T) = \sum_{j=1}^{K} P(A_j)R(A_j). \qquad (3.12)$$

This is the sum over all terminal nodes of the risk associated with each node, each risk first multiplied by the probability of a case falling in that node. It might seem that a reasonable pruning strategy would be to directly minimize Eq. (3.12). What could be better than that? Unfortunately, that would leave a saturated tree untouched. CART would construct enough terminal nodes so that all were homogeneous, even if that meant one node for each observation. With all terminal nodes homogeneous, the risk associated with each would be zero. But, the result would be unstable nodes, serious overfitting of the data, and far too much detail to usefully interpret.

The solution is much like that seen in the previous chapter. A penalty is introduced for complexity. Under the true model perspective in a Level II context, the bias-variance tradeoff reappears, but now as a function of tree size. The penalty is meant to grow a Goldilocks tree of just the right size.

To take complexity into account in CART, a popular solution historically has been to define an objective function for pruning, called "cost complexity," that includes an explicit penalty for complexity. The penalty is not based on the number of parameters, as in conventional regression, or a function of roughness, as in smoothing. For CART, the penalty is a function of the number of terminal nodes, which indirectly addresses both roughness and effective degrees of freedom. More precisely, one attempts to minimize

$$R_\alpha(T) = R(T) + \alpha|T|. \qquad (3.13)$$

Cost complexity, $R_\alpha(T)$, has two parts: the total risk for the tree T, as defined earlier, and a penalty for complexity. For the latter, $\alpha \geq 0$ is the complexity parameter playing much the same role as λ in smoothing splines. In place of some measure of roughness, $|T|$ is the number of terminal nodes in tree T. The larger the value of α, the greater the penalty for each additional terminal node. When $\alpha = 0$, there is no penalty, and a saturated tree results. In short, α provides control over the size of the tree.

Breiman et al. (1984: section 3.3) prove that for any value of the complexity parameter α, there is a unique, smallest subtree of T that minimizes cost complexity. Thus, there cannot be two subtrees of the same size with the same cost complexity. Given α, there is a unique solution.

In many CART implementations, there are ways the software can select a reasonable value for α, or for parameters that play the same role (Zhang and Singer 1999: section 4.2.3). These defaults are often a good place to start, but will commonly lead to results that are unsatisfactory. The tree selected may make a tradeoff between the variance and the bias that is undesirable for the particular analysis being undertaken. For example, there may be far too much detail to be usefully interpreted.

Alternatively, one can specify by trial and error a value of α that leads to terminal nodes, each with a sufficient number of cases, and that can be sensibly interpreted. Interpretation will depend on both the number of terminal nodes and the kinds of cases that fall in each, so a substantial number of different tree models may need to be examined.

More recent thinking on pruning replaces α with cp. Thus,

$$R_{cp}(T) = R(T) + cp * |T| * R(T_1), \tag{3.14}$$

where $R(T_1)$ is the risk for a tree with no splits, $|T|$ is now the number of splits for a tree, and $R(T)$ is the total risk as before. The value of cp ranges from 0 to 1. When $cp = 0$, one has a saturated tree. When $cp = 1$, there are no splits. A key advantage over α is that cp is unit free and easier to work with. It also can be used to pre-prune a tree, much like the minimum bucket size, or can be tuned with procedures such as cross-validation. Sometimes it can be used in both roles for single analysis.

In practice, whether one determines tree complexity by pre-pruning or pruning (or both) seems to make little practical difference. The goal is to construct a useful tree, which is another way to say an appropriate number of splits. How exactly that is accomplished is less important as long as the steps undertaken and the various results evaluated are recorded so that the work can be replicated.

The major difficulty is that for a Level II analysis, snooping has gotten even more aggressive. Beyond the data snooping done by CART itself, there now is a search over trees. As already noted many times, all statistical inference can be badly compromised.[24]

3.11   Missing Data

There are many different kinds of missing data. For our purposes, the plain vanilla kind is sufficient: for any given variable or variables, one or more elements are recorded as a blank, space, or some other character or code (e.g., -99) indicating that desired information is not provided. Sometimes, the data are missing by design. For example, a survey question asking about the ages of children in a household will be skipped for households with no children. Often the data are missing for no apparent reason. In either case, some missing data problems can be circumvented by clever coding (e.g., adding "skipped" as another level for a factor). More commonly, a variety of other remedies need to be considered.

Missing data are a frequent problem for statistical analyses, and CART is no exception. Broadly stated, missing data creates for CART the same kinds of difficulties created for conventional linear regression. There can be a loss of statistical power because of reductions in sample size if entire cases are lost. Bias can be introduced insofar as the information is missing in a systematic manner. IID properties and representativeness of the data can be lost.

There is one and only one ironclad solution to missing data regardless of the form of data analysis: don't have any. The message is that it pays to invest heavily in the data collection so that missing data does not materialize or is very rare. Missing data of a few percent rarely affects a data analysis in an important manner. A fallback position when there are substantial amounts missing data is to try to correct the missing data after the data are collected. For example, the primary documents from which the data were digitized may need to be examined.

But what does one do if neither the best solution nor fallback solution is available? Three kinds of missing data mechanisms are commonly considered that shape possible remedies. For a given variable or sets of variables, there may be no information about certain observations, and that information is "missing completely at random (MCAR)." By "missing completely at random," one means that the mechanism by which the data are lost is equivalent to simple random sampling. One can proceed working only with the complete observations. The primary price is a reduction in the number cases used in the analysis.

A more complicated case is when the information is "missing conditionally at random" or "missing at random (MAR)." Missing data for, say, X_1 depends on, say, X_2. After conditioning on certain variables, the data are now missing completely at random. For example, men may be less likely to report being a crime victim than women. But gender has nothing to do with actually being a crime victim. Perhaps men are just less likely to report being a crime victim. Whether such empirical claims are correct is often difficult to determine, and valid adjustments often depend on having an appropriate adjustment procedure. An essential feature of such procedures here would be including gender as a predictor.

Finally, the information may be "not missing at random" (NMAR). Sometimes this is called "nonignorable nonresponse." For example, individuals who have been crime victims several times may be less likely to report being victimized. The missing data mechanism depends on the variable whose missingness is problematic. This kind of missing data is the most difficult to handle in part because the use of models typically is central.

The easiest response to missing data in a multivariate setting is "listwise deletion." If for any case in the data any variable has a missing entry, that case is removed from the dataset. If the data are missing completely at random, the price primarily is a smaller number of observations.

A related response in a multivariate setting is "pairwise" deletion. The analysis proceeds with listwise deletion but only for each pair of variables. For example, if for least squares regression some of the predictors have missing values, the cross-product matrix of predictors is assembled for all pairs of predictors based on the number of complete observations for each pair. The computed covariances can be based on different numbers of observations.[25]

The most demanding response to missing data is imputation. The basic idea is to replace each missing value with a value that is a good approximation of what the missing value would have been. There are several ways this can be implemented.

For example, using the subset of cases that do not have missing data, one can regress the problematic predictor (e.g., income) on all of the complete predictors. For imputation, the regression fitted values from the variables included as predictors can be used as imputed entries for the missing data. To take a very simple example, for people with a college degree, there is a fitted value for their income that can be used as imputed income when for college graduates income is unknown.

Imputation introduces important complications. To begin, one does not ordinarily want to impute values for the response variable. Artificial relationships between the response and the predictors can be built into the analysis. If there are missing values for the response variable, listwise deletion is usually the prudent choice. But a new joint probability distribution likely has been defined. (e.g., Students with a GPA below 2.0 are excluded.) Estimates of generalization error, for instance, are for this new population.

Imputation for predictors alone is hardly problem free. Because the imputed values are rarely the same as the true values, measurement error is introduced. Even random measurement error in predictors can bias estimation.[26]

Another difficulty is that an imputed value is typically noisy, and that noise should be considered in how the data are analyzed. In practice, this can mean imputing missing data several times and taking any random variation into account. Also, imputed values for a given predictor will often have less variation than the natural variation in that predictor. The reduction in variability can make estimates for regression applications less precise.

Further discussion of missing data in general is beyond the scope of this book, and excellent treatments are easily found (Little and Rubin 2019). But it is important briefly to consider how missing data can affect CART in particular, and what some of the more common responses can be.

3.11.1 Missing Data with CART

Some of the missing data options for CART overlap with conventional practices, and some are special to CART. For the latter, we emphasize the CART options within *rpart*. In either case, there are statistical and subject-matter issues that must be considered in the context of *why* there is missing data to begin with. The "why" helps determine what the best response to the missing data should be.

Just as in conventional practice, listwise deletion is always an option, especially when one can make the case that the data are missing completely at random. If the data are missing conditionally at random, and the relevant conditioning variables are in the dataset, it is sometimes possible to build those conditioning variables into the analysis. Then one is back to missing data by, in effect, simple random sampling.

A second set of options is to impute the data outside of CART itself. Expanding on the earlier example, suppose again that for employed individuals there are some missing data for income. But income is strongly related to education, age, and occupation. For the subset of observations with no missing income data, income is regressed on education, age, and occupation. Then, for the observations that have missing income data, values for the three predictors can be inserted into the estimated regression equation. Predicted values follow that can be used to fill in the holes for the income variable. At that point, CART can be applied as usual.

A useful extension of this strategy is to sample randomly from the regression's predictive distribution to obtain several imputed values for each missing value. CART can then be applied to the data several times with different imputations in place. One can at least get a sense of whether random variation in imputed values makes an important difference (He 2006). If it does, there are averaging strategies derived from procedures addressed in the next chapter.

A third option is to address the missing data for predictors within CART itself. There are a number of ways this might be done. We consider here one of the better approaches, and the one available with *rpart* in R. As before, we only address missing data for predictors.

The first place where missing data will matter is when a split is chosen. Recall that the change in impurity is

$$\Delta I(s, A) = I(A) - P(A_L)I(A_L) - P(A_R)I(A_R), \qquad (3.15)$$

where for split s and node A, $I(A)$ is the value of the parent impurity, $P(A_R)$ is the probability of a case falling in the right daughter node, $P(A_L)$ is the probability of a case falling in the left daughter node, $I(A_R)$ is the impurity of the right daughter node, and $I(A_L)$ is the impurity of the left daughter node. CART tries to find the predictor and the split for which $\Delta I(s, A)$ is as large as possible.

Consider the leading term on the right-hand side. One can calculate its value without any predictors; there are no predictor missing values to worry about. However, to construct the two daughter nodes, predictors are required. Each predictor is evaluated as usual, but using only the predictor values that are not missing. That is, $I(A_R)$ and $I(A_L)$ are computed for each optimal split for each predictor using only the data available for that predictor. The associated probabilities $P(A_R)$ and $P(A_L)$ are re-estimated for each predictor in turn based on the data actually present. This is essentially pairwise deletion.

But determining the split is only half the story. Now, observations have to be assigned to one of the two daughter nodes. How can this be done if the predictor values needed are missing? CART employs a sort of "CART-lite" to impute those missing values by exploiting "surrogate variables."

Suppose there are ten other predictors $X_1 - X_{10}$ that are to be included in the CART analysis, and suppose there are missing observations for X_1 only, which happens to be the predictor chosen to define the split; the split defines two categories for X_1.

The predictor X_1 now becomes a binary response variable for the two classes determined by previously determined split. The coded values might be 1 for cases going in one partition and 0 for cases going in the other partition. CART is applied with binary X_1 as the response and $X_2 - X_{10}$ as potential splitting variables. Just as immediately above, pairwise deletion is employed. Only one partitioning is allowed;

a full tree is not constructed. The nine predictors are then ranked by the proportion of cases in X_1 that are misclassified. Predictors that do not do substantially better than the marginal distribution of X_1 are dropped from further consideration.

The variable with the lowest classification error for X_1 is used in place of X_1 to assign cases to one of the two daughter nodes when the observations on X_1 are missing. That is, a predicted class for X_1 is used when the actual classes for X_1 are missing. If there are missing data for the highest ranked predictor of X_1, the second highest predictor is used instead. If there are missing data for the second highest ranked predictor of X_1, the third highest predictor is used instead, and so on. If each of the variables $X_2 - X_{10}$ has missing data, the marginal distribution of the X_1 split is used. In practice, often this is exactly what happens. Imputation can fail just when it is most needed.

Perhaps the best advice is to avoid the use of surrogate variables. The temptations for misuse are great, and there is no clear missing data threshold beyond which imputation is unlikely to produce misleading results. Imputation of the missing values for the predictors will often be a software option, not a requirement. (But check what the default is.) It should not be implemented without a careful consideration of the consequences.

Alternatively, one should at least look carefully at the results with and without using surrogates. Results that are substantially different need to be reported to whomever is going to use the findings. There then may be a way to choose on subject-matter grounds which results are more sensible. Sometimes neither set will be sensible, which takes us back to where we began. Great efforts should be made to avoid missing data.

3.12 More on CART Instability

Estimation variance is not an issue for a CART Level I analysis because the enterprise is descriptive. Estimation variance is a significant issue for CART Level II analyses. Indeed, one of the reasons why CART is no longer a popular data analysis procedure is that it can be very unstable. And here, test data does not help, as we will soon see.

Perhaps, the most obvious difficulty is the stability in classes assigned to terminal nodes. Each fitted class is determined by a vote within a single terminal node. No estimation strength is borrowed from other nodes. Consequently, when the number of observations in a node is small, the results of the within-node vote could come out very differently in a new realized dataset. The instability can be especially troubling when the within-node votes are close and are coupled with a small number of observations. With slight changes in the composition of a node because of new IID realized data, the assigned class can change. If the assigned classes are unstable, generalization error will be inflated.

Instability can be even a greater problem in the partitioning process. Just as with the assignment of classes to terminal nodes, chance variation in just a few observations can make a critical difference. Moreover, the stagewise process guarantees that when an unstable splitting decisions is made, its consequences cascade through all subsequent splits. Recall also that although the "best" split is chosen at each stage, there may be very little difference in fitting performance between the best split and the second best split. And, just as with conventional stepwise regression, instability in tree structure is exacerbated with predictors that are strongly correlated.

3.13 Summary of Statistical Inference with CART

With extensive material on CART behind us, we now can focus on statistical inference for CART. Many problems and cautions have been discussed. Valid, Level II, statistical inference is now easily summarized.

As usual, one must be able to make a credible case that the data are IID from a substantively relevant joint probability distribution. The case will depend on how the data were obtained and on subject-matter expertise. One should not simply assume the data are IID and proceed.

The estimation target is an approximation of the true response surface. It would be truly remarkable if a classification or regression tree estimated the true response surface in an unbiased, or even asymptotically unbiased, manner — and how would you know? In addition, statistical tests and confidence intervals will almost certainly not get the correct p-values or coverage, respectively.

If one only has training data, usual inferential practice will not perform as advertised, even for the response surface approximation. Should the tuning parameters be determined before the data analysis begins, the adaptive nature of the greedy algorithm still precludes conventional statistical inference: estimation, statistical tests, and confidence intervals. Data snooping is built into the CART algorithm as the "best" splits are determined. An important complication is that CART is not just doing model selection. It is transforming all predictors into indicator variables in an adaptive fashion. It also allows for neighborhoods to be defined as products of indicator variables that are determined inductively. However, if one is satisfied with the earlier regression equation representation using indicator variables for the terminal nodes as predictors, all is not lost (Kuchibhotla et al. 2018a,b).

With training, evaluation and test data, or at least training and test data, and if as before, one is content working with a regression mean function using terminal node indicator variables as predictors, a valid form of statistical inference can be undertaken. The tree grown with the training data defines the terminal nodes, and therefore, specifies the structure of a mean function that can be used as an approximation of the true response surface in the originating joint probability distribution. Linear regression, logistic binomial regression, or logistic multinomial regression can be options depending on the kind of response variable. *This is essentially the formulation discussed in Chap. 1.*[27]

With the specification of the regression mean function now fixed, regression parameters and fitted values can be estimated with *test data* in an asymptotically valid manner because there is no longer any data snooping involved. From the perspective of the test data, the mean function specification is provided before the data analysis begins. One has a linear, binomial, or multinomial approximation of the true response surface whose regression coefficients and measures of fit can be interpreted in the manner discussed in Chap. 1. Standard errors for the regression coefficients can be estimated, as before, with either the sandwich or the nonparametric bootstrap.

With CART, the fitted values are likely to be the main focus. For numeric response variables, the fitted values are conditional means, which in a level II analysis may be treated as estimates of conditional expectations. Estimated measures of fit, such as the MSE, follow directly. For categorical variables, the fitted values are conditional proportions, which in a Level II analysis may be treated as estimates of conditional probabilities. Estimated measures of fit, such as the deviance, follow directly. Outcome classes are determined, as usual, and confusion tables coupled with performance measures are then easily computed. All such summary statistics can be treated as estimates of the corresponding features of the population approximation. Applying the nonparametric bootstrap, using the test data and the specified regression equation, will yield asymptotic valid statistical tests and confidence intervals for the estimated fit measures. In short, this is a conventional application of the nonparametric bootstrap to a regression equation.[28] In the next section, uncertainty in the fitted values themselves is addressed.

The same reasoning can be applied with split samples, although new judgment calls are introduced. The first judgment call is whether to split the data at all. If the dataset has relatively few observations, the risks are considerable. The statistical inference depends on asymptotics and splitting the data makes a small dataset smaller. Unfortunately, there is in practice no line below which the dataset is too small to split. A lot depends on the properties of the data and on how intensive the data search will be (e.g., how large a tree will be grown). But it is likely that datasets with fewer than several hundred observation should not be subdivided. One may well be limited to a Level I analysis.

The second judgment call is how many observations to allocate to each split. Here too, there is little guidance. Probably the most common choice is to construct splits with equal number of observations, but there is typically little formal rationale. Otherwise, relatively more cases should be allocated where precision and asymptotics are more important. One might, for instance, assign greater numbers of cases to the training data and the test data while assigning a smaller number of cases to the evaluation data. Or, one might not have an evaluation dataset at all and rely instead on cross-validation to tune the algorithm. Perhaps the best advice is to consult past studies in which such issues arose and learn from those. One can often get a good sense of what tradeoffs were made and with what consequences.

3.13.1 Summary of Statistical Inference for CART Forecasts

Recall that the manner in which the terminal nodes of a classification or regression tree are related to the fitted values is summarized properly by a conventional regression equation from the generalized linear model. The regression is not a model in itself because the tree on which it is based is not a model. When that mean function specification is used in concert with test data, the approximation framework discussed in Chap. 1 applies along with all of its features. The fitted values can be of interest in themselves and are the foundation for forecasting. The statistical inference required is much the same because the fitted values can be used properly as forecasts.

For forecasting, there are new data that are IID realizations from the joint probability distribution that generated the training data, the evaluation and test data; the same applies to split samples. The predictor variables are the same, but the response is unobserved. One can use the regression results to get a fitted value for each observation using procedures like *predict* in R. More simply, one can use the *predict* procedure directly with CART output. The fitted values can be used for forecasting.

If the response variable is numeric, the usual forecast will be a conditional mean. Split sample, conformal prediction intervals can follow naturally because one has already a split sample, and here too, one can work directly with CART output. An example of split sample, conformal prediction intervals was given in Chap. 2 based on material provided in Chap. 1.

There are more choices to be made when the response variable is categorical. If one is interested in forecasting the probability of an outcome class, the conformal approach still works. G is an indicator variable, usually coded 0 or 1, and the forecasted value is a probability. For each case, subtracting the fitted probability from the indicator variable leads to residuals that can be treated as before. All else plays through. Conformal scores can take a variety of forms.

If one is interested in forecasting an outcome class, the task must be reformulated. When an outcome class is a 1 or a 0, how can an interval around either sensibly be constructed? Only values of 1 or 0 are allowed. Several interesting strategies have been proposed (e.g., Balasubramanian et al. 2014, section 1.3.1) but so far at least, they do not address well what is needed in practice. The position here is reconsider what one wants to know.

Think back to a confusion table. From the columns, one can compute the probability that when a given class is forecasted, that forecasted class is correct. One surely has useful information that goes directly to the role of uncertainty. And when the confusion table is constructed from test data, one has asymptotically valid results, given the population approximation determined by the classification tree. But a confusion table is meant to characterize how the approximation performs for all possible realized cases from the joint probability distribution. In contrast, forecasts usually are made for individual cases. Moreover, one does not know the actual class when forecasts are made.

Useful information is easily found in the terminal node in which a forecasting case falls. Each terminal node is populated with test data and for each case, one knows the actual class and the forecasted class. One also knows the in-node vote proportion for the class assigned, which can be interpreted as the probability that the assigned class is correct. Because the proportion is computed from IID test data, the usual expression for the standard error applies from which, if desired, a confidence interval can be computed.

But one must be clear that uncertainty in the recursive partitioning and the training data are being ignored. *Given* the training data and the tree structure, one can with test data construct a defensible forecast with its associated uncertainty, an estimate of the probability that the forecasted class is correct, and a valid confidence interval around that probability. The uncertainty addressed comes solely from the IID test data. There are many real- life forecasting situations in which this approach corresponds well to actual practice. Forecasting tools are developed, the forecasting tools are treated as fixed, and forecasts are made. Unaddressed is what would happen if the forecasting tools were updated or reconstructed from scratch with new data.

Finally, because all of the data used must be IID from the same joint probability distribution, the fitted values obtained when the response variable value is known have the same statistical properties as the fitted values obtained when the response variable value is unknown. That is, one can think of test data as forecasting data for which the outcome is already in the dataset.

3.14   Overall Summary and Conclusions

CART has the look and feel of an effective statistical learning tool. It is relatively easy to use, builds directly on familiar regression procedures, does not demand great computing power, and generates output that can be presented in an accessible manner. CART also provides a useful way to introduce the costs of classification errors. However, CART has some important limitations.

First, if one wants an unbiased estimate of the true $f(\mathbf{X})$, there is no reason to believe that CART's $\hat{f}(X)$ will provide it, or that it will even come close. Despite the flexible ways in which CART can respond to data, substantial bias is a virtual certainty. All fitting procedures are limited by the data available. Key predictors be absent. But even if the requisite data are provided, the use of step functions and the stagewise estimation procedure are significant complications. Powerful data snooping is also in the mix.

One can always settle for a Level I analysis. A fallback Level II strategy is to work with a best linear approximation of the true response surface computed from test data. Asymptotically valid statistical inference, including statistical tests and confidence intervals, can follow.

Second, each of the splitting decisions can be very unstable. A few observations can in some situations dramatically affect which variables are selected and the values used for partitioning the data. Then, all subsequent partitions can be altered.

This instability is closely related to overfitting, which can substantially limit the generalizability of the results. The findings from the data examined may not generalize well to other random realizations from the same population (let alone to data from other populations). This means that any approximation of the true response surface could have been very different. Treating the training data and fitted tree as fixed and relying on test data for statistical inference is formally correct, but ignores instability in the fitted tree passed on to the test data.

Third, for classification, the classes assigned to terminal nodes by the fitted tree can be unstable too. When the computed proportions for the terminal node classes are about the same, the movement of just a few cases from one side of a proportion threshold to the other can change the assigned class. It can be instructive, therefore, to examine the distributions in each terminal node. If many of the votes from the fitted tree are close, there is even more concern about instability.

Finally, even moderately elaborate tree diagrams will seriously tax substantive understanding. The problem is not just complexity. CART is trying in a single-minded manner to use associations in the data to maximize the homogeneity of its data partitions. How those associations come to be represented may have nothing remotely to do with subject-matter understandings or how subject-matter experts think about those associations. High order interaction effects are a dramatic illustration. The apparent transparency of the tree display is a ruse.

In short, CART is unlikely to be a useful, stand-alone, data analysis procedure. One needs to do better, and one can. With that aspiration, we turn in the next chapter to bagging.

Exercises

Problem Set 1

The purpose of this exercise is to provide an initial sense of how CART compares to conventional linear regression when the response variable is quantitative.

1. To begin, construct a regression dataset with known properties:

```
x1=rnorm(300)
x2=rnrom(300)
error=2*rnorm(300)
y1=1+(2*x1)+(3*x2)+error
```

Apply conventional linear regression using *lm*. Then apply *rpart*, and print the tree using *prp* from the library *rpart.plot*. Compare the regression output to the way in which the data were actually generated. Compare the tree diagram to the way in which the data were actually generated. Compare how well linear regression and CART fit the data. For CART, use *rsq.rpart* from the library *library(rpart.plot)* to consider the fit. What do you conclude about the relative merits of linear regression and CART when the $f(X)$ is actually linear and additive?

2. Now, redefine the two predictors as binary factors and reconstruct the response variable.

```
x11=(x1 > 0)
x22=(x2 > 0)
y=1+(2*x11)+(3*x22)+error
```

Proceed as before comparing linear regression to CART. How do they compare? What do you conclude about the relative merits of linear regression and CART when the $f(X)$ is actually a step function and additive?

3. Under what circumstances is CART likely to perform better than linear regression? Consider separately the matter of how well the fitted values correspond to the observed values and the interpretation of how the predictors are related to the response.

Problem Set 2

The goal of the following exercises is to give you some hands-on experience with CART in comparison with some of the procedures covered in earlier chapters. An initial hurdle is getting R to do what you want. There are lots of examples in the chapter. Also, make generous use of *help* and I have provided a number of hints along the way. However, I have tried to guide you to results in the least complicated way possible and as a consequence, some of the more subtle features of CART are not explored. Feel free to play with these in addition. You can't break anything.

Load the data set called "frogs" from the DAAG library. The data are from a study of ecological factors that may affect the presence of certain frog populations. The binary response variable is pres.abs. Use the help command to learn about the data. For ease of interpretation, limit yourself to the following predictors: altitude, distance, NoOfPools, NoOfSites, avrain, meanmin, and meanmax.

1. Use logistic regression from *glm* to consider how the predictors are related to whether frogs are present. Which predictors seem to matter? Do their signs make sense?

2. Using the procedure *stepAIC* from the *MASS* library with the default for stepwise direction, find the model that minimizes the AIC. Which predictors remain? Do their signs make sense?

3. Using *table*, construct a confusion table for the model arrived at by the stepwise procedure. The observed class is pres.abs. You will need to assign class labels to cases to get the "predicted" class. The procedure *glm* stores under the name "fitted.values" the estimated conditional probabilities of the presence of frogs. If the probability is greater than 0.5, assign a 1 to that case. If the probability is equal to or less than 0.5, assign a 0 to that case. Now cross-tabulate the true class by the assigned class. What fraction of the cases is classified incorrectly? Is

classification more accurate for the true presence of frogs or the true absence of frogs? What is the rationale for using 0.5 as the threshold for class assignment? What is the cost ratio in the table? What are its implications for an overall measure of classification performance? (Hint: some classifications are likely to be relatively more costly than others. This needs to be taken into account for all confusion tables, not just those from CART.)

4. Using your best model from the stepwise procedure, apply the generalized additive model. You can use *gam* in either the *gam* or *mvcv* library. Use smoothers for each predictor. Let the procedure decide how many degrees of freedom to use for each smooth. Look at the numerical output and the smoothed plots. How do the results compare to those from logistic regression?

5. Construct a confusion table for the model arrived at through GAM. Once again, the observed class is pres.abs. Use the same logic as applied previously to *glm* to determine the assigned class. What fraction of the cases is classified incorrectly? Is classification more accurate for the true presence of frogs or the true absence of frogs? How do these results compare to the GLM results? (Hint: don't forget to cost-weight the overall measure of classification accuracy.)

6. Going back to using all of the predictors you began with, apply CART to the frog data via the procedure *rpart* in the library *rpart*. For now, accept all of the default settings. But it is usually a good idea to specify the method (here, method="class") rather than let *rpart* try to figure it out from your response variable. Use the *print* command to see some key numerical output. Try to figure out what each piece of information means. Use *rpart.plot* to construct a tree diagram. What predictors does CART select as important? How do they compare with your results from GLM and GAM? How do the interpretations of the results compare?

7. Use *predict* to assign class labels to cases. You will need to use the help command for *predict.rpart* to figure out how to do this. Then construct a confusion table for the assigned class and the observed class. What fraction of the cases is classified incorrectly? Is classification more accurate for the true presence of frogs or the true absence of frogs? How do these results compare to the GLM and GAM results? If the three differ substantially, explain why you think this has happened. Alternatively, if the three are much the same, explain why you think this has happened.

8. Run the CART analysis again with different priors. Take a close look at the information available for *rpart* using the help command. For example, for a perfectly balanced prior in *rpart* you would include *parms=list(prior= c(0.50,0.50))*. Try a prior of 0.5 for presence and then a prior of 0.30 for presence. (For this *rpart* parameter, the prior probability of 0 comes first and the prior probability of 1 comes second.) What happens to the ratio of false negatives to false positives? What happens to the overall amount of cost-weighted classification error compared to the default?

9. Set the prior so that in the confusion table false negatives are about ten times more costly than false positives (with pres.abs = 1 called a "positive" and pres.abs = 0 called a "negative"). Apply CART. Study the output from *print*,

the tree diagram using *rpart.plot*, and the confusion table. What has changed enough to affect your interpretations of the results? What has not changed enough to affect your interpretations of the results? *rpart.plot*

10. Construct two random samples with replacement of the same size as the dataset. Use the *sample* command to select at random the rows of data you need and use those values to define a new sample with R's indexing capability, *x[r,c]*. For the two new samples, apply CART with the default parameters. Construct a tree diagram for each. How do the two trees compare to each other and to your earlier results with default settings? What does this tell you about how stable your CART results are and about potential problems with overfitting.

11. Repeat what you have just done, but now set the minimim terminal node size to 50. You will need the argument *control=rpart.control (minbucket=50))* in your call to *rpart*. How do the three trees compare now? What are the implications for overfitting in CART?

Problem Set 3

Here is another opportunity to become familiar with CART, but this time with a quantitative response variable. From the library *car*, load the data set "Freedman." The dataset contains for 100 American cities the crime rate, population size, population density, and percent nonwhite of the population. The goal is to see what is associated with the crime rate.

1. Using the *gam* from the library *gam*, regress the crime rate on the smoothed values of the three predictors. Examine the numerical output and the plots. Describe how the crime rate is related to the three predictors.

2. Repeat the analysis using *rpart* and the default settings. Describe how the crime rate is related to the three predictors. How do the conclusions differ from those using the generalized additive model?

3. Plot the fitted values from the GAM analysis against the fitted values from the CART analysis. The fitted values for *gam* are stored automatically. You will need to construct the fitted values for CART using *predict.rpart*. What would the plot look like if the two sets of fitted values corresponded perfectly? What do you see instead? What does the scatterplot tell you about how the two sets of fitted values are related?

4. Overlay on the scatterplot the least squares line for the two sets of fitted values using *abline*. If that regression line had a slope of 1.0 and an intercept of 0.0, what would that indicate about the relationship between the two sets of fitted values? What does that overlaid regression line indicate about how the two sets of fitted values are related?

5. Using *scatter.smooth*, apply a lowess smoother to the scatterplot of the two sets of fitted values. Try several different spans. What do you conclude about the functional form of the relationship between the two sets of fitted values?

6. For the GAM results and the CART results, use *cor* to compute separately the correlations between the fitted values and the observed values for the crime rate. What procedure has fitted values that are more highly correlated with the crime rate? Can you use this to determine which modeling approach fits the data better? If yes, explain why. If no, explain why.

Problem Set 4

1. At a number of places, the bootstrap has been mentioned and applied. The basic idea behind the bootstrap is easy enough in broad brushstrokes. But the details can be challenging even for math-stat types because there are important subtleties and many different bootstrap variants. Fortunately, for many of the applications that have been discussed and that will be discussed, uncertainty in some important features of the output can be usefully addressed with procedures available in R. Currently, *boot* is popular because of its great flexibility. But it has a relatively steep learning curve, and some readers may prefer to write their own bootstrap code.

The code below produces a bootstrap distribution of the proportion of correct classification in a CART confusion table using the Titanic data and the outcome class of survival. From the empirical distribution, one can consider the sampling distribution for the proportion correctly classified and construct a confidence interval.

The code is meant to only be illustrative. As already mentioned, it probably makes little sense to consider a Level II analysis for the Titanic data. However, code like this will work for test data should a Level II analysis be appropriate. The main difference is that there would be no new CART fit for each bootstrap sample. The rpart step shown in the code would not be included. Rather, the rpart-object would be computed outside of the function and called when *predict* was used with test data.

Run the code and consider the output. Then try it with another dataset and test data. Interpret the CART confusion table and the distribution of the proportion of cases correctly classified.

```
# Application of nonparametric bootstrap for CART
library(PASWR)
library(boot)
library(rpart)
data("titanic3")
attach(titanic3)
temp<-data.frame(survived,pclass,sex,age)
# Select variables working1<-na.omit(temp)
# Remove NAs from training data
detach(titanic3)

# Apply CART to training data
```

```
out<-rpart(survived~sex+age+pclass,data=working1,
           method="class")

# Define the function to be bootstrapped
confusion<-function(data,i) # i is the index for
    the bootstrap sample
{
  working2<-working1[i,] # names the bootstrap
    sample for each iteration i
  preds<-predict(out,data=working2) # get fitted
    values
  conf<-table(preds[,2]>.5,working2$survived)
    # Confusion table as usual
  fit<-(conf[1,1]+conf[2,2])/dim(working2)[1]
    # Proportion correct
  return(fit)
}

# Apply the bootstrap and examine the output
fitting<-boot(working1,confusion,R=300) # Look at
    the object
plot(fitting)
quantile(fitting$t,probs=c(.025,.975))
```

Endnotes

[1] There are extensions of CART that go beyond the generalized linear model. A parallel to multinomial logistic regression is one example. But for didactic purposes these extensions are addressed later.

[2] A good *multinomial* regression procedure in R is *multinom* in library *nnet*. Technically, multinomial logistic regression is not a GLM, which is a good reason why it is not included in the *glm* library in R.

[3] Some orders for splits of the same predictor cannot work. For example, age might be first split at 30 and then later at 18. This works for the partition of individuals less than or equal to 30 because there are likely to be some individuals at, above, or below 18. But for the partition including those over 30, there are no 18 year olds on which to further partition the data. In short, only some orders are feasible. But it can be important to appreciate which splits are not chosen and which splits cannot be chosen.

[4] It is easy to confuse the regression equation representation of terminal nodes with a model. It is not a model. It is a summary of how the terminal nodes as predictors are related to the response; it is synopsis of the output from an algorithm, nothing more (or less).

[5] Among the many problems is that the step functions used to grow a tree are discontinuous.

[6]Thanks go to Thomas Cason who updated and improved the existing Titanic data frame using the Encyclopedia Titanica.

[7]The procedure *rpart* is authored by Terry Therneau and Beth Atkinson. The procedure *rpart.plot* is authored by Stephen Milborrow. Both procedures are superb. One can embed *rpart* in procedures from the *caret* library to gain access to a wide variety of handy (if a bit overwhelming) enhancements. A risk is data analysis decisions, which should be informed in part by subject-matter expertise and are dominated by code-automated determinations. Subject-matter nonsense can result. Users should not automatically surrender control to what appear to be labor-saving devices. The *caret* library was written by Max Kuhn.

[8]Here, the use of the class labels "success" and "failure" is arbitrary, so which off-diagonal cells contain "false positives" or "false negatives" is arbitrary as well. What is called a "success" in one study may be called a "failure" in another study.

[9]The use of I in Eq. (3.2) for impurity should not be confused with the use of I to represent an indicator variable. The different meanings should be clear in context.

[10]In statistics, cross-entropy is called the deviance.

[11]There is often a preference for a relatively small number of very homogeneous terminal nodes rather than a much large number of terminal nodes that are not especially homogeneous. This is likely if the kinds of cases in the very homogeneous nodes have a special subject-matter or policy importance. An instance is inmates being considered for release on parole who fall into a terminal node in which most of the parolees are re-arrested for a crime of violence. These inmates may be few in number, but their crimes can be particularly harmful.

[12]Misconduct can be minor offenses like failing to report for a work assignment to offenses that would be serious felonies if committed outside of prison (e.g., aggravated assault). Because of privacy concerns, the data may not be shared.

[13]The tree diagram is formatted differently from the tree diagram used for the Titanic data to emphasize the terminal nodes.

[14]In R, the character variable default order left to right is alphabetical.

[15]The issues are actually tricky and beyond the scope of this discussion. At intake, how an inmate will be placed and supervised are unknown and are, therefore, not relevant predictors. Yet, the training data may need to take placement and supervision into account.

[16]The overfitting may not be serious in this case because the number of observations is large and a small tree was grown.

[17]As Therneau and Atkinson (2015: section 3.3.2) state,"When altered priors are used, they affect only the choice of split. The ordinary losses and priors are used to compute the risk of the node. The altered priors simply help the impurity rule choose splits that are likely to be good in terms of the risk." By "risk" they mean the expected costs from false negatives and false positives.

[18]The argument parms = list(prior = c(0.65,0.35)) sets the marginal distribution of a binary outcome to 0.65 and 0.35. A coded example follows shortly.

[19]Very similar results could be obtained using *minbucket* rather than *cp*, even though they are defined very differently.

[20]These are not options in *rpart*.

[21]These data cannot be shared.

[22]The function defaults to only black and white. If you want color (or something else), you need to get into the source code. It's not a big deal.

[23]The requirement of independence would need to be very carefully considered because some of the applicants may be from the same high schools and may have been influenced in similar ways by a teacher or guidance counselor. Fortunately, the independence assumptions can be relaxed somewhat, as mentioned briefly earlier (Kuchibhotla et al. 2018b). The main price is that a larger number of observations are likely to be necessary.

[24]One might wonder again why CART does not use Eq. (3.14) from the start when a tree is grown instead of some measure of node impurity. $R_{cp}(T)$ would seem to have built in all of the end-user needs very directly. As mentioned earlier, the rationale for not using a function of classification errors as a fitting criterion is discussed in Breiman et al. (1984: section 4.1). As a technical matter, there can be at any given node, no single best split. But perhaps a more important reason is that less satisfactory trees can result.

[25]In a least squares regression setting, this is generally not a good idea because the covariance matrix may no longer be positive definite. And for many algorithmic procedures, this is not a feasible approach in any case.

[26]Consider a conventional regression with a single predictor. Random measurement error (i.e., IID mean 0) will increase the variance of the predictor, which sits in the denominator of slope expression. Asymptotically, $\hat{\beta} = \frac{\beta}{1+\sigma_\epsilon^2/\sigma_x^2}$, where σ_ϵ^2 is the variance of the measurement error, and σ_x^2 is the variance of the predictor. The result is a bias toward 0.0. When there is more than one predictor, each with random measurement error, the regression coefficients can be biased toward 0.0 or away from 0.0.

[27]Data analysts should *not* re-apply CART to the test data, even if the tuning parameter values have been determined. The algorithm is incurably adaptive.

[28]These estimate of fitting performance correspond to neither estimates of generalization error nor expected prediction error, although they are in that spirit. One would need another test dataset to implement either definition.

References

Balasubramanian, V. N., Ho, S.-S., & Vovk, V. (2014). *Conformal prediction for reliable machine learning.* Amsterdam: Elsevier.

Berk, R. A. (2018). *Machine learning forecasts of risk in criminal justice settings.* New York: Springer.

Bhat, H. S., Kumer, N., & Vaz, G. (2011). *Quantile Regression Trees.* Working paper, School of Natural Sciences, University of California, Merced, CA.

Breiman, L., Friedman, J. H., Olshen, R. A., & Stone, C. J. (1984). *Classification and regression trees.* Monterey, CA: Wadsworth Press.

Chaudhuri, P., & Loh, W.-Y. (2002). Nonparametric estimation of conditional quantiles using quantile regression trees. *Bernoulli, 8*(5), 561–576.

Chaudhuri, P., Lo, W.-D., Loh, W.-Y., & Yang, C.-C. (1995). Generalized regression trees. *Statistic Sinica, 5*, 641–666.

Chipman, H. A., George, E. I., & McCulloch, R. E. (1998). Bayesian CART model search. *Journal of the American Statistical Association, 93*(443), 935–948.

Chipman, H. A., George, E. I., & McCulloch, R. E. (1999). Hierarchical priors for Bayesian CART shrinkage. *Statistics and Computing, 10*(1), 17–24.

Chipman, H. A., George, E. I., & McCulloch, R. E. (2010). BART: Bayesian additive regression trees. *Annals of Applied Statistics, 4*(1): 266–298.

Choi, Y., Ahn, H., & Chen, J. J. (2005). Regression trees for analysis of count data with extra poisson variation. *Computational Statistics & Data Analysis, 49*, 893–915.

Grubinger, T., Zeileis, A., & Pfeiffer, K.-P. (2014). evtree: Evolutionary learning of globally optimal classification and regression trees in R. *Journal of Statistical Software, 61*(1). http://www.jstatsoft.org/

He, Y. (2006). *Missing Data Imputation For Tree-Based Models*. PhD dissertation for the Department of Statistics, UCLA.

Hothorn, T., Hornik, K., & Zeileis, A. (2006). Unbiased recursive partitioning: a conditional inference framework. *Journal of Computational and Graphical Statistics, 15*(3), 651–674.

Ishwaran, H. (2015). The effect of splitting on random forests. *Machine Learning, 99*, 75–118.

Kass, G. V. (1980). An exploratory technique for investigating large quantities of categorical data. *Applied Statistics, 29*(2), 119–127.

Kuchibhotla, A. K., Brown, L. D., & Buja, A. (2018a). Model-free study of ordinary least squares linear regression. arXiv: 1809.10538v1 [math.ST].

Kuchibhotla, A. K., Brown, L. D., Buja, A., George, E. I., & Zhao, L. (2018b). A model free perspective for linear regression: uniform-in-model bounds for post selection inference. arXiv:1802.05801.

Lee, S. K. (2005). On generalized multivariate decision tree by using GEE. *Computational Statistics & Data Analysis, 49*, 1105–1119.

Little, R., & Rubin, D. (2019). *The statistical analysis of missing data* (3rd ed.). New York: John Wiley.

Loh, W.-L. (2014). Fifty years of classification and regression trees (with discussion). *International Statistical Review, 82*(3), 329–348.

Meinshausen, N. (2006). Quantile regression forests. *Journal of Machine Learning Research, 7*, 983–999.

Quinlan, R. (1993). *Programs in machine learning*. San Mateo, CA: Morgan Kaufman.

Therneau, T. M., & Atkinson, E. J. (2015). *An Introduction to Recursive Partitioning Using the RPART Routines*. Technical Report, Mayo Foundation.

Wu, Y., Tjelmeland, H., & West, M. (2007). Bayesian CART: Prior specification and posterior simulation. *Journal of Computational and Graphical Statistics, 16*(1), 44–66.

Xiaogang, S., Tianni, Z., Xin, Y., Juanjuan, F., & Song, Y. (2008). Interaction trees with censored survival data. *The International Journal of Biostatistics, 4*(1), Article 2.

Zeileis, A., Hothorn, T., & Hornik, K. (2008). Model-based recursive partitioning. *Journal of Computational and Graphical Statistics, 17*(2), 492–514.

Zhang, H., & Singer, B. (1999). *Recursive partitioning in the health sciences*. New York: Springer.

Chapter 4
Bagging

Summary We have in earlier chapters considered fitting algorithms for which there are a single set of results. Perhaps most important, there is one set of fitted values. These are often unstable and subject to a painful bias – variance tradeoff. In this chapter, we turn to what some call "ensemble" algorithms which can produce many sets of fitted values. These, in turn, can be averaged in a manner that reduces instability, often with no increase in the bias. We begin with a discussion of bagging.

4.1 Introduction

In this chapter, we make a major transition. We have thus far focused on statistical procedures that produce a single set of results: regression coefficients, measures of fit, residuals, classifications, and others. There is but one regression equation, one set of smoothed values, or one classification tree. Most statistical procedures operate in a similar fashion.

The discussion now shifts to statistical learning that builds on many sets of outputs aggregated to produce results. Such algorithms make a number of passes over the data. On each pass, inputs are linked to outputs just as before. But the ultimate results of interest are the collection of all the results from all passes over the data.

Bayesian model averaging may be a familiar illustration from another statistical tradition (Madigan et al. 1996; Hoeting et al. 1999). In Bayesian model averaging, there is an assumed $f(X)$; there is a "true model." A number of potentially true models, differing in the predictors selected, are evaluated. The model output is then averaged with weights determined by model uncertainty. Output from models with greater uncertainty is given less weight. From a statistical learning perspective, Bayesian model averaging has a number of complications, including the dependence that is necessarily built in across model results (Xu and Golay 2006). Also, it is not

© Springer Nature Switzerland AG 2020

R. A. Berk, *Statistical Learning from a Regression Perspective*,
Springer Texts in Statistics, https://doi.org/10.1007/978-3-030-40189-4_4

clear why a model with less uncertainty is necessarily closer to the true model. We address shortly how statistical learning procedures relying on multiple results proceed rather differently.

Aggregate results from many passes over the data can have several important benefits. For example, under the right circumstances, averaging over sets of fitted values can increase their stability and can be seen as a form of regularization. The averaging tends to cancel out results shaped by idiosyncratic features of the data. In turn, generalization error is reduced. An increase in stability permits the use of more complex functions of the predictors when they are needed. As mentioned in Chap. 1, this is a general theme in machine learning: compute a complex set of fitted values and then regularize.

In this chapter, we focus on bagging, which capitalizes on a particular kind of averaging process that can address complexity and stability. In more traditional terms, bagging can have beneficial consequences for the bias–variance tradeoff. Sometimes you can have your cake and eat it too.

Although bagging can be applied to a wide variety of statistical procedures, we will again concentrate on classifiers. The rationale is largely the same: the exposition is more effective and the step to quantitative responses is easy to make. We begin with a return to the problem of overfitting. Although overfitting has been discussed several times in earlier chapters, it needs to be linked more explicitly to CART to help set the stage for a full exposition of bagging and subsequent procedures. In this chapter, we will bag classification and regression trees.

4.2   The Bagging Algorithm

The notion of combining fitted values from a number of fitting attempts has been suggested by several authors (LeBlanc and Tibshirani 1996; Mojirsheibani 1997, 1999). In an important sense, the whole becomes more than the sum of its parts. It is a bit like crowdsourcing.

"Bagging," which stands for "Bootstrap Aggregation," is perhaps the earliest procedure to exploit sets of fitted values over random samples of the data. Unlike model averaging, bagging is not a way to arrive at a model. Bagging is an algorithm that can help improve the performance of fitted values from a given statistical procedure. Breiman's remarkable 1996 paper on bagging is well worth a careful read. We focus, as before, on classification trees with a binary outcome as the "given statistical procedure." We later consider other statistical procedures for which bagging can be helpful.

For training data having N observations and a binary response variable, bagging classification trees takes the following form:

1. Take a random sample of size N *with replacement* from the data. These are sometimes called "bootstrap samples."
2. Construct a classification tree as usual.

3. Assign a class to each terminal node as usual, that determines the class assigned to each case. Store the class attached to each case and the predictor values that define the neighborhood in which each terminal node resides (e.g., males under 30 years of age with a high school diploma).
4. Repeat Steps 1–3 a large number of times.
5. For each observation in the dataset, count the number of times over trees that it is classified in one category and the number of times over trees it is classified in the other category.
6. Assign each observation to a final class by a majority vote over the set of trees. If the outcome has two classes, and more than 50% of the time over a large number of trees a given observation is classified as a 1, that becomes its classification. The same reasoning applies to the 0 class. The winning class is determined by a majority vote.

These steps easily generalize to categorical responses that have more than two classes. All that changes is voting procedure: a plurality, which is not necessarily a majority, wins. However, there can be subtle interpretive issues with pluralities. Suppose the vote over classification trees for each of the three classes A, B, and C is 40%, 30%, 30%, respectively. Class A wins the plurality but B and C combined take the majority of votes. The majority vote is against the winner by a plurality. This issue will be addressed in a bit more depth later. There will be no technical solution. A resolution will depend on stakeholders and how they intend to use the results.

Although there remain important variations and details to consider, these are the key steps to produce bagged classification trees. There is averaging by votes within each terminal node as before, but now there also is averaging by votes over classification trees. The voting outcomes for both steps result in proportions that can be seen as a means for response variables coded as 1 or 0.

The assigned class over trees for each case is used much as it was for CART. Confusion tables are good place to start. But there is no longer a single tree to interpret because there are many trees and no such thing as an average tree. Predictor values are linked to fitted classes, but not in a manner that can be substantively interpreted. We have a true black box statistical learning procedure. There will be more of them.

4.3   Some Bagging Details

The bagging algorithm may seem straightforward. Bagging is just as way to average away unwanted noise. But there are a number of subtleties that we will need to carry forward in this chapter and later chapters.

4.3.1   Revisiting the CART Instability Problem

One good way to motivate bagging is to consider again the instability of classification trees. That instability can be readily apparent even across bootstrap samples that necessarily share large fractions of the data.

Figure 4.1 shows two such classification trees from the Titanic data. Although, as before, the first split for both is on gender, the two trees subsequently part company. The next two splits are the same for both trees, but the thresholds differ. Then, the splits that follow on the right branch differ in some of the predictors selected

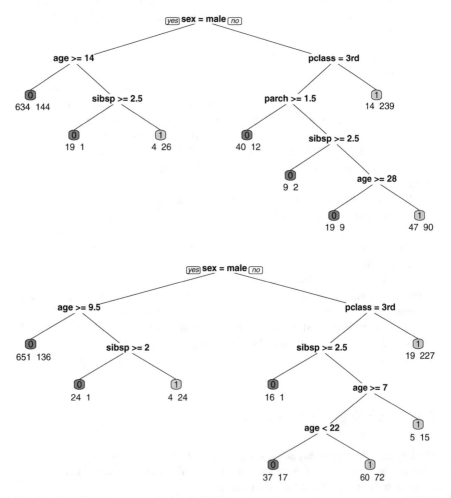

Fig. 4.1 Classification tree analysis of titanic survival for two bootstrap samples of 1309 observations from the same training data (the red nodes are assigned the class of "perished," and the blue nodes are assigned the class of "survived")

as well as thresholds. And the counts in all of the terminal nodes vary across the two trees. All of these differences lead to somewhat different classifications. For example, there are 10 boys between 9.5 and 13 years of age who are excluded from the far left terminal node on the top tree but who are not excluded from the far left terminal node on the bottom tree. Overall, about 10% of the cases common to both trees were classified differently. The bottom tree was more likely to assign the class of "survived" than the top tree. This is a best case scenario in the sense that about 68% of the observations in the two analyses are shared, and the overall sample size is relatively large. More commonly, recursive partitioning is far more unstable.

A classification tree can be used for Level I analyses when all one cares about is characterizing the data on hand. Instability becomes relevant for Level II analyses. For example, instability is a concern for generalization error, which speaks to performance in test data and other realized observations from the generative joint probability distribution. The same reasoning applies to bagging. Because bagging addresses instability, a Level II perspective is foundational.[1]

4.3.2 Resampling Methods for Bagging

The top bagging priority is to reduce instability, and it all begins with resampling. Resampling is a general term meant to convey that one or more new datasets are constructed by chance procedures *from the original dataset on hand*.

Over the past two decades, many resampling procedures have been developed that can provide information about the sampling distributions of data-derived estimates. The bootstrap is perhaps the most well known. Other techniques include the jackknife (Efron and Tibshirani 1993: section10.5) and permutation tests (Edgington and Ongehena 2007). Resampling procedures can provide asymptotically valid tests and confidence intervals making fewer assumptions than conventional methods and can sometimes be applied when there are no conventional methods at all. For a discussion of bagging, we only need a few ideas from the bootstrap, and in particular, how one can generate a very large number of random samples from training data. There are very good and extensive treatments of the bootstrap provided by Efron and Tibshirani (1993) and Hall (1997).

Usually, the bootstrap is seen as a simulation of the frequentist thought experiment and as such, is automatically a Level II formulation. For the frequentist, the data on hand are realized independently from a joint probability distribution or a finite population. In Fig. 4.2, the process is shown by the thick arrow toward the left side. The data on hand are seen as a single set of independent realizations from a limitless number of observations that could be realized. In this theoretical world of limitless datasets from independently realized observations, sample statistics in principle can be computed from each dataset leading to one or more sampling distributions (i.e., one for each feature of the joint probability distribution being estimated). Conventional confidence intervals and statistical tests follow directly.

Fig. 4.2 A schematic for
bootstrap sampling

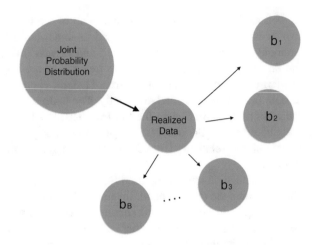

In the real world, one is able to draw $b_1, b_2, \ldots, b_B$ random samples with
replacement that empirically simulate the statistical theory of limitless data realizations. From these, empirically computed confidence intervals and statistical tests
can follow. For example, if the mean were computed from each of the bootstrap
sample, the result would an empirical sampling distribution for the mean. A 95%
confidence interval for the mean might be the next step.

There are many different kinds of bootstrap procedures, and it remains an
important research area. The resampling just described is sometimes called a "pairs"
bootstrap because both Y and X are sampled, or a "nonparametric" bootstrap
because there is no model specified through which the realized data were generated.

Bagging exploits the resampling strategy in the algorithm's first step, but with
an interpretative twist. A total of N observations with replacement is drawn.
Sampling with replacement on the average causes about 37% of cases to be excluded
from a given sample. It follows that a substantial number of cases are selected
more than once. From a frequentist perspective, one has the formal sampling
properties required,[2] but there is less information in such samples than had all of the
observations appeared only once. Some statistical power can be lost, and procedures
that are sample-size dependent can suffer.[3]

But for bagging, the resampling is *not* being used to construct an empirical
sampling distribution. The resampling is an algorithmic device that allows one to
draw a large number of random samples with N observations from the data. Each
sample is used to grow a tree whose fitted values are then averaged case by case over
trees. There is no estimation. There are also no confidence intervals or statistical
tests.

As a result of the sampling with replacement, each tree automatically has about
$0.37 \times N$ "hold-out" observations, often called "out-of-bag" (OOB) observations,
which are not used to grow that tree. The OOB observations are an immediate source
of test data for that tree, and each tree will have its own OOB data created by random
sampling with replacement. Having valid test data as a byproduct of sampling with

replacement is huge. Up to this point, test data had to be obtained as part of the data collection process or constructed from split samples. We will exploit OOB data shortly.

4.3.3 Votes Over Trees and Probabilities

When one bags a set of classification trees, conventional practice relies on CART. That is, each tree is grown in the same manner discussed in the previous chapter: recursive partitioning using a loss function for a categorical response variable to determine the best splits, followed by assigned classes determined by a vote within each terminal node. In this chapter, we take conventional CART as a given.

The bagging innovation is to take for each case a vote over trees to determine the assigned class. The vote for any case can be represented as two or more proportions (e.g., for case i, 0.35 for class A and 0.65 for class B). Because the bagging classifier is grown with an IID sample of *the training data*, the proportions of votes each class musters have the look and feel of probabilities.

Even if the assumptions required for a probability interpretation are met, the probabilities for each case capture *the chances that the bagging algorithm consistently assigns that case to the same class.*[4] The "trial" behind each probability is the application of CART to a new random sample of the training data (Breiman 1996: section 4.2). One has a measure of the algorithm's *reliability*. One does not have a measure of the chances that for that the class assigned is the correct class. There is often confusion on this point.

Here is a simple example. Suppose for a particular neighborhood in the joint probability distribution, the probability of outcome class A is 0.75; a substantial majority of the cases have A as their label. There are a minority of cases whose class label is B. Over bootstrap samples of the data, each analyzed by CART, the As in this neighborhood nearly always win. The bagging reliability is very high for both the As and the Bs because over trees, each case is almost always assigned the same outcome class. For the As, the algorithm consistently assigns the right class. But for the Bs, the algorithm consistently assigns the wrong class. For the Bs, the algorithms reliably get it wrong. Moreover, for the As, the true probability in this neighborhood is 0.75. But the vote over trees is nearly 1.0, giving the misleading impression that the probability of outcome class A is also nearly 1.0, not .75.

At a deeper level, one can properly wonder why votes over trees are used to determine the assigned class. Why not use for each case the average proportions over trees to determine the assigned class? Thus, for case i, the average vote across 100 trees might be 45% for class A and 55% for class B. Class B wins. Could that be a more effective form of regularization?

A simple answer is that votes over trees are, like the median, more resident to outliers. Consider as a toy example a single case and four bagged trees with the votes for class A of 0.78, 0.43, 0.35, and 0.44. The mean proportion is 0.50, and the vote is 1–3. Imagine that the value of 0.78 gradually grows. The mean proportion increasingly exceeds 0.50 and by that value, class A is assigned. Yet, the vote for class A remains 1–3 (25%). Based on the vote, the assigned class is B.

One might counter that with the large samples common in statistical learning anomalous values as large or larger than 0.78 would be very unlikely to materialize. But that would overlook that the class for the case in question is assigned by terminal nodes that may have few cases and because of the unstable recursive partitioning could represent very different neighborhoods from tree to tree. Voting can prove to be a powerful regularizer.

4.3.4 Forecasting and Imputation

Thinking back to CART, each terminal node will contain the mean of values in that node if the response variable is numeric. For a categorical response variable, each node will contain a proportion for each outcome class, with the outcome class determined by the largest proportion. To arrive at a forecast or imputation, a node mean or a derived class is assigned depending on the node in which a case lands.

Bagging builds on how CART does forecasting. Based on the predictor values of each case for which forecasts are needed, each case lands in one terminal node for each of the bagged trees. The forecasted bagged value for a numeric response variable is the average value over the means for the nodes in which a case falls. For categorical response variable, forecasted bagged value is class that wins the vote over the nodes in which the case falls. Forecasts and imputations are nothing more than fitted values for cases in which the response variable values are unknown.

In R, forecasts or imputations are easily obtained. One first applies the bagging algorithm with a procedure such as *ipred*. Then, as before, the *predict* procedure is used with the data from which forecasts or imputations are needed.

4.3.5 Bagging Estimation and Statistical Inference

Statistical inference for bagging is much like statistical inference for CART. Each tree is still an adaptive procedure that bagging does not change. Estimation, statistical tests, and confidence from the training data are all problematic, just as they were for CART. But if one has appropriate test data, the very similar inferential options are available.

There is no longer anything like a simple algebraic expression to summarize the approximation function. The algorithmic structure maps each configuration of predictor values to a fitted value. One has, therefore, the domain of a function represented by the predictor values and the range of a function represented by the fitted values. We just do not know how to formally represent the function. The expression is inside the black box as a consequence of a collection of bagged trees.

So, what might be the estimand? One intuitive way to proceed is to imagine dropping a limitless number of hypothetical observations that could be generated by the joint probability distribution down the bagged algorithmic structure produced with the training data. The fitted values for those hypothetical observations can be treated as estimands for the approximation's response surface. For a numeric response variable, one is estimating the conditional expectations of that approximation. The same reasoning would apply to functionals of those fitted values, such as their variance. For categorical variables, the proportions would constitute an approximation of a true response surface in the form of conditional probabilities. The assigned class could follow as before from an imposed threshold on those conditional probabilities. Then, because in test data the actual outcome values are available, another set of estimands can be various fitting measures taken from a confusion table.

Whether these formally are proper estimands apparently is not clear. But intuitively, the empirical fitted values and functions of those fitted values obtained from test data may be asymptotically unbiased estimates. That is, the test data would be dropped down the bagged trees whose structure was earlier determined with the training data. Fitted values of various kinds can follow. In short, the framework is very much like the framework we used for CART, even though one has no expression for the approximation function.[5]

Just as with CART, one can use the nonparametric bootstrap with test data to capture uncertainty associated with fitted values. However, because there is no linear regression linking inputs to outputs, there are no regression coefficients to be re-estimated using the test data. The very large number of regression coefficients from tree to tree are treated as fixed. We are proceeding with the framework on which the definition of generalization error depends.

In short, as a practical matter, the resampling inferential procedures used with CART may well be appropriate for bagged trees. But the formal justification so far is lacking. And one must be clear that the uncertainty in the training data and the fitted algorithmic structure is ignored. If forecasting applications are anticipated, this may well suffice. But one is not including uncertainty that would follow from new IID training datasets and new applications of bagging. Working from the test data rules out all uncertainty produced before the test data are introduced.

4.3.6 Margins for Classification

The meaning of "margin" in bagging is somewhat different from the meaning of "margin" in margin maximizing forms of statistical learning (e.g., AdaBoost, support vector machines). But the statistical goals are the same: to arrive at stable

classifications. From a bagging perspective, (Breiman 2001a,b) defines the margin
as

$$mg(\mathbf{X}, Y) = av_k I(h_k(\mathbf{X}) = Y) - \max_{j \neq Y} av_k I(h_k(\mathbf{X}) = j), \qquad (4.1)$$

where for randomly realized data and *a given case*, there is an ensemble of K
classifiers denoted by $h_k(\mathbf{X})$. Y is the correct class, j is some other class, and $I(.)$ is
the indicator function as before. The K classifiers might be K classification trees.[6]
In words, over the K classifiers, there is a proportion of times the case is classified
correctly, and a maximum proportion of times the case is classified incorrectly. The
difference in the two proportions is the margin for that case.

The average of an indicator variable is a proportion. The "*max*" allows for
more than two outcome classes with the proper comparison a worst case scenario.
Suppose there are outcome classes A, B, and C. A is the actual class for a given
observation. The votes correctly pick class A 65% of the time, incorrectly pick class
B 30% of the time, and incorrectly pick class C 5% of the time. The margin for that
case is $0.65 - 0.30 = 0.35$, not $0.65 - 0.05 = 0.60$. "The larger the margin, the
more confidence in the classification" (Breimen 2001: 7).

Margins can be negative. Suppose that over all of the bagged trees for a binary
outcome, an observation is correctly classified 75% of the time and incorrectly
classified 25% of the time. The margin is $0.75 - 0.25 = 0.50$. A negative margin
implies that misclassifications dominate the vote. If an observation is correctly
classified 30% of the time and incorrectly classified 70% of the time, the margin
is $0.30 - 0.70 = -0.40$. If for a given case its class is relatively rare, it often is
likely to be misclassified, leading to a negative margin.

A lopsided vote in favor of the correct class conveys that despite noise introduced
by the bagging resampling, most of the time the case is classified correctly. One can
say that the correct classification for that case is highly reliable. A lopsided vote in
favor of an incorrect class is also highly reliable — reliable and wrong.

Reliability is different from validity. Reliability addresses whether the algorithm,
despite its inherent use of randomness, consistently gives the same results. In
contrast, if the vote is very close, the case is just about as likely to be misclassified
as classified correctly. Systematic relationships between the response and the
predictors cannot meaningfully overcome the algorithm-generated noise. One can
say that the classification, whether correct or incorrect, is unreliable.

One can only know when a classification is correct if the actual outcome class is
known. That will be true in training data, evaluation data, and test data. In that
context, margins can be used as diagnostic tools. How reliable are the correct
classifications? How reliable are the incorrect classifications? Ideally, the former
are very reliable and the latter are not. One hopes that in new realizations of the
data, there is then a good chance that many of the incorrect classifications will be
overturned. One might also be able to identify particular types of cases for which
misclassifications are likely and/or unreliable.

Forecasting applications differ because the outcome class is not known. The votes over classifiers still represent reliability, but whether the classification is correct or incorrect is not known. Nevertheless, reliability is important. Suppose for a given case, the vote is close. Because vote is close, bagging the very same data again could easily result in a close vote the other way. The initial forecasted class is not reliable; the forecast could have easily been different. It is usually important for stakeholders who will use the forecast to know the forecast's reliability, even if they do not know whether the forecast is correct. Should the vote be lopsided, the forecasted class is reliable, and even though the true class is not known, the forecast may be given more credibility.

Whatever the level of confidence, it is with respect to the performance of the bagged classifier itself. Was it able to classify particular cases with sufficient reliability? It is not confidence about any larger issues such as whether the fitted values are good approximations of the true response surface. It is nothing like a model diagnostic or model misspecification test. There are often misunderstandings on this point. To address accuracy and related criteria, we return to our old friend: the confusion table.

In summary, large margins can be a major asset. For each case, the margin can be a measure of reliability for the class assigned. Larger margins imply greater bagging reliability. Forecasting is different. In the earlier prison inmate instance, housing decisions at intake were based on an inmate's forecasted misconduct class. If the vote for a given inmate is equivocal, prison staff properly might decide to base the housing decision on other information. If the vote is decisive, prison staff properly might base the housing decision primarily on the class assigned. But justification for proceeding in this manner also would depend on a confusion table constructed from test data showing that the misconduct projections are likely to be correct. In this instance, reliability and validity work as a team.

4.3.7 Using Out-of-Bag Observations as Test Data

In conventional CART software, a classification tree is grown with training data, and the training data used to grow the tree are used again to compute the number of classification errors. The training data are dropped down the tree to determine how well the tree performs. The training data are said to be "resubstituted" when tree performance is evaluated.

In some implementations of bagging, out-of-bag observations from each tree can be treated as a test dataset and dropped down the tree. There need be no resubstitution. A record is kept of the class with which each out-of-bag observation is labeled, as well as its values on all of the predictors. Then in the averaging process, only those class labels are used. In other words, the averaging for a given case over trees is done only using the trees for which that case was *not* used to grow the tree. This leads to more honest fitted values, more honest votes, and more honest confusion tables than produced by conventional bagging when there are no actual test data.[7] The same logic and benefits apply to regression trees, but the OOB averaging results in the average mean over relevant terminal nodes.

4.3.8   Bagging and Bias

Although the major target of bagging is the variance of fitted values, there can be in certain situations a reduction in the bias as well with respect to the true response surface. Figure 4.3 illustrates how bagging can affect the bias. To keep the graph simple, there is a smooth nonlinear $f(X)$ linking a single predictor to a quantitative response Y. The true response function is shown and is comprised of conditional expectations.

Imagine that a regression tree is applied one time to each of the three different bootstrap samples of the data. Each time, only one break in the predictor is allowed. (Such trees are sometimes called "stumps.") Three step functions that could result are overlaid as in Fig. 4.3 open rectangles. One has a very rough approximation of the $f(X)$. If that function is the estimation target, there is substantial bias.

Suppose now that there are eleven bootstrap samples and eleven stumps. Eleven step functions that could result are shown with the light blue rectangles. Clearly, the approximation is better and bias is reduced. Because in bagging there are often hundreds of trees, there is the possibility of approximating complex functions rather well. The same reasoning applies to categorical outcomes for which the response surface is comprised of conditional probabilities. In short, bagging can reduce bias by what is, in effect, smoothing (Bühlmann and Yu 2002).[8]

In addition, noted earlier was an indirect impact that bagging can have on bias. Because of the averaging in bagging, one can employ more complex functions of the data with less worry about the impact of overfitting on generalization error. For example, bagging gives more license to grow very larger trees with fewer observations in terminal nodes. The larger trees can lead to less bias, while bagging increases the stability of fitted values.

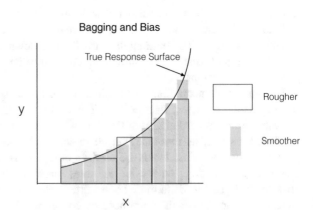

Fig. 4.3 How bagging smooths using a set of step functions to approximate the true response surface

4.4   Some Limitations of Bagging

In general, bagging is a reasonably safe procedure. But it is hardly a panacea. Sometimes it does not help and on occasion it can make things worse. There are better statistical learning procedures ahead.

4.4.1   Sometimes Bagging Cannot Help

Bagging only returns averages of fitted values that are different from those that could be obtained from one pass over the original data if the fitting procedure is a nonlinear or an adaptive function of the data (Hastie et al. 2009: 282). For example, there is no reason to apply bagging to conventional linear regression. The average of the fitted values over a large number of bootstrap samples would be effectively the same as the fitted values obtained from conventional linear regression applied once to the training data. In contrast, there can be useful differences for smoothing splines when the value of λ is determined empirically. This point helps to underscore an earlier discussion about the bootstrap samples used in bagging: in bagging, the goal is not to approximate a sampling distribution but to exploit many passes over the data to improve the performance of fitted values.

4.4.2   Sometimes Bagging Can Make the Estimation Bias Worse

Look again at Fig. 4.3. Suppose $f(X)$ is really very jagged, much like a step function. For a Level I descriptive analysis, the fitted response surface then may be misleading. Important regime changes or discontinuities may be obscured. For example, fitted values of personal income may smooth over a sharp discontinuity between men and women.

For a Level II analysis the risk is an increase in bias with respect to the true response surface. This can materialize as an increase in some form of generalization error, which can degrade forecasting performance. In many situations, however, the threat of degraded Level II performance does not materialize. We may gain in trade a substantial reduction in the estimation variance for whatever is being estimated.

Weak classifiers can also create problems, especially when the distribution of the response distribution is highly unbalanced. Weak classifiers are sometimes defined as those that do not do materially better than the marginal distribution. Suppose the marginal distribution of the response is unbalanced so that it is very difficult for a fitting procedure using the predictors to perform better than that marginal distribution. Under those circumstances, the rare class will likely be misclassified most of the time because votes will be typically won by the class that is far more common. The margin is strongly negative for such cases.[9]

To illustrate, suppose there is a binary response variable, and for the moment, we are interested in a single observation that actually happens to be a "success." Over K classification trees, that observation is classified as a success about two times out of ten. So, the classification for that observation will be wrong about 80% of the time. But if one classifies by majority vote, the class assigned would be a failure, and that would be wrong 100% of the time. Because the K classifiers do a poor job, the majority vote makes things worse. Stronger classifiers typically would place that observation in terminal nodes where the majority of the cases were successes. Then the vote over trees would help.

In practice, such problems will be rare if the data analyst pays attention to how the classifier performs before bagging is applied. If it performs very poorly, bagging risks making things worse. We show in later chapters that if one has a set of weak classifiers, alternative procedures can help.

4.4.3 Sometimes Bagging Can Make the Estimation Variance Worse

Bagging sometimes can perform poorly with respect to the Level II variance (Grandvalet 2004). Figure 4.4 shows a scatterplot with a binary outcome. The observations are represented by filled circles. The light blue circles represent the mass of the data. The dark blue circle and the red circle are high leverage observations because they are outliers in the x-direction. Consider now their impact on the fitted values.

Fig. 4.4 Good and bad influence in bagging. (The blue observation is helpful. The red observation is harmful)

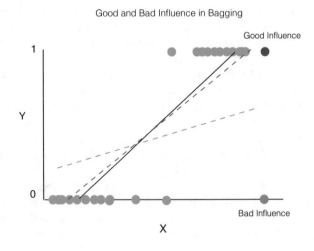

To keep the exposition simple, suppose that within the range of X, true response surface approximation is a linear function of the X. The solid black line shows the fitted values with both the blue circle and the red circle excluded from the dataset. When the red circle is added to the dataset, the fitted values are rotated clockwise and the red dashed line results. It is, therefore, very influential. With the red circle excluded, suppose the blue circles are added. The blue dashed line indicates that very little changes because the blue observation falls very close to the solid black line. Therefore, the blue observation is not influential.

In the bagging resampling process, whether the red observation is sampled increases the variance of the fitted values over bagged trees. This observation makes bagging less effective. In contrast, whether the blue observation is sampled makes little difference. The variance of the fitted values over bagged trees is not increased, and even decreased a bit when the blue observation is sampled. It helps stabilize the fitted values.

These issues have their analogues for quantitative responses. Bagging is at its best when the problem to overcome is instability. But bagging may not help if there are "bad" influence points that can increase the variance in the fitted values depending on whether such points are sampled.

4.5   A Bagging Illustration

In practice, bagging is not used much as a stand-alone procedure. There are far better statistical learning tools. But like classification and regression trees, it can be a key component of more effective approaches and many of the details need to be understood.

Consider bagging applied to the Titanic data, largely to show some R code. The library in R is *ipred* and bagging procedure itself is *bagging*.[10] We use the same classification tree specification as before, which assumes symmetric costs for classification errors. Table 4.1 is the confusion table constructed solely from the training data and Fig. 4.5 shows bagging the code responsible. By all of the performance measures shown in the table, the fit is quite good, but the table is constructed from in-sample data. Also, there is no tree to interpret.

It is not clear that bagging is appropriate for these data that were characterized earlier as a "one-off." There is no instability over samples to worry about; it is not

Table 4.1 Bagged classification tree confusion table for survival on the titanic (N= 1309)

	Classify perished	Classify survived	Classification error
Perished	759	50	0.05
Survived	100	400	0.21
Prediction error	0.12	0.10	Overall error = 0.12

```
## Bagging
library(PASWR) # Where the data are
data("titanic3") # Load data
library(ipred) # Load library

# Bag Classification trees
out1<-bagging(as.factor(survived)~sex+age+pclass+sibsp+parch,
              data=titanic3,coob=T, keepX=T, nbagg=50,
              minsplit=10, cp=.05, xval=0)

fitted<-predict(out1, newdata=titanic3,
                type="class") # fitted class
tab<-table(titanic3$survived,fitted) # confusion table
prop.table(tab,1) # use error
prop.table(tab,2) # model error
```

Fig. 4.5 R code for bagging titanic data

even apparent what instability means in this setting. Again, bagging is essentially a
Level II procedure.

4.6   Summary and Conclusions

Bagging is an important conceptual advance and on occasion can be a useful tool
in practice. The conceptual advance is to aggregate fitted values made possible by
a large number of bootstrap samples. Ideally, many sets of fitted values, each with
low bias but high variance, may be averaged in a manner than can effectively reduce
the bite of the bias–variance tradeoff. Thanks to bagging, there can be a way to
usefully address this long-standing dilemma in statistics. Moreover, the ways in
which bagging aggregates the fitted values is the basis for other statistical learning
developments.

In practice, bagging can generate fitted values that often reproduce the data well
and forecast with considerable accuracy. Both masters are served without making
unrealistic demands on available computing power. Bagging can also be usefully
applied to a wide variety of fitting procedures. However, bagging is not much used
as a stand-alone procedure because there are statistical learning procedures readily
available that import the best features of bagging, add some new wrinkles, and then
perform better.

In addition, bagging also suffers from several problems. Perhaps most important,
there is no way within the procedure itself to depict how the predictors are related to
the response. With test data or OOB data, one can obtain a more honest set of fitted

values and a more honest evaluation of how good the fitted values really are. But as an explanatory aid, bagging is pretty much a bust. This is an inherent feature in all statistical learning. We will make some progress in later chapters supplementing statistical learning with other algorithms.

A second problem is that because so much of the data are shared from tree to tree, the fitted values are not independent. The common set of available predictors can build in additional dependence. Consequently, the averaging is not as effective as it could be. This too is addressed shortly.

Third, bagging may not help much if the fitting function is consistently and substantially inappropriate. Large and systematic errors in the fitted values are just reproduced a large number of times and do not, therefore, cancel out in the averaging process. For categorical response variables, bagging a very weak classifier can sometimes make things worse.

Fourth, the bootstrap sampling can lead to problems when categorical predictors or outcomes are highly unbalanced. For any given bootstrap sample, the unbalanced variable can become a constant. Depending on the fitting function being bagged, the entire procedure may abort.

Finally, bagging can actually increase instability if there are outliers that can dramatically alter the fit. Such outliers will be lost to some of the bootstrap samples but retained in others. It can be difficult in practice to know whether this is a problem or not.

Bagging can be extended so that many of these problems are usefully addressed, even if full solutions are not available. We turn to some of these potential solutions in the next chapter. They are found in another form of statistical learning, still farther away from conventional regression analysis.

Exercises

Problem Set 1

The sampling done in bagging must be with replacement. Run the following code and compare the tables. How many duplicate observations are there in s1 compared to s2? Write code to find out. Run the code a second time. Again, how many duplicate observations are there in s1 compared to s2? Write code to find out. What have you learned about the differences between the samples drawn by the two methods?

```
x<-1:100
s1<-sample(x,replace=T)
table(s1)
s2<-sample(x,replace=F)
table(s2)
```

Problem Set 2

The goal of this exercise is to compare the performance of linear regression, CART, and bagging applied to CART. Construct the following dataset in which the response is a quadratic function of a single predictor.

```
x1=rnorm(500)
x12=x1^2
y=1+(2*(x12))+(2*rnorm(500))
```

1. Plot the $1 + (2 \times x12)$ against x1. This is the "true" relationship between the response and the predictor without the complication of the disturbances. This is the $f(X)$ you hope to recover from the data.
2. Proceed as if you know that the $f(X)$ is quadratic. Fit a linear model with x12 as the predictor. Then plot the fitted values against x1. You can see how well linear regression does when the functional form is known.
3. Now suppose that you do not know that the $f(X)$ is quadratic. Apply linear regression to the same response variable using x1 (not x12) as the sole predictor. Construct the predicted values and plot the fitted values against x1. How do the fitted values compare to what you know to be the correct $f(X)$? (It is common to assume the functional form is linear when the functional form is unknown.)
4. Apply CART to the same response variable using *rpart* and x1 (not x12) as the sole predictor. Use the default settings. Construct the predicted values, using *predict*. Then plot the fitted values against x1. How do the CART fitted values compare to what you know to be the correct $f(X)$? How do the CART fitted values compare to the fitted values from the linear regression with x1 as the sole predictor?
5. Apply bagging to the same response variable using *bagging* from the *ipred* library, and x1 as the sole predictor. Use the default settings. Construct the predicted values using *predict*. Then plot the fitted values against x1. How do the bagged fitted values compare to the linear regression fitted values?
6. You know that the relationship between the response and x1 should be a smooth parabola. How do the fitted values from CART compare to the fitted values from bagging? What feature of bagging is highlighted?

Problem Set 3

Load the dataset "Freedman" from the *car* library. For 100 American cities, there are four variables: the crime rate, the population, population density, and proportion nonwhite. As before, the crime rate is the response and the other variables are predictors.

1. Use *rpart* and its default values to fit a CART model. Compute the root mean square error for the model. One way to do this is to use *predict.rpart* to obtain the fitted values and with the observed values for the variable "crime," compute

the root mean square error in R. Then use *bagging* from the library *ipred* and the out-of-bag observations to obtain a bagged value for the root mean square error for the same CART model. Compare the two estimates of fit and explain what you see. Keep in mind that at least two things are going on: (1) in-sample v. out-of-sample comparisons and (2) the averaging that bagging provides.

2. Using *sd*, compute the standard deviation for the CART fitted values and the bagged fitted values. Compare the two standard deviations and explain what you see.

Problem Set 4

Load the dataset "frogs" from the library *DAAG*. Using "pres.abs" as the response build a CART model under the default settings.

1. Construct a confusion table with "pres.abs" and the predicted classes from the model. Now, using *bagging* from the library *ipred*, bag the CART model using the out-of-bag observations. Construct a confusion table with "pres.abs" and the bagged predicted classes from the model. Compare the two confusion tables and explain why they differ. Keep in mind that at least two things are going on: (1) in-sample v. out-of-sample comparisons and (2) the averaging that bagging provides.

Endnotes

[1] One certainly applies bagging when working at Level I. It is not clear, however, what the gain will be. For a Level I analysis of a classification tree, there is no concern about what might happen with a new realized dataset.

[2] Imagine a total of N draws. For any given draw, each observation has the same probability of being selected. A key consequence is that each possible sample of size N has the same probability of being realized.

[3] If one draws random samples *without* replacement with $0.50 \times N$ observations, one has on the average a dataset with about the same information content as N observations drawn at random with replacement (Buja and Stuetzle 2006). Still, sampling with replacement is the usual approach.

[4] Actually, the trees over bootstrap samples are not independent which is problematic for any probability interpretation. We will do better in the next chapter.

[5] This is one reason why deriving the formal properties of the fitted values is challenging. The reasoning depends on the properties of bagged trees as a plug-in estimator which are hard to pin down with no expression for the approximation function.

[6] Breiman's notation is somewhat different from the notation we have been using, but should be clear. We will see this notation again in the next chapter. His work is so important that it is worth some exposure to his notation.

[7] The process of using the OOB observations can seem confusing. Think about it one tree at a time. For a given tree, an OOB case follows a path down the tree depending on its predictor values and the structure of the splits until the case lands in a terminal node and is assigned the class of

that terminal nodes. For all other trees not grown using that OOB observation, the same process is repeated. Then all of the assigned classes are tallied to produce a vote. The number of trees used in the averaging for a given case may be somewhat smaller than the total number of trees.

[8] In practice, the step functions would likely overlap at least somewhat whether for conditional expectations or conditional probabilities.

[9] Moreover, sometimes the procedure will fail because none of the rare cases is included in a given bootstrap sample.

[10] The package *ipred* is written by A. Peters, T. Hothorn, B.D. Ripley, T. Therneau, and B. Atkinson. There are number of bagging-related procedures in *ipred*.

References

Breiman, L. (1996). Bagging predictors. *Machine Learning, 26*, 123–140.

Breiman, L. (2001a). Random Forests. *Machine Learning, 45*, 5–32.

Breiman, L. (2001b). Statistical modeling: two cultures (with discussion). *Statistical Science, 16*, 199–231.

Bühlmann, P., & Yu, B. (2002). Analyzing bagging. *The Annals of Statistics, 30*, 927–961.

Buja, A., & Stuetzle, W. (2006). Observations on bagging. *Statistica Sinica, 16*(2), 323–352.

Edgington, E.S., & Ongehena, P. (2007). *Randomization tests* (4th ed.). New York: Chapman & Hall.

Efron, B., & Tibshirani, R. (1993). *Introduction to the bootstrap*. New York: Chapman & Hall.

Grandvalet, Y. (2004). Bagging equalizes influence. *Machine Learning, 55*, 251–270.

Hall, P. (1997). *The bootstrap and edgeworth expansion*. New York: Springer.

Hastie, T., Tibshirani, R., & Friedman, J. (2009). *The elements of statistical learning* (2nd ed.). New York: Springer.

Hoeting, J., Madigan, D., Raftery, A., & Volinsky, C. (1999). Bayesian Model Averaging: A Practical tutorial. *Statistical Science, 14*, 382–401.

LeBlanc, M., & Tibshirani, R. (1996). Combining estimates on regression and classification. *Journal of the American Statistical Association, 91*, 1641–1650.

Madigan, D., Raftery, A. E., Volinsky, C., & Hoeting, J. (1996). Bayesian Model Averaging. In *AAA Workshop on Integrating Multiple Learned Models* (pp. 77–83), California: AAAI Press.

Mojirsheibani, M. (1997). A consistent combined classification rule. *Statistics & Probability Letters, 36*, 411–419.

Mojirsheibani, M. (1999). Combining classifiers via discretization. *Journal of the American Statistical Association, 94*, 600–609.

Xu, M., & Golay, M. W. (2006). Data-guided model combination by decomposition and aggregation. *Machine Learning, 63*(1), 43–67.

Chapter 5
Random Forests

Summary This chapter continues to build on the idea of ensembles of statistical learning procedures. Random forests is introduced, which is an extremely useful approach that extends and improves on bagging. As before, there is an ensemble of classification or regression trees and votes over trees to regularize. Additional randomness is introduced when at each potential partitioning for each tree, a random subset of prediction is selected for evaluation. This has a variety of benefits, some of which can be quite subtle. Also discussed are supplementary algorithms to random forests that allow a peek into the black box.

5.1 Introduction and Overview

Just as in bagging, imagine growing a large number of classification or regression trees with bootstrap samples from training data. But now, as each tree is grown, take a random sample of predictors before each node is split. For example, if there are 20 predictors, choose a random five as candidates for defining the split. Then construct the best split, as usual, but selecting only from the five chosen. Repeat this process for each prospective split. Do not prune. Thus, each tree is produced from a random sample of cases, and at each split a random sample of predictors. Compute the mean or proportion for each tree's terminal nodes just as in bagging. Finally, for each case, average over trees as in bagging, but only when that case is out-of-bag. Breiman calls such a procedure as "random forest" (Breiman 2001a).

The random forest algorithm is very much like the bagging algorithm, but there are some important differences in detail to which we now turn. Let N be the number of IID observations in the training data and assume for now that the response variable is binary.

1. Take a random sample of size N *with* replacement from the data.
2. Take a random sample *without* replacement of the predictors.

© Springer Nature Switzerland AG 2020   233
R. A. Berk, *Statistical Learning from a Regression Perspective*,
Springer Texts in Statistics, https://doi.org/10.1007/978-3-030-40189-4_5

3. Construct the first recursive partition of the data as usual.
4. Repeat Step 2 for each subsequent split until the tree is as large as desired. Often this leads to one observation in each terminal node. Do not prune. Compute each terminal node proportion as usual.
5. Drop the *out-of-bag* (OOB) data down the tree. Store the class assigned to each observation along with each observation's predictor values.
6. Repeat Steps 1–5 a large number of times (e.g., 500).
7. Using only the class assigned to each observation when that observation is OOB, count the number of times over trees that the observation is classified in one category and the number of times over trees it is classified in the other category.
8. Assign each case to a category by a majority vote over the set of trees when that case is OOB. Thus, if 51% of the time over a large number of trees a given case is classified as a 1, that becomes its assigned class. If 51% of the time over a large number of trees a given case is classified as a 0, that becomes its assigned class. The assigned class along with the actual class can be used, as before, in a confusion table.
9. If forecasts are needed, the new IID cases from the same joint probability distribution are dropped down each tree and depending on the terminal node in which a case falls, a class is assigned as usual. There is then a vote over trees, as before, through which the winning class becomes the forecasted class. For numeric response variables, or if forecasted conditional proportions are desired, one simple averages over the terminal node conditional means or conditional proportions. These averages serve as forecasts.

The major differences between the bagging algorithm and the random forests algorithm are the sampling of predictors at each potential split of the training data, and using only the out-of-bag data when fitted values or classes are assigned to each case. Both are in the service of making the output from each tree in the random forest more independent, but there are additional benefits addressed below.

For categorical outcomes, a key output from random forests is the assigned classes. Because the assigned classes and the actual classes are for out-of-bag observations, the resulting confusion table effectively is constructed from test data. Still, the black box produced is every bit as opaque as the bagging black box. There are other algorithms that can be used in concert with random forests to provide a peek at what may be going on inside the box. That too is addressed below.

Finally, even when random forests is being used solely to describe associations in the data, there is more going on than a Level I analysis. The use of OOB data to obtain honest fitted values implies Level II concerns broadly and concerns about generalization error in particular. Most discussions of random forests consider results from a dataset as estimates although it can be unclear exactly what is being estimated and where that estimand resides. We will return to these issues toward the end of this chapter, but much of the Level II perspective from bagging carries over.

5.1.1 Unpacking How Random Forests Works

Just like for CART and bagging, beneath a simple algorithm are a host of important details and subtleties. To begin, random forests uses CART as a key building block but in this new setting, CART can be made far more effective. Large trees can produce fitted values and assigned classes less biased with respect to the true response surface. With large trees necessarily comes a more complex $\hat{f}(\mathbf{X})$. Ordinarily, however, an increase in the number of terminal nodes leads to a smaller number of observations in each. The fitted values are more vulnerable to instability. From a Level II perspective, the bias–variance tradeoff remains a serious problem for estimates to the true response surface. But by averaging over trees, the fitted values case-by-case are made more stable. Ideally, both the bias and the variance can be reduced.[1]

Another way to make CART more effective is to sample predictors. One benefit is that the fitted values across trees are more independent. Consequently, the gains from averaging over a large number of trees can be more dramatic. Another benefit is that in part because only a few predictors are considered for each potential partitioning, there can be overall more predictors than observations; p can be very large and even larger than N. This is a major asset in the era of big data. In principle, having access to a very large number of predictors legitimately can help to improve the fit and any forecasting that might follow.

A third benefit can be understood by revisiting the rationale used by CART to determine whether a particular split is to be made for a given tree. Different sets of predictors are evaluated for different splits so that a wide variety of mean functions are evaluated, each potentially constructed from rather different basis functions. Recall the CART splitting criterion for binary response variables:

$$\Delta I(s, A) = I(A) - P(A_L)I(A_L) - P(A_R)I(A_R), \tag{5.1}$$

where $I(A)$ is the value of the parent impurity, $P(A_R)$ is the probability of a case falling in the right daughter node, $P(A_L)$ is the probability of a case falling in the left daughter node, $I(A_R)$ is the impurity of the right daughter node, and $I(A_L)$ is the impurity of the left daughter node. The CART algorithm tries to find the predictor and the split for which $\Delta I(s, A)$ is as large as possible.[2]

The usefulness of a potential split is a function of the two new impurities and the probability of cases falling into either of the prospective daughter nodes. Suppose there is a predictor that could produce splits in which one of the daughter nodes is very homogeneous but has relatively few observations, whereas the other node is quite heterogeneous but has relatively many observations. Recall, that this often is a useful split. Suppose there is another predictor that could generate two nodes of about the same size, each of which is only moderately homogeneous. This split usually is less desirable. If these two predictors were competing against each other, the second predictor might well be chosen, and the small, relatively homogeneous, region that the first predictor would exploit be ignored. However, if the second predictor were not in the pool of competitors, the first might be selected instead.

Similar issues arise with predictors that are substantially correlated. There may be little difference empirically between the two. When they compete to be a splitting variable, one might be chosen almost as readily as the other. But they would not partition the data exactly in the same way. The two partitions that could be defined would largely overlap with each partition having unique content as well. The unique content defined by the predictor not chosen would be excluded.

Moreover, with the shared variability for the two predictors now removed from consideration, the chances that the neglected predictor would be selected later for that tree are significantly reduced because its relationship with the response variable has been eroded. But all is not lost. There will be other trees in the forest and other chances to compete. For one or more subsequent trees, the slighted variable will be competing against others, but not the one with which it is strongly correlated.

In practice, the opportunity for weak predictors to contribute is huge. One by one, they may not help much but in the aggregate, their impact can be substantial. Conventional regression models typically exclude such variables by design. The associations with the response one by one are too small to be interesting in subject-matter terms. In practice, weak predictors are treated as noise and swept into the disturbance term. But a *large number* of small associations, when considered as a group, can lead to much better fitted values and much more accurate imputations and forecasts.

5.2   An Initial Random Forests Illustration

Random forests has its roots in CART and bagging. One might expect, therefore, that when random forests is used for classification, a confusion table will be a key output. But for random forests, the confusion table is conventionally constructed from the OOB observations so that out-of-sample performance is highlighted. Such confusion tables are sometimes called "honest."[3]

We revisit the domestic violence example described earlier with an analysis that shows some of the complexities of working with very challenging data. The data are so challenging that some readers may be underwhelmed with how well random forests performs; this is a hype inoculation.[4] More definitive performance is illustrated later. The primary goal for the moment is to raise important application issues. The secondary goal is to undercut some of the hype that many associate with the procedures covered in this and the next three chapters. The procedures are very good to be sure. But, compelling results are never guaranteed.

There are a little over 500 observations, and even if just double interactions are considered, there are well over 100 predictors. This time, the goal is not to forecast new calls for service to the police department that likely involve domestic violence, but only those calls in which there is evidence that felony domestic violence has actually occurred. Such incidents represent about 6% of the cases. They are very small as a fraction of all domestic violence calls for service. As such, they would normally be extremely difficult to forecast with better skill than could be obtained using the marginal distribution of the response alone. One would make only six mistakes in 100 households if one classified all households as not having new incidents of serious domestic violence.

Using the response variable as the only source of information would in this case mean never correctly identifying any serious domestic violence households. The policy recommendation might be for the police to assume that the domestic violence incident to which they had been called would be the last serious one for that household. This would almost certainly be an unsatisfactory result, which implies that there are significant costs from false negatives. The default cost ratio of 1 to 1 is not responsive to the policy setting.

With a target cost ratio of 10–1 for false negatives to false positives favored by the police department, one obtains the results in Table 5.1.[5] The empirical cost ratio of false positives to false negatives is 146/15. The cost ratio value of 9.7 to 1 means that each false negative is worth nearly 10 times more than each false positive. This is effectively the 10 to 1 cost ratio sought and in practice, it is very difficult to hit the target cost ratio exactly. In practice, moreover, the differences between a confusion table with a 10 to 1 cost ratio and a confusion table with a 9.7 to 1 cost ratio will usually not matter.

Table 5.1 shows that random forests incorrectly classifies households 31 times out of 100 overall. The value of 31 can be interpreted as the overall average cost of a classification error. But noted earlier, the usual overall error gives all errors equal weight. Having decided from policy considerations that the proper cost ratio is 10 to 1, the proper average cost is 0.46 (i.e., $[(10 \times 15) + 146]/516 - 15 + 150)]$. The increase compared to 0.31 makes sense because the relatively few false negatives are very costly. Still, the overall measure of cost-weighted generalization error neglects some very instructive features of the table more relevant to real decision-making.

From the classification error, one can see that about 30% of the cases with no subsequent, serious DV are classified incorrectly and about 52% of the cases with subsequent serious DV are classified incorrectly. That this application of random forests correctly classifies only about half the DV cases may be disappointing, but

Table 5.1 Confusion table for a serious domestic violence incidents using a 10–1 target cost ratio (N = 516)

	No serious DV fitted	Serious DV fitted	Classification error
No serious DV	341	146	0.30
Serious DV	15	14	0.52
Prediction error	0.04	0.91	Total error = 0.31

without using any of the predictors, no DV cases whatsoever would be correctly classified.[6]

If the results from Table 5.1 are to be used to inform real decisions, prediction error is especially instructive. When a forecast is for no subsequent serious DV, the assigned class is incorrect only about 4% of the time. When a forecast is for subsequent serious DV, the assigned class is incorrect about 91% of the time. The large difference in forecasting skill results substantially from the 10 to 1 cost ratio. Implicit is a policy preference to accept a relatively large number of false positives (i.e., 146) so that the number of false negatives is relatively low (i.e., 15). The 146 false positives lead to poor accuracy with the DV class that is predicted. But the fewer true serious DV cases are missed.

At the same time, the policy preference means that classification accuracy when no DV is the assigned class is improved compared to the baseline. Recall, that if the marginal distribution of the response is used, all 516 cases are predicted to be arrest-free, and 6% of the cases are not arrest-free. From Table 5.1, 69% of the cases are predicted to be arrest-free, and 4% of those cases are not arrest-free. Because the base of 6% is very small, it is impossible to obtain large improvements in percentage units; even perfect forecasting would only reduce the forecasting errors by 6 percentage points. In such circumstances, it is common to report ratios, and then the forecasting errors is reduced by one-third (2%/6%).

In short, because false positives have been deemed relatively inexpensive, the procedure accepts much weaker evidence to assign the serious DV class than to assign the no serious DV class. In this illustration, it takes very strong statistical evidence for a case to be classified as no serious DV. High accuracy follows for forecasts of no serious DV.

Although confusion tables using OOB data are an essential feature of random forests output, there are other kinds of output that can be very helpful. These are derived from additional algorithms that will be discussed shortly. In preparation and to help provide readers with better access to the technical literature, we turn to a few formalities.

5.3   A Few Technical Formalities

With some initial material on random forests behind us, it is useful to take a somewhat more formal look at the procedure. We build on an exposition by Breiman (2001a). The abstractions considered make more rigorous some ideas that we have used in the past two chapters and provide important groundwork for material to come. We also consider whether random forests overfits as the number of trees in the forest increases. As before, we emphasize categorical, and especially binary, response variables.

It will be important to differentiate between randomness introduced by the algorithm and randomness introduced by the data. One can undertake a Level I analysis despite randomness from algorithm because it has nothing to do with how the data were generated. The moment interest includes generalizing beyond the data on hand, randomness in the data is in play, and a Level II analysis must follow. Most formal expositions of random forests emphasize Level II issues.

In order to help readers who may wish to read Breiman's treatment of random forests or subsequent work that draws directly from it, Breiman's notation is adopted. Bold type is used for vectors and matrices. Capital letters are used for random variables. The terms "predictor" and "input" are used interchangeably.

5.3.1   What Is a Random Forest?

With categorical response variables, a random forest is an ensemble of classifiers. The classifiers are K classification trees, each based in part on chance mechanisms. Like CART, these classifiers can work with more than two response categories. The goal is to exploit the ensemble of K trees to assign classes to observations using information contained in a set of predictors. As such, it is an algorithm that seeks to classify cases accurately, very much in the spirit of bagging.

One can formally represent a random forest as a collection of K tree-structured classifiers $\{f(\mathbf{x}, \Theta_k), k = 1, \ldots\}$, where $\mathbf{x}$ is a vector of p input variables used to assign a class, and k is an index for a given tree. "Each tree casts a unit vote for the most popular class at input $\mathbf{x}$" (Breiman 2001a: 6). As an ensemble of classifiers, a random forest is also a classifier.

Θ_k is a random vector constructed for the kth tree so that it is independent of past random vectors $\Theta_1, \ldots, \Theta_{K-1}$ and is generated from the same distribution. For bagging, it is the means by which observations can be selected at random with replacement from the training data. For random forests, it also includes the means by which subsets of predictors are sampled without replacement for each potential split. In both cases, Θ_k is a collection of integers. The integers serve as indices determining which cases and which predictors, respectively, are selected. Integers for both sampling procedures can be denoted by Θ_k. The training data are treated as fixed. Uncertainty comes solely from the algorithm. Uncertainty from the IID realized data is not addressed by Θ_k.

The paramount output from a random forest is an assigned class for each observation i determined at its input values $\mathbf{x}_i$. In CART, for example, the class assigned to an observation i is the class associated with the terminal node in which an observation falls. With random forests, the class assigned to each observation is determined by a vote over the set of tree classifiers when OOB data are used. Classes are assigned to observations just as they are in bagging when OOB data are used. It remains important conceptually to distinguish between the class by the vote assigned by the kth tree and the class assigned by the vote over a forest. It is also important to appreciate that when used as a classifier, random forests does *not* produce probabilities for the response variable classes. There is no analogy to the fitted values from logistic regression.

5.3.2 Margins and Generalization Error for Classifiers in General

Consider first *any* ensemble classifier, not random forests in particular. Suppose there is a training dataset with input values and associated values for a categorical response. As before, each observation in the training dataset is realized at random and independently. The set of inputs and a response are random variables.

There is an ensemble of K classifiers, $f_1(\mathbf{x}), f_2(\mathbf{x}), \ldots, f_K(\mathbf{x})$. For the moment, we do not consider how these different classifiers are constructed. The margin function at *the data point* $\mathbf{X}, Y$ is then defined as

$$mg(\mathbf{X}, Y) = av_k I(f_k(\mathbf{X}) = Y) - \max_{j \neq Y} av_k I(f_k(\mathbf{X}) = j), \qquad (5.2)$$

where $I(.)$ is an indicator function, j is an incorrect class, av_k denotes averaging over the set of classifiers for a single realized data point, and max denotes the largest value. We earlier used this approach for bagging. For a given set of x-values and the associated observed class, the margin is the average number of votes over classifiers for the correct observed class minus the maximum average number of votes over classifiers for any other class. The term "data point" for this discussion is for a row in the dataset. Because Eq. (5.2) applies to any row, it applies to all rows.[7]

From the definition of the margin function, generalization error is then,

$$g = P_{\mathbf{X},Y}(mg(\mathbf{X}, Y) < 0), \qquad (5.3)$$

where P means probability. In words, Breiman's generalization error is the probability over realizations of a row of the data that the vote will be won by an incorrect class: the probability that the margin will be negative. Because Eq. (5.3) applies to any row, it applies to realizations for all rows. There are no test data in this formulation of generalization error, and the training data are not fixed. Recall that when Hastie et al. (2009: 220) define generalization error, the training data are fixed and performance is evaluated over realizations of test data. One is, of course, free to define concepts as one wants, but for both definitions, generalization error should be small.

5.3.3 Generalization Error for Random Forests

Now, suppose for the kth classifier $f_k(\mathbf{X}) = f(\mathbf{X}, \Theta_k)$. There are K tree classifiers that comprise a random forest. Breiman proves (2001a) that as the number of trees increases, the estimated generalization error converges to the true generalization error, which is

$$P_{\mathbf{X},Y}(P_\Theta(f(\mathbf{X}, \Theta) = Y) - \max_{j \neq Y} P_\Theta(f(\mathbf{X}, \theta) = j) < 0). \qquad (5.4)$$

$P_\Theta(f(\mathbf{X}, \Theta) = Y)$ is the probability of a correct classification of a data point over trees that differ randomly because of the sampling of the training data with replacement and the sampling of predictors without replacement. One can think of this as the proportion of times a classification is correct over a limitless number of trees grown from the same dataset. Parallel reasoning for an incorrect classification applies to $P_\Theta(f(\mathbf{X}, \theta) = j)$.[8] Then, we are essentially back to Eq. (5.3). As before, $P_{\mathbf{X},Y}$ introduces the probability of an incorrect classification over realizations of the data themselves. We address the uncertainty that is a product of random forests and then the uncertainty that is a product of the random variables. Breiman proves that as the number of trees increases without limit, all of these sources of randomness cancel out leaving the true generalization error shown in Eq. (5.4).

What does one mean in this context by "true" generalization error? Just as in bagging, one imagines classifying potential, realized cases with the classification structure built using random forests with the training data. These hypothetical realized cases are processed as if they were test data. A population confusion table can result. With this confusion table, generalization error is defined. This is the "true generalization error" that is being estimated. It is the product of a random forest acknowledged to be imperfect. The approximation framework is still applied.

The importance of the convergence is that demonstrably random forests does not overfit as more trees are grown. One might think that with more trees, one would get an increasingly false sense of how well the results generalize. Breiman proves that this is not true. Given all of the concern about overfitting, this is an important result.

There is some work addressing random forests statistical consistency for what appears to be the true response surface. Even if all of the needed predictors are available, there can be situations in which random forests is not consistent (Biau et al. 2008; Biau and Devroye 2010). However, because this work is somewhat stylized, it is not clear what the implications for practice may be. Work that is more recent and somewhat less stylized proves consistency but among other things, requires sparsity (Biau 2012). This means that only a "very few" of the large set of potential predictors are related to the response (Biau 2012: 1067). We are apparently back to the conventional linear regression formulation in which there are two kinds of predictors: those that matter a lot and those that do not matter at all. A look at the variable importance plots reported later in this chapter shows no evidence of sparsity. There may well be other kinds of data for which sparsity can be plausibly defended (e.g., for genomics research).

Another assumption that all of the recent theoretical work seems to share is that the trees in a random forest are "honest" (Wager 2014: 7). By "honest," one means that the data used to determine the fitted value for each terminal node are not the data used to determine the data partitions. By this definition, the trees in Breiman's random forests are *not* honest, so the theoretical work does not directly apply. Moreover, "... the bias of CART trees seems to be subtle enough that it does not affect the performance of random forests in most situations" (Wager 2014: 8). It is probably fair to say that the jury is still out on the formal properties of random forests, but that in practice, there is a consensus that it performs well.

5.3.4 The Strength of a Random Forest

The margin function for a given realized data point in a random forest (not just any classifier) is defined as

$$mr(\mathbf{X}, Y) = P_\Theta(f(\mathbf{X}, \Theta) = Y) - \max_{j \neq Y} P_\Theta(f(\mathbf{X}, \Theta) = j), \qquad (5.5)$$

where $f(\mathbf{X}, \Theta)$ denotes random forest classifications for a given row that can vary because of the chance mechanisms represented by Θ. Because of the randomness build into the random forest algorithm, the margin function is defined using the probability of a correct vote and the probability of an incorrect vote over forests grown from the same dataset. It appropriates a piece the definition of random forests generalization error.

It is a short step from a random forest margin function to a definition of the "strength" of a random forest. We take the expectation over realizations of the data. That is, the expected value of Eq. (5.5) is

$$s = E_{\mathbf{X},\mathbf{y}} mr(\mathbf{X}, Y). \qquad (5.6)$$

The strength of a random forest is an expected margin over all possible realizations of the data. And no surprise, strong is good.

5.3.5 Dependence

As previously noted, the effectiveness of averaging over trees using votes depends in part on the independence of the trees. But, how does one think about that independence in this setting? There is apparently some confusion in the literature (to which I plead guilty). Breiman, (2001a: 9) explains that "$\bar{\rho}$ is the correlation between two different members of the forest averaged over the Θ, Θ' distribution." Recall that Θ represents the sources of randomness in a random forest.

This correlation is a theoretical construct (Hastie et al. 2009: section 15.4). Imagine repeated IID realizations of the training data from the generative joint probability distribution. For each training dataset, a random forest is grown and then for each, a random pair of trees is chosen. We focus on a given set of predictor values for the two trees. For these random pairs, how large is the correlation between the fitted values for the given predictor values? The correlation will be smaller insofar as different splitting variables are used. Hence, we have an important part of the reason for sampling predictors.

Dependence is important because Breiman shows (Breiman 2001a: 6) that the upper bound for the generalization error is

$$g^* = \frac{\bar{\rho}(1 - s^2)}{s^2}, \qquad (5.7)$$

where $\bar{\rho}$ is the expected correlation, and s is the strength of the random forest. Ideally, the former is small and the latter is large.

Equation (5.7) implies that both the sizes of margins and that ways in which the random forest algorithm introduces randomness are critical. The random forest algorithm already does a pretty good job reducing the expected correlation. But in practice, random forest sometimes can be tuned to help. For example, sampling fewer inputs at each splitting opportunity can in some situations improve performance, and the random forest software in R emphasized here (i.e., *randomForest*) has a default function for determining the number of predictors that seems to work quite well.[9]

5.3.6 Putting It Together

Why does random forests work so well as a classifier? Although there are not yet any formal proofs, recent work by Wyner and colleagues (2017) provides a conceptual framework coupled with simulations that support some very instructive intuitions. We will see later that their thinking applies to boosting and neural nets as well.

5.3.6.1 Benefits From Interpolation

It has become common practice, and often the default practice, to grow trees as large as the data will allow. Terminal nodes are often perfectly homogeneous. Indeed, sometimes tuning parameters are set so that each terminal node can contain a single observation. Consequently, in the bootstrap sample used to grow each tree, the fit to the training data can be perfect; for each observation, the tree assigns the correct class. When this happens, one has an interpolating classifier (Wyner et al. 2017: 9).

Figure 5.1 provides a very simple illustration for a single classification tree. One has a 3-dimensional scatter plot for a realized training dataset. There are two numerical predictors X and Z, and a binary outcome represented as red, blue, or purple. The red and blue outcome classes are noiseless in the sense that no matter what the realization of the data, observations in their particular predictor locations always are either red or blue; all realized cases in that neighborhood always will be that one color. In contrast, the purple circles can be either red or blue depending on the realization. In other words, realized cases in those neighborhoods can change color.

The box in the upper left-hand corner results from a single, classification tree terminal node with $X < 2$ and $Z > 12$. The node has one observation and, therefore, is necessarily classified correctly. With sufficiently fine-grained partitioning of X and Z using a sufficiently large tree, each circle in Fig. 5.1 can reside in its own terminal node. Each would be classified correctly, and its terminal nodes would be perfectly homogeneous. One would have what Wyner and his colleagues call an interpolation of the data. The fit in the training data is perfect.

Fig. 5.1 Visualization of
interpolation for a single
classification tree with blue
and red outcomes having no
noise and purple outcomes
having some noise

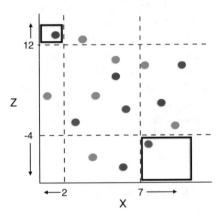

Things are more complicated in the lower right-hand box. For observations with $X > 7$ and $Z < -4$, the outcome class can vary over realizations. It could be a blue outcome for one data realization and a red outcome for another data realization. In the joint probability distribution responsible hypothetical cases in that neighborhood can be red or blue. Suppose in one realization of the training data, the color is red, and the case is classified as red. One still has an interpolation of the realized data. But if in the corresponding true predictor space in the generative distribution the outcome class can be red or blue, one may have misclassification and generalization error can be introduced.

But there is some good news too. Because of the interpolation, one has "local robustness" (Wyner et al. 2017: 9–10). Whatever the error in the fit caused by the purple circle, that error is confined to its own terminal node. That is, all of the classifications for the other circles are made separately from the noisy circle. Consequently, the damage is very localized. In an important sense, overfitting can have some demonstrable benefits.

5.3.6.2   Benefits from Averaging

Interpolation does not by itself solve the overfitting problem. It just helps to limit the damage. Enter random forests. Each tree is grown with a random sample of the training data. The terminal node neighborhoods will likely vary from tree to tree because of the instability discussed earlier, and from tree to tree each OOB will land a single terminal node. Regardless of how the neighborhood of these terminal nodes is defined, a vote for each case is taken. The plurality wins.

Just as in bagging, voting is an averaging process that reduces generalization error from a single tree. Although each tree will overfit, averaging over trees compensates. Noise tends that can affect the fit for a single tree tends to cancel out when averaging over many trees. Because many (most?) neighborhoods for a given case will be purple, the averaging is essential as a form of regularization.

5.3.6.3   Defeating Competition Between Predictors

Striving to interpolate is helped by the sampling of predictors. Imagine that in Fig. 5.1 one location has a red circle right on top of a blue circle. There is no way with X and Z alone to arrive at an interpolation point at that location. As discussed in Chap. 1, there might be a solution in some linear basis expansion of X and Z.

Another solution is to come upon a variable, W, that in combination with X and Z could define two terminal nodes, one with the blue circle and one with the red circle. But, looking back to Eq. (5.1), suppose that for a given prospective partitioning of the data, W does not make a sufficient contribution to homogeneity to be selected as the next partitioning variable. Even if it is strongly related to the response, it is also too strongly related to X. An opportunity to distinguish between a red circle and a blue circle is lost. This problem can be solved by sampling predictors. Suppose, there is a predictor U that, like X, is strongly related to the response, but unlike X is only moderately related to Z. If for some split, X is not available as a potential partitioning variable but U is, U, W, and Z can participate sequentially in the partitioning process.

5.3.6.4   All Together Now

Although all of the mechanisms just described are always in play, challenges from real data are substantial. In practice, all of the class labels are noisy so that the circles in Fig. 5.1 would all be purple. A perfect fit in the training data will not lead to a perfect fit in the test data. Moreover, a perfect fit is certainly no guarantee of obtaining unbiased estimates of the true response surface. There will typically be omitted predictors, and the classification trees are still limited by the ways splits are determined and the greedy nature of the tree algorithm. It remains true, however, that "random forests has gained tremendous popularity due to robust performance across a wide range of datasets. The algorithm is often capable of achieving best-in-class performance with respect to generalization error and is not highly sensitive to choice of tuning parameters, making it an ideal off-the-shelf tool of choice for many applications" (Wyner et al. 2017: 9).

5.4   Random Forests and Adaptive Nearest Neighbor Methods

A conceptual link was made earlier between CART and adaptive nearest neighbor methods. Not surprisingly, similar links can be made between random forests and adaptive nearest neighbor methods. But for random forests, there are a number of more subtle issues (Meinshausen 2006; Lin and Jeon 2006). These are important not just for a deeper understanding of random forests, but for recent theoretical treatments (Scornet et al. 2015; Wager 2014; Wager et al. 2014; Wager and Walther 2015).

Recall that in CART, each terminal node represents a region of nearest neighbors. The boundaries of the neighborhood are constructed adaptively when the best predictors and their best splits are determined. With the neighborhood defined, all of the observations inside are used to compute a mean or proportion. This value becomes the measure of central tendency for the response within that neighborhood. In short, each terminal node and the neighborhood represented has its own conditional mean or conditional proportion.

Consider the case in which equal costs are assumed. This makes for a much easier exposition, and no key points are lost. The calculations that take place within each terminal node implicitly rely on a weight given to each value of the response variable. For a given terminal node, all observations not in that node play no role when the mean or proportion is computed: Consequently, each such observation has a weight of zero. For a given terminal node, all of its observations are used when the mean or proportion is computed. Consequently, each value of the response variable in that node has a weight equal to $1/n_\tau$, where n is the number of observations in terminal node τ. Once the mean or proportion for a terminal node is computed, that mean or proportion can serve as a fitted value for all cases that fall in that terminal node.

Figure 5.2 shows a toy rendering. The tree has a single partitioning of the data. There happen to be three values of the response variable in each terminal node. Consider terminal node A. The mean for terminal node A is 2.33, computed with weights of 1/3 for the values in that node and weights of 0 otherwise; the values of the response variable in terminal node B play no role when the mean of node A is computed. Each of the three observations landing in terminal node A is assigned

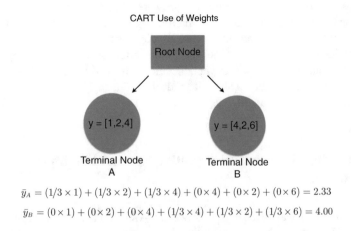

$$\bar{y}_A = (1/3 \times 1) + (1/3 \times 2) + (1/3 \times 4) + (0 \times 4) + (0 \times 2) + (0 \times 6) = 2.33$$

$$\bar{y}_B = (0 \times 1) + (0 \times 2) + (0 \times 4) + (1/3 \times 4) + (1/3 \times 2) + (1/3 \times 6) = 4.00$$

Fig. 5.2 CART weighting used to assign a mean or proportion to a terminal node A or B

a value of 2.33 as their fitted value. If the response variable had been binary, the numbers in the two terminal nodes would have been replaced by 1s and 0s. Then a conditional proportion for terminal node A would be the outcome of the weighted averaging. And from this, an assigned class could be determined as usual. The same reasoning applies to terminal node B.

A bit more formally, a conditional mean or proportion for any terminal node τ is

$$\bar{y}_\tau | x = \sum_{i=1}^{N} w_{(i,\tau)} y_i, \tag{5.8}$$

where the sum is taken over the *entire* training dataset, and w_i is the weight for each y_i. The sum of the weights over all observations for a given terminal node is 1.0. In practice, most of the weights for the calculations in any terminal will be zero because they are not associated with the terminal node τ. This is no different from the manner in which nearest neighbor methods can work when summary measures of a response variable are computed.

There are two important features of the weighting terminal node by terminal node. First, each terminal node defines a neighborhood. The x-values for each observation determine in which neighborhood the observation belongs. It will often turn out that observations with somewhat different sets of x-values land in the same neighborhood. For example, a partition may be defined by a threshold of 25 years of age. All ages less than 25 are sent to one neighborhood and all ages of 25 and above are sent to another.

Second, for any given tree, each of the N observations will have a single, nonzero weight because each observation must land in one (and only one) of the terminal nodes. It is in that node that the single weight is determined as the reciprocal of the number of observations. In our toy example, each of the six observations happens to have a weight of 1/3 because both terminal nodes have three observations.

Now imagine that the tree is grown as a member of a random forest. The form of the calculations shown for terminal nodes A and B still applies with the fitted values, in this instance, a conditional mean or proportion. However, there are now a large number of such trees. For each observation, random forests averages the weights obtained from each tree (Lin and Jeon 2006: 579–580). Consequently, the ith fitted value from a random forest is a weighted average of N_{OOB_i} values of the response, much like in Fig. 5.2, but using average weights.[10] That is,

$$\hat{y}_i = \sum_{i=1}^{N_{OOB_i}} \bar{w}_i y_i, \tag{5.9}$$

where $\bar{w}_i$ is the average weight.

The weights can serve another important purpose. Suppose for a given neighborhood defined by x_0, there are 10 observations and, therefore, 10 values for a numeric response. A numeric response is used because it best illustrates the use of average

Table 5.2 Weights and
cumulative weights for a
target value $\mathbf{x}_0$

Average weight	Response value	Cumulative weight
0.10	66	0.10
0.11	71	0.21
0.12	74	0.33
0.08	78	0.41
0.09	82	0.50
0.10	85	0.60
0.13	87	0.73
0.07	90	0.80
0.11	98	0.91
0.09	99	1.0

weights. There are also 10 average weights. If one orders the response values from
low to high, the weights, conceptualized as probabilities, can be used to compute
other summary measures than the mean. Table 5.2 can be used to illustrate.

From left to right, there are ten average weights that sum to 1.0, ten response
values available for $\mathbf{x}_0$, listed in order, and then cumulative weights. The terminal
node mean is computed by multiplying each response by its average weight and
adding the products. In this case, the mean is 83. Quantiles are also available. The
10th percentile is 66. The 50th percentile (the median) is 82. The 90th percentile is
a little less than 98. In short, one is not limited to the mean of each $\mathbf{x}_0$.

Suppose one has a random forest and a variety of predictor profiles of x-values.
When the response is quantitative, there routinely is interest in determining the fitted
conditional mean for each profile. But sometimes, there will be interest in fitted
conditional medians to "robustify" random forest results or to consider a central
tendency measure unaffected by the tails of the distribution. Sometimes, there is
subject-matter interest in learning about a conditional quantile such as the 25th
percentile or the 90th percentile.

For example, in today's world of school accountability based on standardized
tests, perhaps students who score especially poorly on standardized tests respond
better to smaller classroom sizes than students who excel on standardized tests.
The performance distribution on standardized tests, conditioning on classroom
size, differs for good versus poor performers. Building on work of Lin and Jeon
just discussed, Meinshausen (2006) alters the random forests algorithm so that
conditional quantiles can be provided as fitted values. An application is provided
later in this chapter using the R library *quantregForest*.[11]

But there are caveats. In particular, each tree is still grown with a conventional
impurity measure, which for a quantitative response is the error sum of squares
(Meinshausen 2006: section 3). If one is worried about the impact of a highly
skewed response variable distribution, there may well be good reason to worry about
the splitting criterion too. For example, one might prefer to minimize the sum of
the absolute values of the residuals (i.e., L_1 loss) rather than the sum of squared
residuals (i.e., L_2 loss) as an impurity measure. This was originally proposed by

Breiman and his colleagues in 1984 (Chap. 8), and there have been interesting efforts to build on their ideas (Chaudhuri and Loh 2002; Loh 2014). But L_1 loss does not seem to have yet been incorporated into random forests. We will see later that L_1 loss has been implemented in stochastic gradient boosting.

5.5   Introducing Misclassification Costs

Just as in CART, there is a need when random forests is used as a classifier to consider the relative costs of false negatives and false positives. There are four approaches that have been seriously considered for the binary class case. They differ by whether costs are imposed on the data before each tree is grown, as each tree is grown, or at the end when classes are assigned. Although binary outcomes will be emphasized, the lessons for response variables with more than two categories will be covered as well.

1. Just as in CART, one can use a prior distribution to help capture relative misclassification costs as each tree is grown. This has the clear advantages of being based on the mechanics of CART and capitalizing on a trial-and-error way to translate the target cost ratio into the empirical cost ratio.
2. After all of the trees are grown, one can differentially weight the classification votes over trees. For example, one vote for classification in the less common category might count the same as two votes for classification in the more common category. This has the advantage of being easily understood.
3. After all of the trees are grown, one can abandon the majority vote rule and use thresholds that reflect the relative costs of false negatives and false positives. For instance, rather than classifying as a 1 all observations when the vote is larger than 50%, one might classify all observations as a 1 when the vote is larger than 33%. The implicit cost ratio is now 2–1. This too is easy to understand.
4. When each bootstrap sample is drawn before a tree is grown, one can over-sample cases from one class relative to cases from the other class, in much the same spirit as disproportional stratified sampling used for survey data collection (Thompson 2002: Chapter 11). Before a tree is grown, one over-samples the cases for which classification errors are relatively more costly. Conceptually, this is a lot like altering the prior distribution directly and can be seen as a form of weighting.

All four approaches share the problem that initially, the empirical ratio of false negatives to false positives in the confusion table probably will not sufficiently correspond to the target cost ratio. In practice, this means that whatever method is used to introduce relative costs, that method is a way to tune the results. With some trial and error, an appropriate ratio of false negatives to false positives can usually be achieved.

Although experience suggests that in general all four methods can tune the results as needed, one probably should favor tuning by the prior or by stratified bootstrap sampling. Both of these methods will affect the confusion table through the trees themselves. Changing the way votes are counted or which thresholds are used only affects the classes assigned and leaves the trees unaltered. Consequently, other output from a random forest to be considered shortly is not responsive to stakeholder cost preferences. At a deeper level, one has to wonder how valid the votes really are if they are taken in terminal nodes produced by trees with incorrect misclassification costs.

There is one very important situation in which the stratified sampling approach is likely to be demonstrably superior to the other three approaches. If the response variable is highly unbalanced (e.g., a 95–5 split), any given bootstrap sample may fail to include enough observations for the rare category. Then, a useful tree will be difficult to grow because it will often be difficult to move beyond the marginal distribution of the response. Oversampling rare cases when the bootstrap sample is drawn will generally eliminate this problem. Using a prior that makes the rare observations less rare can also help, but that help applies in general and will be ineffective if a given bootstrap sample makes the rare cases even more rare.

We consider some applications in depth shortly. But a very brief illustration is provided now to prime the pump.

5.5.1   A Brief Illustration Using Asymmetric Costs

Table 5.3 was constructed by random forests using data from the prison misconduct study described earlier. In this example, the response is incidents of very serious misconduct, not the garden-variety kind. Such misconduct is relatively rare. Less than about 3% of the inmates had such reported incidents. So, just as for the domestic violence data shown in Table 5.1, it is extremely difficult to do better than the marginal distribution under the usual statistical learning defaults. In addition, there is simply not a lot misconduct cases from which the algorithm can learn. Trees in the forest will be unable to isolate the rare cases as often as might be desirable; tree depth may be insufficient.

Suppose that the costs of classification errors for the rare cases were substantially higher than the costs of classification errors for the common cases. These relative costs can be introduced effectively by drawing a stratified bootstrap sample, oversampling the rare cases. And by making the rare cases less rare, problems

Table 5.3 Random forest confusion table for forecasts of serious prison misconduct with a 20 to 1 target cost ratio (N = 4806)

	Forecast no misconduct	Forecast misconduct	Classification error
No misconduct	3311	1357	0.29
Misconduct	58	80	0.42
Prediction error	0.02	0.94	Overall error = 0.29

that might follow from the highly unbalanced response variable can sometimes be overcome.

For Table 5.3, the bootstrap samples for each of the response categories were set to equal 100.[12] The "50–50" bootstrap distribution was selected by trial and error to produce an empirical cost ratio of false negatives to false positives of about 20 to 1 (actually 23 to 1 here). The cost ratio may be too high for real policy purposes, but it is still within the range considered reasonable by prison officials.

Why 100 cases each? Experience suggests that the sample size for the less common response category should equal about two-thirds of the number of cases in that class. If a larger fraction of the less common cases is sampled, the out-of-bag sample size for that class may be too small. The OOB observations may not be able to provide the quality of test data needed.

With the number of bootstrap observations for the less common category determined to be 100, the 50–50 constraint leads to 100 cases being sampled for the more common response category. In practice, one determines the sample size for the less common outcome and then adjusts the sample size of the more common outcome as needed.

Table 5.3 can be interpreted just as any of the earlier confusion tables. For example, the overall proportion of cases incorrectly identified is 0.29, but that fails to take the target costs of false negatives to false positives (i.e., 20 to 1) into account. Random forests classifies 42% of the incidents of misconduct incorrectly and 29% of the no misconduct cases incorrectly. Were prison officials to use these results for forecasting, a forecast of no serious misconduct would be wrong only 2 times out of 100, and a forecast of serious misconduct would be wrong 94 times out of 100. The very large number of false positives results substantially from the target 20 to 1 cost ratio. But, for very serious inmate misconduct, having about 1 true positive for about 17 false positives (1357/80) may be an acceptable tradeoff. The misconduct represented can include homicide, assault, sexual assault, and narcotics trafficking. If not, the cost ratio could be made more symmetric.

To summarize, random forests provides several ways to take the relative costs of false negatives and false positives into account. Introducing stratified bootstrap sampling seems to work well in practice. Ignoring the relative costs of classification errors does not mean that costs are not affecting the results. The default is using the marginal distribution of the response variable as the empirical prior, and then one is stuck with the empirical costs that materialize in a confusion table, even if they are inconsistent the facts or the preferences of stakeholders.

5.6   Determining the Importance of the Predictors

Just as for bagging, random forests leaves behind so many trees that collectively they are useless for interpretation. Yet, a goal of statistical learning can be to explore how inputs are related to outputs. Exactly how best to do this is currently unresolved, but there are several useful options available. We begin with a discussion of "variable importance."

5.6.1   Contributions to the Fit

One approach to predictor importance is to record the improvement in the fitting measure (e.g., Gini index, mean square error) each time a given variable is used to define a split. The sum of these reductions for a given tree is a measure of importance for that variable when that tree is grown. For random forests, one can average this measure of importance over the set of trees. Sometimes the improvement is standardized. For example, all of the average predictor contributions to the fit are summed, and each predictor's importance is reported as a percentage of that total.

One difficultly with these conventional measures of fit is that they are in-sample. Moreover, as with conventional variance partitions, reductions in the fitting criterion ignore the *prediction* skill of an algorithm, which many statisticians treat as the gold standard. Why should one care about fit unless the primary interpretative goal is explanation?

It also can be difficult to translate contributions to fit statistic into practical terms. Simply asserting that a percentage contribution to a fit statistic is a measure of importance is circular. Importance must be defined outside of the procedure used to measure it. And what is it about contributions to fit that makes a predictor more or less important? Even if an external definition is provided, is a predictor important if it can account for, say, 10% of the reduction in impurity?

Finally, one must be fully clear that contributions to the fit by themselves are silent on what would happen if in the real world a predictor is manipulated. Causality can only be established by how the data were generated, and causal interpretations depend on there being a real intervention altered independently of all others predictors (Berk 2003).

5.6.2   Contributions to Prediction

Breiman (2001a: section 10) has suggested an application of randomization to assess the role of each predictor. This method is implemented in *randomForest* and is based on the reduction in what Breiman calls prediction accuracy when a given predictor is randomly shuffled. Shuffling precludes any predictor, on the average, from making a systematic contribution to a prediction. For categorical response variables, importance is defined as the increase in *classification* error within the OOB data. One conditions on an actual outcome to determine the proportion of times the wrong class is assigned. For numeric response variables, the standard approach is to use the increase in mean squared error for the OOB data. One is again conditioning on the actual value of Y. The term "prediction" can be a little misleading, but to be consistent with Breiman, we will stick with it here. Rather than prediction accuracy, the proper term is classification accuracy.

Breiman's approach has much in common with the concept of Granger causality (Granger and Newbold 1986: section 7.3). Imagine two times series, Y_t and X_t. If the future conditional distribution of Y given current and past values of Y is the same as the future conditional distribution of Y given current and past values of Y and X, X does not Granger-cause Y.[13] If the two future conditional distributions differ, X is a Granger-cause of Y.

These ideas generalize so that for the baseline conditional distribution, one can condition not just on current and past values of Y but on current and past values of other predictors (but not X). Then X Granger-causes Y, conditional on the other predictors, if including X as a predictor changes the future conditional distribution of Y. In short, the idea of using forecasting performance as a way to characterize the performance of predictors has been advanced in both the statistical and econometrics literature.

Breiman's importance measure of prediction accuracy differs perhaps most significantly from Granger-cause in that Breiman does not require time series data and randomly shuffles the values of predictors rather than dropping (or adding) predictors from (to) a procedure. The latter has some important implications discussed shortly.

For Breiman's approach, the following algorithm is used to compute each predictor's importance. It is a supplement to random forests.

1. Construct a measure prediction error v for each tree as usual by dropping the out-of-bag (OOB) data down the tree. This is an out-of-sample measure because data not used to grow the tree are used to evaluate its predictive skill.
2. If there are p predictors, repeat Step 1 p times, but each time with the values of a given predictor randomly shuffled. The shuffling makes that predictor on the average unrelated to the response and all other predictors. All predictors other than the shuffled predictor are fixed at their empirical values in the OOB data. For each shuffled predictor j, compute new measure of prediction error, v_j.
3. For each of the p predictors, average over trees the difference between the prediction (i.e., classification) error with no shuffling and the prediction (i.e., classification) error with the jth predictor shuffled.

The average increase in prediction error when a given predictor j is shuffled represents the importance of that predictor. That is,

$$I_j = \sum_{k=i}^{K} \left[\frac{1}{K} (v_j - v) \right], \quad j = 1, \ldots, p, \tag{5.10}$$

where there are K trees, v_j is the prediction error with predictor j shuffled, and v is the prediction error with none of the predictors shuffled. It is sometimes possible for prediction accuracy to improve slightly when a variable is shuffled because of the randomness introduced. A negative measure of predictor importance follows.

Negative predictor importance can be treated as no decline in accuracy or simply can be ignored.

As written, Eq. (5.10) is somewhat open-ended. The measures of prediction error (v and v_j) are not defined. For a quantitative response variable, the MSE is an obvious choice. There are more options for categorical response variables: the deviance, percentage of cases classified incorrectly, average change in the margins, or some other measure. Currently, the preferred measure is the proportion (or percentage) of cases misclassified. This has the advantage of allowing direct comparisons between the increases in misclassification and all of the row summaries in a confusion table. For a binary response, one is considering the increase in the false positive rate and the false negative rate. All of the other measures considered to date have been found less satisfactory for one reason or another. For example, some measures are misleadingly sensitive; small changes in the number of classification errors can lead to large changes in the importance measure.

When used with categorical response variables, a significant complication is that Eq. (5.10) will almost always produce different importance measures for any given predictor for different categories of the response. Because one is conditioning on different outcome classes, there will be for any given predictor, a measure of importance for each outcome class, and the measures will not generally be the same. For example, if there are three response classes, there will be three measures of importance for each predictor that will generally differ. This can lead to different importance rankings of predictors depending on which response category is being considered. A detailed illustration is presented shortly.

Partly in response to such complications, one can standardize the declines in performance. The standard deviation of ($v_j - v$) over trees can be computed. In effect, one has a bootstrap estimate over trees of the standard deviation associated with the increase in classification error, which can be used as a descriptive measure of stability. Larger values imply less stability.

In addition, one can divide Eq. (5.10) by this value. The result can be interpreted as a z-score so that all importance measures over predictors are now all on the same scale. And with a bit of a stretch, confidence intervals can be computed and conventional hypothesis tests performed. It is a stretch because the sampling distribution of the predictor importance measure is usually not known. Perhaps more important, the descriptive gains from standardization are modest at best, as the illustrations that follow make clear.

One of the other drawbacks of the shuffling approach to variable importance is that only one variable is shuffled at a time. There is no role for joint importance over several predictors. This can be an issue when predictors are correlated. There will be a contribution to prediction accuracy that is uniquely linked to each predictor and joint contributions shared between two or more predictors. Also, there are closely related difficulties when a single categorical predictor is represented by a set of indicator variables. The importance of the *set* is not captured.

It might seem that Granger's approach of examining forecasting skill with and without a given predictor included is effectively the same as Breiman's shuffling approach. And if so, one might consider, for instance, dropping sets of predictors to document their joint contribution. Actually, the two strategies are somewhat different. In Granger's approach, dropping or adding predictors to the model means that the model itself will be re-estimated each time. So, the comparisons Granger favors are the result of different predictors being included *and different models*. The impact of neutralizing a predictor and changing the model are confounded. Under Breiman's approach, the algorithm is not re-applied. The shuffling is undertaken as an additional procedure with the algorithmic results fixed.

In summary, for many scientists the ability to predict accurately in Breiman's sense is an essential measure of an algorithm's worth. If one cannot predict well, it means that the algorithm cannot usefully reproduce the empirical world. It follows that the algorithmic results have little value. The take-home message is simple: if prediction skill is the gold standard (or even just a very important criterion by which to evaluate an algorithm), then a predictor's contribution to that skill is surely one reasonable measure of that predictor's importance.

5.6.2.1 Some Examples of Importance Plots with Extensions

Consider now a random forests analysis of data from an educational and job training program for homeless individuals. Because providing such services to homeless individuals is expensive, administrators wanted to know in advance which individuals referred to the program would likely not be helped. For example, such individuals may have had more fundamental needs such as treatment for drug dependence. At the same time, the administrators wanted to make a special effort to identify individuals with promise and were prepared to accept a substantial number of individuals who would not find a steady job when predicted to do so. A provisional cost ratio of 4 to 1 was determined. It was four times worse to overlook a promising individual than to mistakenly decide that an individual was promising.

Random forests was applied to training data on a little less than 7000 individuals who had gone through their program. One of the primary outcomes was whether after finishing the program, steady employment followed. It did for about 27% of the graduates of the program. The response variable is still unbalanced, but not nearly as severely as in the past two examples.

Table 5.4 shows the confusion table that resulted. Consistent with stakeholder preferences, there are about four false positives for every false negative (i.e.,

Table 5.4 Random forests confusion table for the employment after training with a 4 to 1 target cost ratio (N=6723)

	Fitted		Classification
	Not employed	Employed	error
Not employed	2213	2626	0.54
Employed	606	1278	0.32
Prediction error	0.21	0.67	Overall error = 0.48

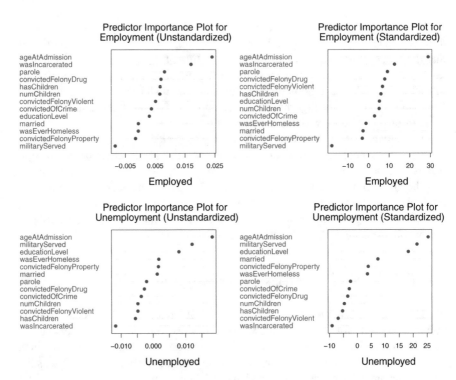

Fig. 5.3 Variable importance plots for employment outcome with a 4 to 1 target cost ratio (N=6723)

2626/606). 68% of those who would find employment were accurately classified. However, because of the imposed 4 to 1 cost ratio, a prediction of success on the job market would be wrong 67% of the time. As before, this lack of accuracy results substantially for the lower cost of false positives determined by stakeholders.

Variable importance plots are shown in Fig. 5.3. Reduction in prediction accuracy is shown on the horizontal axis. The code for the random forest analysis and the subsequent importance plots are shown in Fig. 5.4. Although we are still using Breiman's term "prediction accuracy," we are actually considering classification accuracy in OOB data.

The upper left figure shows unstandardized reductions in prediction accuracy for employment when each predictor is in turn randomly shuffled. The age at which an individual enters the program is the most important input. When that variable is shuffled, prediction accuracy declines about 2.5 percentage points (i.e., from 68% to 65.5%). The importance of all of the other predictors can be interpreted in the same fashion. The bottom four predictors make no contribution to predictive accuracy. Recall that contributions less than 0.0 result from the noise built into the random forests predictor importance algorithm and in practice, are taken to be equal to 0.0.

```
library(randomForest)
# random forests
rf1<-randomForest(Employed~ageAtAdmission+
convictedOfCrime+convictedFelonyViolent+
convictedFelonyProperty+convictedFelonyDrug+
wasIncarcerated+numChildren+parole
married+hasChildren+educationLevel+
wasEverHomeless+militaryServed,
data=TestData,importance=T,sampsize=c(1200,1100))

par(mfrow=c(2,2))

# Variable Importance Plots
varImpPlot(rf1,type=1,scale=F,class="Employed",
main="Forecasting Importance Plot for Employment
(Unstandardized)",col="blue",cex=1,pch=19)

varImpPlot(rf1,type=1,scale=T,class="Employed",
main="Forecasting Importance Plot for Employment
(Standardized)", col="blue",cex=1,pch=19)

varImpPlot(rf1,type=1,scale=F,class="Unemployed",
main="Forecasting Importance Plot for Unemployment
(Unstandardized)", col="blue",cex=1,pch=19)

varImpPlot(rf1,type=1,scale=T,class="Unemployed",
main="Forecasting Importance Plot for Unemployment
(Standardized)", col="blue",cex=1,pch=19)

# Partial Dependence Plots
part1<-partialPlot(rf1,pred.data=TestData,x.var=ageAtAdmission,
rug=T,which.class="Employed")

par(mfrow=c(2,1))

scatter.smooth(part1$x,part1$y,span=1/3,xlab="Age at Admission",
ylab="Centered Log Odds of Employment", main="Partial
Dependence Plot for Employment on Age",col="blue",pch=19)

part2<-partialPlot(rf1,pred.data=TestData,x.var=educationLevel,
rug=T,which.class="Employed", main="Partial Dependence
Plot for Employment on Education", xlab="Educational Level,
ylab="Centered Log Odds of Employment"),ylim=c(-.05,.25))
```

Fig. 5.4 R code for random forests analysis of employment outcome

Predictor importance does not show *how* an input is related to the response. The functional form is not revealed, nor are any of the likely interaction effects with other inputs. Going back to the bread baking metaphor, each input is but an ingredient in a recipe. One can learn the importance of an input for prediction, but nothing more. Also not shown is prediction accuracy that is shared among inputs. Consequently, the sum of the individual contributions can be substantially less than 68%.

The upper right figure shows the standardized contributions to employment prediction accuracy in standard deviation units. The ordering of the inputs in the upper right figure has changed a bit because of the standardization, and as a descriptive summary, it is not clear what has been gained. It may be tempting to use each input's standard deviation, which can be easily extracted from the output, to construct confidence intervals. But, for a variety of technical reasons, this is not a good idea (Wager et al. 2014).

The bottom two figures repeat the same analyses, but using unemployment as the outcome. One might think that the figures in the bottom row would be very similar to the figures in the top row. Somewhat counterintuitively, they are not. Recall how classification is accomplished in random forests. For a binary outcome, the class is assigned by majority vote. Two important features of those votes are in play here: the voting margin and the number of actual class members.

Consider a simple example in which there are 500 trees in the random forest. Suppose a given individual receives a vote of 251 to 249 to be assigned to the employment class category. The margin of victory is very small. Suppose that in fact that individual does find a job; the forecast is correct. Now a predictor is shuffled. The vote might be very different. But suppose it is now just 249 to 251. Only two votes over trees have changed. Yet, the individual is now placed incorrectly in the unemployed class. This increases the prediction error by one individual.

Is that one individual increase in misclassifications enough to matter? Probably not given the usual sample sizes. But if a substantial number of the votes over trees is close, a substantial increase in the number of classification errors could result. And if the sample size is relatively small, the accuracy decline in units of percentage points could be relatively large. Such results are potentiated if the votes in terminal nodes within trees are close as well. Perhaps the key point is that these processes can differ depending on the outcome class, which explains why predictor importance can vary by the outcome class.

In Fig. 5.3, the prediction contributions are generally larger for the upper two figures than for the lower two figures. This is substantially a consequence of the marginal distribution of the response. There are more than twice as many individuals who do not find work compared to individuals who do. As a result, it would take many more classification changes after shuffling for the smaller prediction accuracy declines shown in the lower figures to approximate the larger predictor accuracy declines shown in the upper figures. It is more difficult to move the needle.

5.7 Input Response Functions

Predictor importance is only part of the story. In addition to knowing the importance of each input, it can be very instructive to have a description of how each predictor is related to the response. The set of response functions needs to be described.

One useful solution based on an earlier suggestion by Breiman and his colleagues (1984) is "partial dependence plots" (Friedman 2001; Hastie et al. 2009: section 10.13.2). For tree-based approaches, one proceeds as follows.

1. Grow a forest.
2. Suppose x_1 is the initial predictor of interest, and it has v distinct values in the training data. Construct v datasets as follows.

   (a) For each of the v distinct values of x_1, make up a new dataset where x_1 only takes on that value, leaving all other variables untouched.
   (b) For each of the v datasets, predict the response for each tree in the random forest. There will be for each tree a single response value averaged over all observations. The observations can come from the full dataset, the data used to grow the tree, test data, or some other dataset. For numeric response variables, the predicted value is a conditional mean. For categorical response variables, the predicted value is a conditional proportion or some functional of a conditional proportion.
   (c) Average these predictions over the trees. The result is an average conditional mean, an average conditional proportion, or an average of some conditional functional (e.g., a logit) over trees.
   (d) Plot the average prediction for each value for each of the v datasets against the v values of x_1

3. Go back to Step 2 and repeat for each predictor.

There is a lot going on in this algorithm that may not be immediately apparent. Partial dependence plots show the average relationship between a given input and the response within the empirical, joint distribution of the other inputs. For each of the v values, the values of all other inputs are always the same. Therefore, variation in these other inputs cannot explain an empirically determined response function for those v values.

Suppose the selected input is age. One asks what would the average outcome be if everyone were 21 and nothing else changed? Then one asks, what would the average outcome be if everyone were 22 and nothing else changed? The same question is asked for age 23, age 24, and so on. All that changes are for the single age assigned to each case: 21, 22, 23, 24 . . . .

Now in more detail, suppose the response is binary and initially everyone is assigned the age of 20. Much as one would do in conventional regression, the outcome for each case is predicted using all of the other inputs as well. Those fitted values can then be averaged. For a binary outcome, the average is a conditional proportion or more likely, just as in logistic regression, an average conditional logit.[14]

Next, everyone is assigned the age of 21, and the same operations are undertaken. For each age in turn, the identical procedure is applied. One can then see how the outcome class proportions or logits change with age alone because as age changes, none of the other variables do. Should the response be quantitative, each fitted average is a conditional mean. One can then see how the conditional mean changes with age alone.

The partial dependence is usually plotted. Unlike the plots of fitted values constructed from smoothers (e.g., from the generalized additive model), partial dependence plots usually impose no smoothness constraints, and the underlying tree structure tends to produce somewhat bumpy results. In practice, one usually overlays an "eyeball" smoother when the plot is interpreted. Alternatively, it is often possible to overlay a real smoother if the software stores the requisite output. In R, *randomForest* does.

For quantitative response variables, the units on the vertical axis usually are the natural units of the response, whatever they happen to be (e.g., wages in dollars). For categorical response variables, the units of the response on the vertical axis are usually *centered* logits. The details are important. Consider first the binary case.

Recall that logistic regression equation commonly is written as

$$\log\left(\frac{p}{1-p}\right) = \mathbf{X}\boldsymbol{\beta}, \tag{5.11}$$

where p is the probability of a success. The term on the left-hand side is the log of the odds of a success, often called a logit. The term on the right-hand side is the usual linear combination of predictors and a constant.

When there are more than two outcome classes, the most common approach is to build up from the familiar binary formulation. If there are K response classes, there are $K - 1$ equations, each of the same general form as Eq. (5.11). One equation of the K possible equations is redundant because the response categories are exhaustive and mutually exclusive. Thus, if an observation does not fall in categories $1, \ldots, K - 1$, it must fall in the Kth category. Perhaps the most popular identifying restriction is to choose a single outcome class as the reference category, just as in the binomial case (i.e., there are two possible outcomes and one equation). Then, for each of the $K - 1$ equations, the logit is the log of the odds for a given class compared to the reference class.

Suppose there are four response categories, and the fourth is chosen as the reference outcome class. There would then be three equations with three different responses, one for $\log(p_1/p_4)$, one for $\log(p_2/p_4)$, and one for $\log(p_3/p_4)$. The predictors would be the same for each equation, but each equation would have its own set of regression coefficients likely differing in values across equations.

One might think that partial dependence plots would follow a similar convention. But they do not. The choice of the reference outcome class determines which logits will be used, and the logits used affect the regression coefficients that result. Although the overall fit is the same whatever the reference category, and although one can compute from the set of estimated regression coefficients the correct regression coefficients should another reference category be used, the set of regression coefficients reported differ depending on the reference class.

There is usually no statistical justification for choosing one reference class over another. The choice is usually made on subject-matter grounds to make interpretations easier, and the choice can easily vary from data analyst to data analyst. So, the need for a reference class can complicate interpretations of the results and means that a user of the results has to undertake additional work if regression coefficients using another reference category are desired.

In response to these and other complications, partial dependence plots are based on a somewhat different approach. There are K, rather than $K - 1$, response functions, $f_k(\mathbf{X})$, one for each response variable class. For the logistic model and class k, these take the form of

$$p_k(\mathbf{X}) = \frac{e^{f_k(\mathbf{X})}}{\sum_{k=1}^{K} e^{f_k(\mathbf{X})}}. \tag{5.12}$$

Equation (5.12) has the conditional proportion (or probability depending on Level I v. Level II) as the left-hand term. For the right-hand term, the numerator is for class k the exponentiated response function (i.e., an exponentiated logit). The denominator is the sum of all such K expressions (i.e., all exponentiated logits). If there are logits empirically available for each outcome class, one can get back to conditional proportions or probabilities through Eq. (5.12).

There is still a redundancy problem to solve. The usual solution employed in partial dependence plots is to constrain $\sum_{k=1}^{K} f_k(\mathbf{X}) = 0$. This leads to the multinomial deviance loss function and to the use of a rather different kind of baseline.

Instead of using a given outcome class as the reference, the unweighted mean of the logged proportions or probabilities for the K categories is used as the reference. In much the same spirit as analysis of variance, the response variable units are then in deviations from a mean. More specifically, we let

$$f_k(\mathbf{X}) = \log[p_k(\mathbf{X})] - \frac{1}{K} \sum_{k=1}^{K} \log[p_k(\mathbf{X})]. \tag{5.13}$$

Thus, the response function is the difference between the logged proportion for class k and the average of the logged proportions for all K response classes. The units are essentially logits but with the mean over the K classes as the reference. Consequently, each response class can have its own equation and, therefore, its own partial dependence plot. This approach is applied even when there are only two response classes, and the conventional logit formulation might not present interpretive problems.

To illustrate, consider once again the employment data. Suppose age in years is the predictor whose relationship with the binary employment response variable is of interest. And suppose for an age of, say, 25, the proportion of individuals finding a job is 0.20 (computed using the partial dependence algorithm). The centered logit is $\log(0.2) - [\log(0.2) + \log(0.8)]/2 = -0.693$ (using natural logarithms). This is the value that would be plotted on the vertical axis corresponding to 25 years of age on the horizontal axis. It is the log of the odds with mean logged proportion over the K response classes as the reference.

The same approach can be used for the proportion of 25-year-old individuals who do not find a job. That proportion is necessarily 0.80, so that value plotted is $\log(0.8) - [\log(0.2) + \log(0.8)]/2 = 0.693$. In the binary case, essentially the same information is obtained no matter which response class is examined.

As required, $0.693 - 0.693 = 0$. This implies that one response function is the mirror image of the other. Thus, one partial dependence plot is the mirror image of the other partial dependence plot, and only one of the two is required for interpretation.

In the binary case, it is especially easy to get from the centered log odds to more familiar units. The values produced by Eq. (5.13) are half the usual log of the odds. From that, one can easily compute the corresponding proportions. For example, multiplying -0.693 by 2 and exponentiating yields an odds of 0.25. Then, solving for the numerator proportion results in a value of 0.20. We are back where we started.[15]

Equation 5.13 would be applied for each year of age. Thus, for 26 years, the proportion of individuals finding a job might be 0.25. Then the value plotted on the horizontal axis would be 26, and the value on the vertical axis would be $\log(0.25) - [\log(0.25) + \log(0.75)]/2 = -0.549$.

The value of -0.549 is in a region where the response function has been increasing. With one additional year of age, the proportion who find work increases from 0.20 to 0.25, which becomes log odds of -0.693 and -0.549, respectively. All other values produced for different ages can be interpreted in a similar way. Consequently, one can get a sense of how the response variable changes with variation in a given predictor, all other predictors held constant. The same reasoning carries over when there are more than two response classes, as we will soon see.

5.7.1 Partial Dependence Plot Example

Figure 5.5 shows two partial dependence plots constructed from the employment data with code that can be found toward the bottom of Fig. 5.4. The upper plot shows the relationship between the input age and the centered log odds of employment.[16] Age is quantitative. Employment prospects increase nearly linearly with age until about age 50 at which time they begin to gradually decline. The lower plot shows the

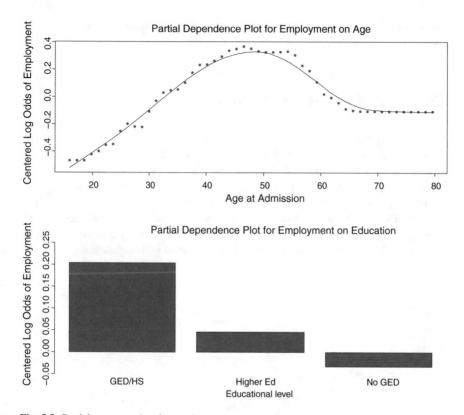

Fig. 5.5 Partial response plots for employment on age and education (N=6723)

relationship between the input education and the centered log odds of employment. Education is a factor. The employment prospects are best for individuals who have a high school or GED certificate. They are worst for individuals who have no high school degree or GED. Individuals with at least some college fall in between.[17] Program administrators explained the outcome for those with at least some college as a result of the job market in which they were seeking work. The jobs were for largely unskilled labor. There were not many appealing jobs for individuals with college credits.

In order to get a practical sense of whether employment varies with either input, it can be useful to transform the logits back to proportions. Suppose that one were interested in the largest gap in the prospects for employment. From the upper plot, the largest logit is about 0.39, and the smallest logit is about −0.42. These become proportions of 0.69 and 0.30, respectively. The proportion who find work increases by 39 percentage points. Age seems to be strongly associated with employment.

It is important not to forget that the response functions displayed in partial dependence plots reflect the relationship between a given predictor and the response, conditioning on all other predictors. All other predictors are being "held constant" in the manner discussed above. The code in Fig. 5.4 shows that there are a substantial number of such predictors.

5.7.2   More than Two Response Classes

When the response has more than two outcome categories, there are no longer the symmetries across plots that are found for binary outcomes. For a binary response variable, it does not matter which of the two categories is used when the partial dependence plot is constructed. One plot is the mirror image of the other. Figure 5.6 shows what can happen with three outcome categories.

The three employment outcomes in Fig. 5.6 are "no salary," "hourly salary," "yearly salary." The first category means that no job was found. For those who found a job, a yearly salary is for these individuals associated with higher status positions

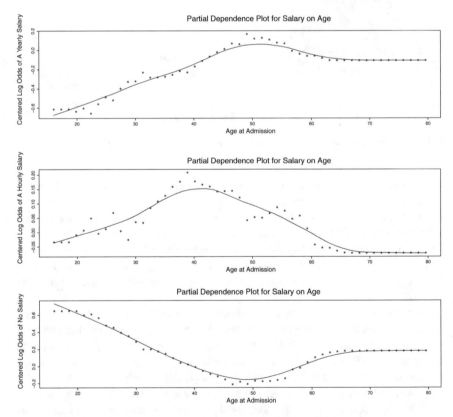

Fig. 5.6 Partial response plots for employment on yearly salary, weekly salary, or no salary on age (N= 6723)

compared to positions offering an hourly salary. The plot at the top, for the yearly salary outcome, looks rather like the plot for finding any job. Prospects are bleak for those under 20, peak around 50 and then gradually taper off. The plot in the middle, for the hourly salary outcome, has the same general shape, but peaks around 40 and then falls off far more abruptly. The plot at the bottom for no salary looks much like the top plot, but with a sign reversal. No plot is the mirror image of another because if the outcome in question does not occur, one of *two* other categories will. Moreover, the two other categories change depending on the single outcome whose centered logits are plotted.

In practice, each plot can have a story to tell. For example, comparing the top two plots, being over 50 years old is associated with a small decline in prospects for higher status jobs. In contrast, being over 50 years old is associated with a dramatic decline in prospects for lower status jobs. Part of the explanation can probably be found in the nature of the job. Hourly jobs will often require more physical capabilities, which can decrease dramatically starting around age 50. (As I know from personal experience.)

When there are more than two classes, extracting numeric interpretations is more difficult. One can always compare logits. As before, working with proportions or probabilities is usually easier. Suppose there are, say, three classes, k_1, k_2, and k_3 with three logits represented by logit_1, logit_2, and logit_3. Simplifying the notation a bit, the proportion or probability associated with k_1 is

$$p(k_1) = \frac{e^{\text{logit}_{k1}}}{(e^{\text{logit}_{k1}} + e^{\text{logit}_{k2}} + e^{\text{logit}_{k3}})}. \tag{5.14}$$

For example, the largest logit in the top figure is for 50 years olds and, reading off of the graph, is about 0.19. The other logits, approximated in the manner, are about 0.12 and -0.1. Using Eq. (5.14), the associated proportion or probability is about 0.37. Proceeding in the same way, the smallest logit is the top figure is for 18 year olds and is about -0.6. The other logits are approximately -0.03 and 0.6. The associated proportion or probability is 0.16. The difference is about 20 percentage points, which is a large enough effect to care about.

Just as with variable importance plots, one never knows for partial dependence plots how each input is linked to the outcome. In particular, variation in an input may well be partitioned between a large number of interaction effects. In econometric language, something akin to reduced form relationships are being represented.[18]

5.8 Classification and the Proximity Matrix

It can be interesting to determine the degree to which individual observations tend to be classified alike. Rather than the usual practice of examining associations between variables, attention is turned to associations between observations. For example, which students in a high school tend to fall in the same terminal nodes?

In random forests, this information is contained in the "proximity matrix." The proximity matrix is constructed as follows.

1. Grow a classification tree as usual.
2. Drop all the training data (in-bag and out-of-bag) down the tree.
3. For all possible pairs of cases, if a pair lands in the same terminal node, increase their proximity value by one.
4. Repeat Steps 1 to 4 until the designated number of trees has been grown.
5. Normalize by dividing by the number of trees.

The result is an $N \times N$ matrix with each cell showing the proportion of trees for which each pair of observations lands in the same terminal node. The higher that proportion, the more alike those observations are in how the trees place them, and the more "proximate" they are.

As noted earlier, working with a very large number observation can improve how well random forests performs because large trees can be grown. Large trees can reduce bias. For example, working with 100,000 observations rather than 10,000 can improve classification accuracy substantially. However, because a proximity matrix is $N \times N$, storage can be a serious bottleneck. Storage problems can be partly addressed by only storing the upper or lower triangle, and there are other storage-saving procedures that have been developed. But large datasets still pose a significant problem.

Little subject-matter sense can be made of an $N \times N$ matrix of even modest size. Consequently, additional procedures usually need to be applied. We turn to one popular option: multidimensional scaling. There are many kinds of multidimensional scaling, some dating back to the 1950s. Computer scientists now call multidimensional scaling a form of unsupervised learning.

5.8.1   Clustering by Proximity Values

The proportions in a proximity matrix can be seen as measures of similarly, and the matrix is symmetric with 1s along the main diagonal. Consequently, a proximity matrix can be treated as a similarity matrix in much the same spirit as some kernel matrices discussed earlier. As such, it is subject to a variety of clustering procedures with multidimensional scaling (MDS) the one offered by *randomForests* in *R*.

It is common to work with dissimilarities rather than similarities. For a proximity matrix, this means subtracting all of the proportions from 1.0. The scaling task is to map the dissimilarities into a lower dimensional space (i.e., smaller than $N \times N$) that nevertheless approximates the dissimilarities well. That is, the Euclidian distances between the points in the lower dimension space correspond as closely as possible to the dissimilarities. There are many ways such an objective can be tackled (de Leeuw and Mair 2009), but the common approach is to minimize the sum of the squared differences between the dissimilarities and their corresponding Euclidian distances in the lower dimensional space. In practice, the results are displayed in a 2-

dimensional plot, which means that the dissimilarities in N dimensions are projected onto 2 dimensions.

Within *randomForests*, the calculations are done by *cmdscale*, and the plotting is done by *MDSplot*. However, with more than several hundred observations, there is so much overplotting that making sense of the results is very difficult. Labeling the points could help, but not with so much overplotting. Also, the computational challenges are substantial.[19] This is unfortunate because many machine learning procedures work best with large number of observations.

Figure 5.7 shows a 2-D MDS plot from the proximity matrix constructed for the employment analysis. There are discernible pattens. The red dots are for individuals who found employment, and the blue dots are for individuals who did not. Ideally,

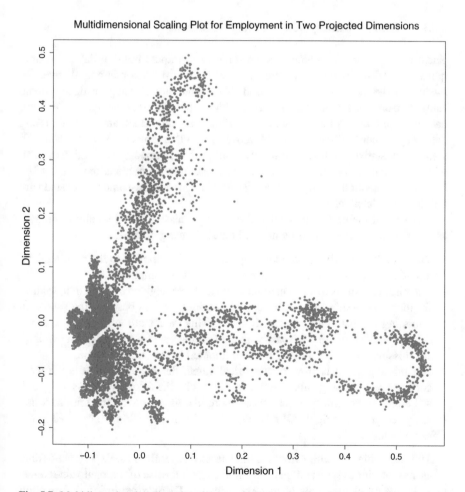

Fig. 5.7 Multidimensional scaling plot of the proximity matrix from the employment analysis in 2-D: red dots for employed and blue dots for unemployed

the individuals who found employment would tend to be alike, and the individuals who did not find employment would tend to be alike. That is, there would be lots of terminal nodes dominated by either employed individuals or unemployed individuals so that they would tend to fall in similar neighborhoods. However, it is difficult to extract much from the figure because of the overplotting. Working with a small random sample of cases would allow for a plot that could be more easily understood, but there would be a substantial risk that important patterns might be overlooked.

In short, better ways need to be found to visualize the proximity matrix. Multidimensional scaling has promise, but can be very difficult to interpret with current graphical procedures and large Ns.[20]

5.8.1.1   Using Proximity Values to Impute Missing Data

There are two ways in which random forests can impute missing data. The first, quick method relies on a measure of location. If a predictor is quantitative, the median of the available values is used. If the predictor is categorical, the modal category from the available data is used. Should there be small amounts of missing data, this method may be satisfactory. But if there are only small amounts of missing data, why bother to impute at all? Moreover, recall that replacing missing data with a summary statistic will reduce the variability of the variables with missing data, which can undermine statistical inference. There are also implications for any IID claims made about how the data were generated. One must assume that the data are missing completely at random.

The second method assumes that the data are missing conditionally at random and capitalizes on the proximity matrix in the following manner.

1. The "quick and dirty" method of imputation is first applied to the training data, a random forest is grown, and the proximity values computed.
2. If a missing value is from a quantitative variable, a weighted average of the values for the non-missing cases is used. The proximity values between the case with a missing value and all cases with non-missing values are used as the weights. Cases that are more like the case with the missing value are given greater weight. All missing values for that variable are imputed in the same fashion.
3. If a missing value is from a categorical value, the imputed value is the most common non-missing value for the variable, with the category counts weighted, as before, by proximity. Again, cases more like the case with the missing value are given greater weight. All missing values for that variable are imputed in the same fashion.

The step using proximity values is then iterated several times. Experience to date suggests that four to six iterations are sufficient. But the use of imputed values tends to make the OOB measures of fit too optimistic. There is really less information being brought to bear in the analysis than the random forest algorithm knows. The computational demands are also quite demanding and may be impractical for many datasets until more efficient ways to handle the proximities are found. Finally, imputing a single weighted value for each missing observation papers over chance variation in the imputation. This the same problem raised for the quick and dirty method.

5.8.1.2 Using Proximities to Detect Outliers

The proximity matrix can be used to spot outliers in the space defined by the predictors. The basic idea is that outliers are observations whose proximities to all other observations in the data are small. The procedures in *randomForest* to detect outliers are not implemented for quantitative response variables. For categorical response variables, outliers are defined within classes of the response variable. Within each observed outcome class, each observation is given a value for its "outlyingness" computed as follows.

1. For a given observation, compute the sum of the squares of the proximities with all of the other observations in the same outcome class. Then take the inverse. A large value will indicate that on the average the proximities are small for that observation; the observation is not much like other observations. Do the same for all other observations in that class. One can think of these values as unstandardized.
2. Within each class, compute the median and mean absolute deviation around the median of the unstandardized values inverse proximities.
3. Subtract the median from each of the unstandardized values and divide by the mean absolute deviation. In this fashion, the unstandardized values are standardized.
4. Values less than zero are set to 0.0.

These steps are then repeated for each class of the response variable. Observations with values larger than 10 can be considered outliers. Note that an observation does not become suspect because of a single atypical x-value. An outlier is defined by *how it is classified*, which is a function of all of its x-values. An outlier typically lands in terminal nodes where it has little company.

Figure 5.8 is an index plot of outlier values for the employment data, with employed cases represented by red spikes and unemployed cases represented as blue spikes. The R code is shown in Fig. 5.9.

For this analysis, there are perhaps 4–6 observations of possible concern, but their outlier measures are close to 10 and with over 9000 observations overall, they would make no material difference in the results if dropped. It might be different if the outlier measures were in the high teens, and there were only a few hundred observations in total.

When the data analyst considers dropping one or more outlying cases, a useful diagnostic tool can be a cross-tabulation of the classes assigned for the set of observations that two random forest analyses have in common: one with all of the data and one with the outliers removed. If the common observations are, by

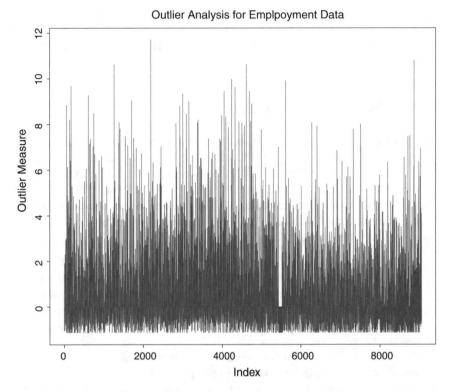

Fig. 5.8 Index plot of outlier measures for employment data with values greater than 10 candidates for deletion (Red spikes are for employed and blue spikes are for unemployed)

```
plot(outlier(rf1),type="h", ylab="Outlier Measure",
     main="Outlier Analysis for Employment Data",
     col=c("red","blue")[as.numeric(TestData$Employed)])
```

Fig. 5.9 R code for index plot of outlier measures

and large, classified in the same way in both analyses, the outliers do not make an important difference to the classification process.

5.9   Empirical Margins

Recall Breiman's definition of a margin: the difference between the proportion of times over trees that an observation is correctly classified minus the largest proportion of times over trees that an observation is incorrectly classified. That

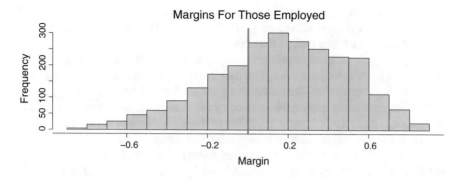

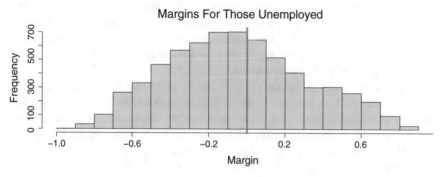

Fig. 5.10 Distribution of margins for employed and unemployed individuals (The red vertical line is located at a margin value of 0.0)

definition can be used for each observation in a dataset. Positive values represent correct classifications, and negative values represent incorrect classifications.

Figure 5.10 shows histograms for two empirical margins. The upper plot is for individuals who were employed. The lower plot is for individuals who are not employed. We are conditioning on the actual response class much as we do for rows of a confusion table. For both histograms, the red, vertical line is located at a margin value of 0.0.

For employed individuals, the median margin is 0.18, which translates into a solid majority vote or more for half of the correctly classified cases. Moreover, 68% of the employed individuals are correctly classified. For unemployed individuals, the median margin is −0.07. About 55% of the unemployed individuals are incorrectly classified, although many by close votes.

The margins can serve an additional performance diagnostic to supplement the rows of a confusion table. In addition to classification accuracy computed from each row, one can learn how definitive both the correct and incorrect classifications are. Ideally, the votes are decisive for the correctly classified cases and razor thin for the incorrectly classified cases. The results in Fig. 5.10 have some of this pattern, but only weakly so.

Perhaps the major use of margins is to compare the stability of results from different datasets. One might have results from two datasets that classify with about the same accuracy, but for one of those, the classifications are more stable. The results from that dataset should be preferred because they are less likely to be a result of a random forest luck of the draw.

The stability is with respect to the random forest algorithm itself because margins are derived from votes over trees. The data are fixed. If a new random forest were grown with the same data, the classes assigned to all cases would not likely be the same. The uncertainty captured is created by the random forest algorithm itself. As such, it represents the in-sample reliability of the algorithm and says nothing about accuracy. Indeed, it is possible to have results that are reliably wrong.

There can be no margins in forecasting settings because the outcomes are not yet known. But the votes are easily retrieved by *randomForest* and can be very instructive. More decisive votes imply more reliable forecasts. For example, a school administrator may be trying to project whether a particular student will drop out of high school. If so, there may be good reason to intervene with services such as tutoring. The case for intervening should be seen as more credible if the dropout forecast is coupled with high reliability.

There is no clear threshold beyond which reliability is automatically high enough. That will be a judgment call for decision-makers. Moreover, that line may be especially hard to draw when there are more than two outcome classes. Suppose the vote for three response classes proportions are 0.25, 0.30, and 0.45. The class with 45% of the votes wins by a substantial plurality. But the majority of votes is cast against that class. Which reliabilities should be evaluated?

For real world settings in which forecasts from a random forest are made, the best advice may be to use the votes to help determine how much weight should be given to the forecast compared to the weight given to other information. In the school dropout example, an overwhelming vote projecting a dropout may mean discounting a student's apparent show of contrition and promises to do better. If the vote is effectively too close to call, the show of contrition and promises to do better carry the day.

5.10 Quantitative Response Variables

There is not very much new that needs to be said about quantitative response variables once one appreciates that random forests handles quantitative response variables much as bagging does. Even through for each tree there are still binary partitions of the data, there are no response variable classes and no response class proportions from which to define impurity. Traditionally, impurity is defined as the within-node error sum of squares. A new partition of the data is determined by the split that would most reduce the sum, over the two prospective subsets, of the within-partition error sums of squares. Predicted values are the mean of the response variable in each of the terminal nodes. For each OOB observation, the average of its terminal node means is the fitted value assigned.

For regression trees, therefore, there are no classification errors, only residuals. Concerns about false negatives and positives and their costs are no longer relevant. There are no confusion tables and no measures of importance based on classification errors. To turn a regression tree into a fully operational random forest, the following steps are required.

1. Just as in the classification case, each tree is grown from a random sample (with replacement) of the training data.
2. Just as in the classification case, for each potential partitioning of the data, a random sample (without replacement) of predictors is used.
3. The value assigned to each terminal node is the mean of the response variable values that land in that terminal node.
4. For each tree in the random forest, the fitted value for each OOB case is the mean previously assigned to the terminal node in which it lands.
5. As before, random forest averages OOB observations over trees. For a given observation, the average of the tree-by-tree fitted values is computed using only the fitted values from trees in which that observation was not used to grow the tree. This is the fitted value that random forest returns.
6. Deviations between these averaged, fitted values and the response variable observed values are used to construct the mean squared error reported for the collection of trees that constitutes a random forest. The value of the mean square error can be used to compute a "pseudo" R^2 as $(1 - MSE)/Var(Y)$.
7. Construction of partial dependence plots is done in the same manner as for classification trees, but now the fitted response is the set of conditional means for different predictor values, not a set of transformed fitted proportions.
8. Input variable importance is computed using the shuffling approach as before. And as before, there is a "resubstitution" (in-sample) measure and an OOB measure. For the resubstitution measure, each time a given variable is used to define a partitioning of the data for a given tree, the reduction in the within-node error sum of squares is recorded. When the tree is complete, the reductions are summed. The result is a reduction in the error sum of squares that can be attributed to each predictor. These totals, one for each predictor, are then averaged over trees. The out-of-sample importance measure is also an average over trees. For a given tree, the OOB observations are used to compute each terminal node's error sum of squares. From these, the mean squared error for that tree is computed. Then a designated predictor is shuffled, and mean square error for that tree is computed again. An increase in this mean square error is a decrease in accuracy. The same steps are applied to each tree, and the accuracy decreases are averaged over trees to get an average decrease in accuracy for that predictor. The standard deviation of these decreases over trees can be used to standardize the average decrease, if that is desirable. The same process is employed for each predictor.

Despite the tight connection between regression trees and random forests, there are features found in some implementations of regression trees that have yet to be introduced into random forests, at least within R. But change is underway.

Extensions to Poisson regression seem imminent (Mathlourthi et al. 2015), and Ishwaran and colleagues (2008) provide in R a procedure to do survival analysis (and lots more) with random forests using *randomForestSRC*. Both alter the way splits within each tree are determined so that the reformulation is fundamental. For example, *randomForestSRC* can pick the predictor and split that maximizes the survival difference in the two offspring nodes. There is also the option to do the analysis with competing risks (Ishwaran et al. 2014) and various weighting options that can be applied to the splitting rule (Ishwaran 2015).

Alternatively, *quantregForest* only changes how values in each terminal node are used. The intent is to compute quantiles. Instead of storing only the mean of each terminal node as trees are grown, the entire distribution is stored. Recall the earlier discussion surrounding Table 5.2. Once the user decides which quantiles are of interest, they can be easily computed.

If one is worried about the impact of within-node outliers on the conditional mean, the conditional median can be used instead. If for substantive reasons there is interest in, say, the first or third quartile, those can be used. Perhaps most importantly, the quantile option provides a way to take the costs of forecasting errors into account. For example, if the 75th quantile is chosen, the consequences of underestimates are three times more costly than the consequences of overestimates (i.e., $75/25 = 3$).

However, such calculations only affect what is done with the information contained in the terminal nodes across trees. They do not require that the trees themselves be grown again with a linear loss function, let alone a loss function with asymmetric costs. In other words, the trees grown under quadratic loss are not changed. If there are concerns about quadratic loss, they still apply to each of the splits. All of the usual random forests outputs (e.g., variable importance plots) also are still a product of a quadratic loss function.

5.11   A Random Forest Illustration Using a Quantitative Response Variable

Several years ago, an effort was made to count the number of homeless in Los Angeles County (Berk et al. 2008). There are over 2000 census tracts in the county, and enumerators were sent to a sample of a little over 500. Their job was to count "unsheltered" homeless, who were not to be found in shelters or other temporary housing. Shelter counts were readily available. The details of the sampling need not trouble us here, and in the end, the overall county total was estimated to be about 90,000. We focus here on the street counts only.

In addition to countywide totals, there was a need to have estimated counts for tracts not visited. Various stakeholders might wish to have estimates at the tract level for areas to which enumerators were not sent. Random forests was used with tract-level predictors to impute the homeless street counts for these tracts. Here, we focus on the random forests procedure itself, not the imputation. About 21% of the variance in the homeless street counts were accounted for by the random forests application with the follow inputs.[21]

1. MedianInc — median household income
2. PropVacant — proportion of vacant dwellings
3. PropMinority — proportion of minority
4. PerCommercial — percentage of land used for commercial purposes
5. PerIndustrial — percentage of the land used for industrial purposes
6. PerResidential — percentage of the land used for residential purposes.

Figure 5.11 is a plot of the actual street totals against the fitted street totals in the data. One can see that there are a number of outliers that make any fitting exercise challenging. In Los Angeles county, the homeless were sprinkled over most census tracts, but a few tracts had very large homeless populations. The green 1-to-1 line summarizes what a good fit would look like. Ideally the fitted street counts and the actual street counts should be much the same. The red line summarizes with a least squares line the quality of the fit actually obtained. Were the horizontal axis

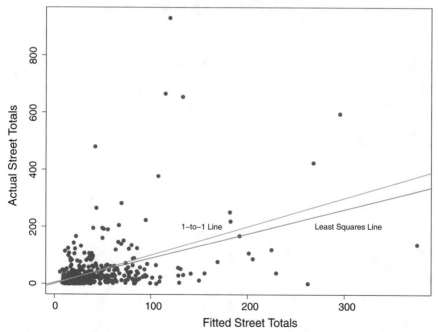

Fig. 5.11 For Los Angeles county census tracts a plot of actual homeless street counts against the random forest fitted homeless street counts (Least squares line is in red, the 1-to-1 line in green, N=504)

extended to allow for fitted counts with the same large values as the actual counts, the two lines would diverge dramatically.

The counts in the highly populated census tracts are often badly underestimated. For example, the largest fitted count is around 400. There are 5 census tracts with actual street counts over 400, one of those with a count of approximately 900. From a policy point of view this really matters. The census tracts most in need of services are not accurately characterized by random forests. Several important inputs were not available, and it shows. Statistical learning is no panacea.

Figure 5.12 shows two variable importance plots. On the left, the increase in average OOB mean squared error for each predictor is plotted. On the right, the increase in the average in-sample node impurity for each predictor is plotted. For example, when the percentage of land that is commercial is shuffled, the OOB mean squared error increases by about 7%, and the proportion of the residential population that is minority has no predictive impact whatsoever. When household median income is shuffled, average node impurity increases by 6e+05, and all of the predictors have some impact on the fit. The ranking of the variables changes depending on the importance measure, but for the reasons discussed earlier, the out-of-sample measures is preferable, especially if forecasting is an important goal.

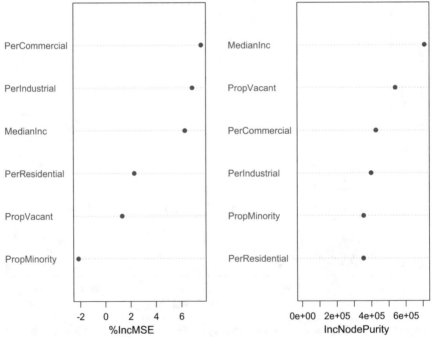

Fig. 5.12 Variable importance plots for street counts (On the left is the percent increase in the OOB mean squared error, and on the right is the in-sample increase in node impurity. N=504)

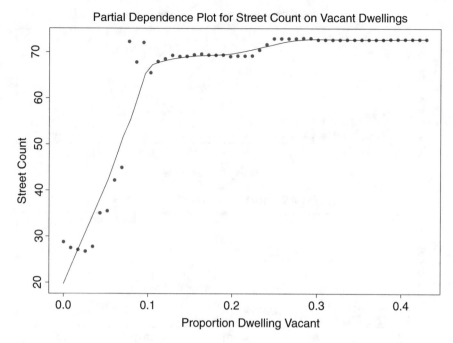

Fig. 5.13 The partial dependence plot for street counts on the proportion of vacant dwellings in a census tract (N=504)

Figure 5.13 is a partial dependence plot showing a positive association between the percentage of the residential dwellings that are vacant and the number of homeless counted. When vacancy is near zero, the average number of homeless is about 20 per tract. When the vacancy percent is above approximately 10%, the average count increases to between 60 and 70 (with a spike right around 10%). The change is very rapid. Beyond 10% the relationship is essentially flat. At that point, perhaps the needs of squatters are met.

In response to the poor fit for the few census tracts with a very large number of homeless individuals, it is worth giving *quantregForest* a try. As already noted, a random forest is grown as usual, but the distributions in the terminal nodes of each tree are retained for analysis. We will consider the impact of using three different quantiles: 0.10, 0.50, and 0.90. For these data, quantiles substantially larger than 0.50 would in practice usually be the focus. The code used in the analyses to follow is shown in Fig. 5.16.[22]

Figure 5.14 shows three plots laid out just like Fig. 5.11, for the conditional quantiles of 0.10, 0.50, and 0.90. All three fit the data about equally well if the adjusted R^2 is the measure because the outliers are very few. But should there be special concerns about the half dozen or so census tracts with very large homeless counts, it may make sense to fit the 90th percentile. For example, the largest fitted value for conditional 10th percentile is about 37. The largest fitted value for

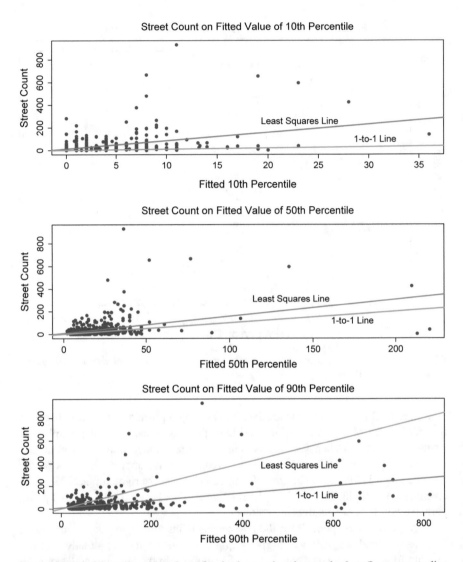

Fig. 5.14 Plot of Quantile random forest fitted values against the actual values (Least squares line in red and 1-to-1 line in green. Quantiles = 0.05, 0.50, 0.90. N=504)

conditional 50th percentile is about 220. The largest fitted value for conditional 90th percentile is nearly 700. Several tracts with large homeless counts are still badly underestimated, but clearly, the small number of tracts with substantial number of homeless is better approximated. Whether this is appropriate depends on the relative costs of underestimates to overestimates. We are again faced with the prospect of asymmetric costs, but for quantitative response variables.

When for the homeless data the 90th percentile is used, the cost of underesti-mating the number of homeless in a census tract is nine times more costly than

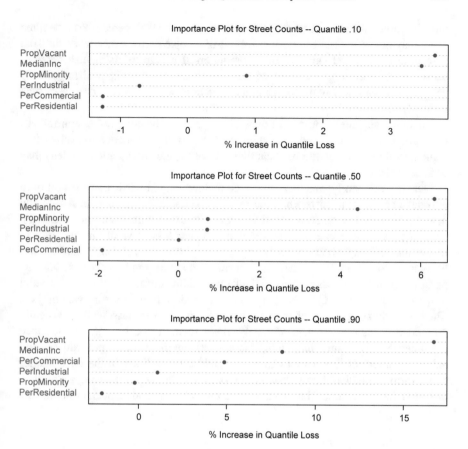

Fig. 5.15 Street count variable importance plots for quantiles of 0.10, 0.50, and 0.90 (Importance is measured by the OOB increase in the quantile loss after shuffling. N=504)

overestimating the number of homeless in a census tract (i.e., $0.90/0.10 = 9$). Whether the 9-to-1 cost ratio makes sense is a policy decision. What are the relative costs of underestimating the number of homeless compared to overestimating the number of homeless? More will be said about these issues when quantile boosting is discussed in the next chapter. But just as for classification, there is no reason to automatically impose symmetric costs.

Figure 5.15 shows three variable importance plots, one for each of the three quantiles being used: 0.10, 0.50, 0.90. The percentage point increase in quantile (linear) out-of-sample loss is the measure of importance. For example, for the conditional 90th percentile, the most important input is the proportion of vacant dwellings, which when shuffled increased the out-of-sample L_1 loss by about 16 percentage points. As before, negative values are treated as 0.0.

Perhaps the most important message is that by this measure of importance, the order of the variables can vary by the conditional quantile estimated. Inputs that are most important for out-of-sample performance when the 90th percentile is the fitted value may not be the most important for out-of-sample performance when the 10th percentile is the fitted value. That is, predictors that help to distinguish between census tracts with large numbers of homeless may be of no help distinguishing between census tracts with small numbers of homeless. Different processes may be involved.

There are apparently no partial dependence plots of quantile regression forests. It seems that relatively modest changes in the partial dependence plot algorithm could accommodate conditional quantiles. However, the computation burdens may be substantially increased.

Quantile random forests has some nice features and in particular, the ability to introduce asymmetric costs when the response variable is quantitative. As already noted, however, the random forest is grown as usual with each split based on quadratic loss. Were one truly committed to linear loss, it would make sense to revise the splitting criterion accordingly. More recently, *randomForestSRC* has become available in R, which has a form of quantile random forests that can partition with linear loss.[23] This variant on random forests is but one of several in the randomForestSRC package, including a random forest for survival analysis. There is a dizzying array of options, but the defaults for classification basically reproduce *randomForest*. Unfortunately, there seems to be no way to introduce asymmetric costs using the tuning parameters in the various procedures, and extracting interpretative output can be a struggle. We will see in the next chapter that a form of gradient boosting is even more wide ranging in the analysis options provided, has a theoretical basis that is far more coherent, and is much easier to use.

5.12 Statistical Inference with Random Forests

As long as users of random forests are content to describe relationships in the data on hand, random forests is a Level I procedure. But the use of OOB data to get honest performance assessments and measures of predictor performance speaks to Level II concerns, and generalization error in particular. If forecasting is an explicit goal, a Level II analysis is being undertaken.

Taking Level II analyses a step farther, there have been some recent efforts to provide a rationale and computational procedures for random forests statistical inference including for such output as variable importance (Wager 2014; Wager et al. 2014; Wager and Walther 2015; Mentch and Hooker 2015; Ishwaran and Lu 2019). The issues are beyond the scope of our discussion in part because the work is at this point still very much in progress. Key complications are a lack of clarity about the proper estimand, the inductive nature of random forests, tree depth dependence on sample size, the sampling of predictors, and summary values for terminal nodes computed from the same data used to grow the trees.

However, if one has test data, one can proceed in the same spirit as in bagging. The estimation target is the fitted values from the very same random forest grown with the training data. The test data can be used to estimate generalization error or other features of a confusion table. One can then apply the pairwise (nonparametric) bootstrap to the test data in the fashion discussed in earlier chapters. For example, one can construct confidence intervals around the fitted values. One often can also construct conformal prediction intervals around forecasts.[24] But as before, the training data and trained algorithmic structure are treated as fixed. Uncertainty from those sources is not considered.

5.13 Software and Tuning Parameters

In this chapter, all empirical work has been done with the R procedure *random-Forest*, which works well even for large datasets. But there are some disciplines in which the datasets are extremely large (e.g., 1,000,000 observations and 5000 predictors) and working with subsets of the data can be counter-productive. For example, in genomics research there may be thousands of predictors.

Over the past few years, new implementations of random forests have be written for R, and some are remarkably fast (Ziegler and König 2014). A recent review by Wright and Ziegler (2017) confirms that *randomForest* is "feature rich and widely used." But the code has not been optimized for high dimensional data.

Wright and Ziegler describe their own random forests implementation, *ranger*, in some depth. It is indeed very very fast, but currently lacks a number of features that can be important in practice. All of the other implementations considered are either no more optimized than *randomForest*, or run faster but lack important features (e.g., partial dependence plots). No doubt, at least some of these packages will add useful features over time. One possible candidate in R is *Rborist* (Seligman 2015). *Willows* (Zhang et al. 2009) and *Random Jungle* (Schwarz et al. 2010) are also candidates, but neither is currently available in R.[25] There are, in addition, efforts to reconsider random forests more fundamentally for very high dimensional data. For example, Xu and colleagues (2012) try to reduce the number of input dimensions by taking into account information much like that assembled in the *randomForest* proximity matrix. Readers intending to use random forests should try to stay informed about these developments. Here, we will continue with *randomForest*.

Despite the complexity of the random forest algorithm and the large number of potential tuning parameters, most of the usual defaults work well in practice. If one tunes from information contained in the OOB confusion table, the OOB data will slowly become tainted. For example, if for policy or subject- matter reasons one needs to tune to approximate a target asymmetric cost ratio in a confusion table, model selection is in play once again. Still, when compared to the results from true test data, the OOB results usually hold up well if the number of cost ratios estimated is modest (e.g., <10) and the sample size is not too small (e.g., >1000). The same holds if on occasion some of the following tuning parameters have to be tweaked.

1. *Node Size*—Unlike in CART, the number of observations in the terminal nodes of each tree can be very small. The goal is to grow trees with as little bias as possible. The large variance that would result can be tolerated because of the averaging over a large number of trees. In the R implementation *randomForest*, the default sample sizes for the terminal nodes are one for classification and five for regression. These seem to work well. But, if one is interested in estimating a quantile, such as in quantile random forests, then terminal node sizes at least twice as large will often be necessary for regression. If there are only five observations in a terminal node, for instance, it will be difficult to get a good read on, say, the 90th percentile.

2. *Number of Trees*—The number of trees used to constitute a forest needs to be at least several hundred and probably no more that several thousand. In practice, 500 trees is often a good compromise. It sometimes makes sense to do most of the initial development (see below) with about 500 trees and then confirm the results with a run using about 3000 trees. But, the cost is primarily computational time and only if the number of inputs and number of observations is large do computational burdens become an issue. For example, if there are 100 inputs and 100,000 observations, the number of trees grown becomes an important tuning parameter.

3. *Number of Predictors Sampled*—The number of predictors sampled at each split would seem to be a key tuning parameter that should affect how well random forests performs. Although it may be somewhat surprising, very few predictors need to be randomly sampled at each split, and within sensible bounds on the number sampled, it does not seem to matter much for the OOB error estimates. With a large number of trees, each predictor will have an ample opportunity to contribute, even if very few are drawn for each split. For example, if the average tree in a random forest has ten terminal splits, and if there are 500 trees in the random forest, there will be 5000 chances for predictors to weigh in. Sampling two or three each time should then be adequate.

   But a lot depends on the number of predictors and how strongly they are related. If the correlations are substantial, it can be useful to reduce the number of predictors sampled for each partitioning decision. In the original manual for the FORTRAN version of random forests, Breiman recommended starting with the number of predictors sampled equal to the square root of the number of predictors available. Then, trying a few more or a few less as well can be instructive.

The feature of random forests that will usually make the biggest difference in the results is how the costs of false negatives and false positives are handled, or for quantile random forests, the quantile used. Even through asymmetric costs are introduced by altering one or more of the arguments in *randomForest*, one should not think of the target cost ratio as a tuning parameter. It is a key factor in the fitting process determined in advance from substantive and policy considerations. However, to arrive at a good approximation of the target cost ratio, some tuning of one or more arguments will usually be necessary (e.g., *sampsize*).

Finally, computational burdens can be an issue when the training data have a very larger number of observations (e.g., $>100,000$), when the number of inputs is large (e.g., >100), and when a substantial number of inputs are categorical with many classes.[26] It is difficult to tune one's way out of letting the algorithm grind for hours in part because with each new set of tuning values, the algorithm has to run again. Sometimes a better strategy is to work with a random, modest sized subset of training data for tuning, saving the bulk of the data for results that will be used. Doing some initial screening of the predictors to be used can also help, as long as one is aware of the risks. Combining some of the categories for factors with many levels is worth a try. Finally, many of the computational steps in random forests are easily parallelized and will run well on computers with multiple processors. Soon, software with these capabilities and others that increase processing speed will be routinely available and be richly endowed with desirable features.

Also, a cautionary note. Random forests is not designed to be a variable selection procedure. Nevertheless, it can be tempting to use the variable importance plots to discard weak predictors. There are at least four problems with this approach. First, there is rarely any need to reduce the number of predictors. The way in which splits are determined for each tree in the forest is a kind of provisional, variable selection method that performs well. In other words, there is almost never a need to drop the unimportant variables and re-run random forests. Second, some argue that if multicollinearity is a serious problem, random forests results can be unstable. But that concern refers primarily to estimates of variable importance. Should that form of instability become an issue, any dimension reduction in the set of predictors is probably best done before the random forests analysis begins. However, one is back in the model selection game. Third, if the goal is to use variable importance to determine the predictors to be introduced into some other procedure, performance in prediction may not be what is needed. For example, prediction importance may be unrelated to causal importance. Finally, as discussed earlier, there are lots of worthy procedures designed for variable/model selection as long as one is prepared to address the damage usually done to Level II analyses.

5.14 Bayesian Additive Regression Trees (BART)

Random forests has a Bayesian cousin called Bayesian additive regression trees (BART). It comes out of a very different statistical tradition and has yet to gain much traction in practice, but it can perform very well. We turn briefly to brief exposition.

Bayesian additive regression trees (Chipman et al. 2010) is a procedure that capitalizes on an ensemble of classification or regression trees in the spirit random forests. Random forests generates an ensemble of random trees by treating the tree parameters as fixed while sampling the training data and predictors. The statistical traditions are frequentist. Parameters such as tree depth are treated as fixed, and the data are treated as a set random realizations from a joint probability distribution of random variables. Bayesian additive regression trees turns this upside down. Just as in Bayesian traditions more generally, the data are treated as fixed, and parameters characterizing the ensemble of trees are treated as random.

Each tree in the BART ensemble is realized at random in a manner that is determined by three kinds of hyperparameters:

1. Two hyperparameters for determining the probability that a node will to be split;
2. A hyperparameter determining the probability any given predictor to be selected for the split; and
3. A hyperparameter determining the probability that a particular split value for the selected predictor will be used.

The probability of a split is determined by

$$p(\text{split}) = \alpha(1 + d)^{-\beta}, \tag{5.15}$$

where d is the tree "depth," defined as the number of stages beyond the root note; 0 for the root node (i.e., $d = 0$), 1 for the first split (i.e., $d = 1$), 2 for the two splits that follow (i.e., $d = 2$), 3 for the next set of splits (i.e., $d = 3$), and so on. The values of α and β affect how large a given tree will be. For a given value of β, smaller values for α make a split less likely. For a given value of α, smaller values of β make the penalty for tree depth more binding so that a split for a given value of d is less likely. The probability of a split also declines as the value of d increases. Possible values of α range from 0 to 1 with 0.95 a common choice. Possible values for β are non-negative, but small values such too often work well and can be treated as sensible defaults (Kapelner and Bleich 2014).

If there is to be a split, a predictor is chosen at random. For example, if there are p predictors, each predictor can have a probability of $1/p$ of being selected. In a similar manner, the split value for the selected predictor can be chosen with equal probably. It is possible to alter either random selection strategy if the situation warrants it. For example, if on subject-matter grounds some predictors are thought to be more important than others, they may be chosen with a higher probability than the rest.

The hyperparameters define a very large Bayesian forests composed of potential trees that can be realized at random. Each tree is grown from a linear basis expansion of the predictors. Over trees, one has a very rich menu of possible expansions, a subset of which is realized for any given data analysis. In other words, the role of the hyperparameters is to produce a rich dictionary of linear basis expansions.

Figure 5.17 is meant to provide a sense how this works in practice. Imagine a ball rolling down an inclined plane. In Fig. 5.17, the ball is shown in red at the top. The ball hits the first nail and its path is displaced to the left or to the right in a manner that cannot be predicted in advance. The first nail is analogous to the first random split. Each subsequent nail is a subsequent potential split that can shift the path of the ball to the left or to the right in the same unpredictable fashion. After the

```
library(quantregForest)
X<-as.matrix(HData[,2:7]) # predictors as matrix
Y<-as.numeric(as.matrix(HData[,1])) # response as vector

# Quantile Random Forests
out2<-quantregForest(x=X,y=Y,nodesize=10,importance=T,
                     quantiles = c(.10))
preds<-predict(out2) # Fitted OOB values

# Fitted value plots
par(mfrow=c(3,1))
plot(preds[,1],Y,col="blue",pch=19,
     xlab="Fitted 10th Percentile",
     ylab="Street Count",
     main="Street Count on Fitted Value of 10th Percentile")
abline(lsfit(preds[,1],Y),col="red",lwd=2)
abline(0.0,1.0,lwd=2,col="green")
text(22,220,"Least Squares Line",cex=1)
text(30,90,"1-to-1 Line",cex=1)

plot(preds[,2],Y,col="blue",pch=19,
     xlab="Fitted 50th Percentile",
     ylab="Street Count",
     main="Street Count on Fitted Value of 50th Percentile")
abline(lsfit(preds[,2],Y),col="red",lwd=2)
abline(0.0,1.0,lwd=2,col="green")
text(130,300,"Least Squares Line",cex=1)
text(170,110,"1-to-1 Line",cex=1)

plot(preds[,3],Y,col="blue",pch=19,
     xlab="Fitted 90th Percentile",
     ylab="Street Count",
     main="Street Count on Fitted Value of 90th Percentile")
abline(lsfit(preds[,3],Y),col="red",lwd=2)
abline(0.0,1.0,lwd=2,col="green")
text(500,370,"Least Squares Line",cex=1)
text(550,110,"1-to-1 Line",cex=1)

# Importance Plots
par(mfrow=c(3,1))
imp10<-sort(out2$importance[,1])
dotchart(imp10,col="blue",pch=19,xlab="% Increase
         in Quantile Loss",
         main="Importance Plot for Street Counts -- Quantile .10")
imp50<-sort(out2$importance[,2])
dotchart(imp50,col="blue",pch=19,xlab="% Increase
         in Quantile Loss",
         main="Importance Plot for Street Counts -- Quantile .50")
imp90<-sort(out2$importance[,3])
dotchart(imp90,col="blue",pch=19,xlab="% Increase
         in Quantile Loss",
         main="Importance Plot for Street Counts -- Quantile .90")
```

Fig. 5.16   R code for Quantile random forests

Fig. 5.17 Cartoon
illustration of a pinball
process (The ball is at the top,
the nails are the splits, and the
cups at the bottom are the
terminal nodes

Pinball Metaphor

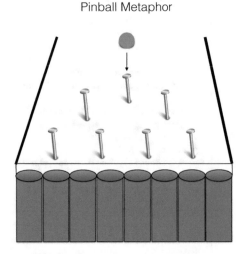

third set of nails, the ball drops into the closest canister. The canisters at the bottom
represent terminal nodes.

Imagine now that 25 balls are sequentially rolled down the plane. The 25 balls
constitute the cases constituting a dataset. Some of the balls are red and some are
blue. The balls will follow a variety of paths to the canisters, and the proportions
of red and blue balls in each canister will likely vary. The exercise can be repeated
over and over with the same 25 balls. With each replication, the proportion of red
balls and blue balls in each canister will likely change.

In Fig. 5.17, there are two sets of nails after the first nail at the top. To be more
consistent with BART, the number of nail rows can vary with each replication. In
addition, the rows can vary in the number of nails and where they are placed.
For example, the two left most nails in the bottom row of Fig. 5.17 might not be
included. The result is a large number of inclined planes, with varying numbers
of nail rows, nail placements, and proportions of red and blue balls in each canister.
One has a fixed collection of red and blue balls that does not change from replication
to replication, but what happens to them does.[27]

Unlike random forests, the realized trees are not designed to be independent, and
the trees are used in a linear model (Chipman et al. 2010):

$$Y = \sum_{j=1}^{m} g(x; T_j, M_j) + \varepsilon,$$ (5.16)

and as usual,

$$\varepsilon \sim N(0, \sigma^2).$$ (5.17)

Y is numerical, and there are m trees. Each tree is defined by the predictors x, T_j, which represents the splits made at each interior node, and M_j, which represents the set of means over terminal nodes. The trees are combined in a manner something like conventional backfitting such that each tree's set of conditional means is related to the response by a function that has been adjusted for the sets of conditional means of all other trees.

We are not done. First, we need a prior for the distribution of the means of Y over terminal nodes conditional on a given tree. That distribution is taken to be normal. Also, Y is rescaled in part to make the prior's parameters easier to specify and in part because the rescaling shrinks the conditional means toward 0.0. The impact of individual trees is damped down, which slows the learning process. Details are provided by Chipman and colleagues (2010: 271). Second, we need a prior distribution for σ^2 in Eq. (5.17). An inverse χ^2 distribution is imposed that has two hyperparameters. Here too, details are provided by Chipman and colleagues (2010: 272).

The algorithms used for estimation involve a complicated combination of Gibbs sampling and Markov Chain Monte Carlo methods that can vary somewhat depending on the software (Kapelner and Bleich 2014). In R, there is *bartMachine* written by Adam Kapelner and Justin Bleich, and *BayesTree* written by Hugh Chipman and Robert McCulloch. Currently, *bartMachine* is the faster in part because it is parallelized, and it also has a richer set of options and outputs. For example, there is a very clever way to handle missing data.

A discussion on the estimation machinery is beyond the scope of this short overview and requires considerable background on Bayesian estimation. Fortunately, both procedures can be run effectively without that background and are actually quite easy to use. In the end, one obtains the posterior distributions for the conditional means from which one can construct fitted values. These represent the primary output of interest. One also gets "credibility intervals" for the fitted values.

BART is readily applied when the response is binary. Formally,

$$p(Y = 1|x) = \Phi[G(x)], \tag{5.18}$$

where

$$G(x) \equiv \sum_{j=1}^{m} g(x; T_j, M_j), \tag{5.19}$$

and $\Phi[G(x)]$ is the probit link function used in probit regression. When used as a classifier, the classes are assigned in much the same way they are for probit regression. A threshold is applied to the fitted values (Chipman et al. 2010: 278). Otherwise, very little changes compared to BART applications with a numerical response.

It is difficult to compare the performance of BART to the performance of random forests, stochastic gradient boosting, and support vector machines. The first three procedures have frequentist roots and make generalization error and expected pre-diction error the performance gold standards. Because within a Bayesian perspective the data are fixed, it is not clear what sense out-of-sample performance makes. If the data are fixed, where do test data come from? If the test data are seen as a random realization of some data generation process, uncertainty in the data should be taken into account, and one is back to a frequentist point of view. Nevertheless, if one slides over these and other conceptual difficulties, BART seems to perform about as well as random forests, stochastic gradient boosting, and support vector machines. Broadly conceived, this makes sense. BART is "just" another way to construct a rich menu of linear basis expansions to be combined in a linear fashion.

BART's main advantage is that statistical inference is an inherent feature of the output; a Level II analysis falls out automatically. But one has to believe the model. Are there any omitted variables, for example? Does one really want to commit to a linear combination of trees with an additive error term. One also has to be make peace with the priors. Most important, one has to be comfortable with Bayesian inference. But, even for skeptics, Bayesian inference might be considered reasonable option given all of the problems discussed earlier when frequentist inference is applied to statistical learning procedures. It is also possible to use BART legitimately as a Level I tool. The hyperparameters and priors distributions can be seen as tuning parameters and given no Bayesian interpretations. BART becomes solely a data fitting exercise.

BART has some limitations in practice. At the moment, only binary categorical response variables can be used. There is also no way to build in asymmetric costs for classification or fitting errors. And if one wants to explore the consequences of changing the hyperparameters parameters (e.g., α and β), it not clear that conventional resampling procedures such as cross-validation makes sense with fixed data.

In summary, BART is a legitimate competitor to random forests. If one wants to do a Level II analysis within a Bayesian perspective, BART is the only choice. Otherwise, it is difficult to see why one would pick BART over the alternatives. On the other hand, BART is rich in interesting ideas and for the more academically inclined, can be great fun.

5.15   Summary and Conclusions

There is substantial evidence that random forests is a very powerful statistical learning tool. If forecasting accuracy is one's main performance criterion, there are no other tools that have been shown to consistently perform any better for data of sort most common in the behavioral, social, and biomedical sciences.[28] Moreover, random forests comes with a rich menu of post-processing procedures and simple means with which to introduce asymmetric costs. We consider a chief competitor in the next chapter.

But a lot depends on data analysis task. We will later briefly address deep learning, which has enormous power, especially with very high dimensional image and speech data when great precision in the fitted values is needed. One is still working with conditional distributions, but many of the tools are very different from those associated with traditional statistical learning.

To apply many of the deep learning variants, one must be prepared to invest substantial time (e.g., weeks) in tuning, even when there is access to a very large number of CPUs and GPUs. As some advertisements warn,"don't try this at home." The most powerful desktop and laptop computers often will be overmatched by deep learning. Deep learning can be seen as industrial strength statistical learning for certain kinds of data. We will return to these issues later.

Random forests seems to get its leverage from five features of the algorithm:

1. growing large, low bias trees;
2. using bootstrap samples as training data when each tree is grown;
3. using random samples of predictors for each partitioning of the data;
4. constructing fitted values and output summary statistics from the out-of-bag data; and
5. averaging over trees.

At the same time, very few of random forest's formal properties have been proven. At a deeper level, the precise reasons why random forests performs so well are not fully understood. There is some hard work ahead for theoretical statisticians. Nevertheless, random forests is gaining in popularity because it seems to work well in practice, provides lots of flexibility, and in R at least, comes packaged with a number of supplementary algorithms that provide a range of useful output.

Exercises

Problem Set 1

The goal of this first exercise is to compare the performance of linear regression, CART, and random forests. Construct the following dataset in which the response is a quadratic function of a single predictor.

```
x1=rnorm(500)
x12=x1^2
y=1+(-5*x12)+(5*rnorm(500))
```

1. Plot the $1 + (-5 \times x12)$ against x1. This is the "true" relationship between the response and the predictor without the complication of the disturbances. This is the $f(X)$ you hope to recover from the data.
2. Proceed as if you know that the relationship between the response and the predictor is quadratic. Fit a linear model with x12 as the predictor. Then plot

the fitted values against x1. The results show how the linear model can perform when you know the correct function form.

3. Now suppose you do not know that the relationship between the response and the predictor is quadratic. Apply CART to the same response variable using *rpart* and x1 as the sole predictor. Use the default settings. Construct the predicted values, using *predict*. Then plot the fitted values against x1. How do the CART fitted values compare to the linear regression fitted values? How well does CART seem to capture the true $f(X)$?

4. Apply random forests to the same response variable using *randomForests* and x1 as the sole predictor. Use the default settings. Construct the predicted values using *predict*. Then plot the fitted values against x1. How do the random forest fitted values compare to the linear regression fitted values? How well does random forests seem to capture the true $f(X)$?

5. How do the fitted values from CART compare to the fitted values from random forests? What feature of random forests is highlighted?

6. Construct a partial dependence plot with x1 as the predictor. How well does the plot seem to capture the true $f(X)$?

7. Why in this case does the plot of the random forest fitted values and the partial dependence plot look so similar?

Problem Set 2

Load the dataset SLID from the *car* library. Learn about the dataset using the *help* command. Treat the variable "wages" as the response and all other variables as predictors. The data have some missing values you will want to remove. Try using *na.omit*.

1. Using the default settings, apply random forests and examine the fit quality.

2. Set the argument *mtry* at four. Apply random forests again and examine fit quality. What if anything of importance has changed?

3. Now set ntrees at 100 and then at 1000 applying random forests both times. What if anything of importance has changed?

4. Going back to the default settings, apply random forests and examine the variable importance plots with no scaling for each predictor's standard deviation. Explain what is being measured on the horizontal axis on both plots when no scaling for the standard deviation is being used. Interpret both plots. If they do not rank the variables in the same way, why might that be? Now scale the permutation-based measure and reconstruct that plot. Interpret the results. If the ranks of the variables differ from the unscaled plot, why might that be? Focusing on the permutation-based measures (scaled and unscaled) when might it be better to use one rather than the other?

5. Construct partial dependence plots for each predictor and interpret them.

Problem Set 3

Load the *MASS* library and the dataset called Pima.tr. Read about the data using *help*.

1. Apply random forests to the data using the diagnosis of diabetes as the response. Use all of the predictors and random forest default settings. Study the confusion table.

   (a) How accurately does the random forests procedure forecast overall?
   (b) How accurately does the random forests procedure forecast each of the two outcomes separately (i.e., *given* each outcome)? (Hint: you get this from the rows of the confusion table.)
   (c) If the results were used to forecast either outcome (i.e., *given* the forecast), what proportions of the time would each of the forecasts be incorrect? (Hint: you get this from the columns of the confusion table.)

2. Construct variable importance plots for each of the two outcomes. Use the unscaled plots of forecasting accuracy. Compare the two plots.

   (a) Which predictors are the three most important in forecasts of the presence of diabetes compared to forecasts of the absence of diabetes? Why might they not be the same?

3. Construct and interpret partial dependence plots of each predictor.
4. Suppose now that medical experts believe that the costs of failing to identify future cases of diabetes are four times larger than the costs of falsely identifying future cases of diabetes. For example, if the medical treatment is to get overweight individuals to lose weight, that would likely be beneficial even if the individuals were not at high risk for diabetes. But failing to prescribe a weight loss program for an overweight individual might be an error with very serious consequences. Repeat the analysis just completed but now taking the costs into account by using the stratified bootstrap sampling option in random forests.

   (a) How has the confusion table changed?
   (b) How have the two variable importance plots changed?
   (c) How have the partial dependence plots changed?

5. Plot the margins to consider the reliability of the random forests classifications. You will need at least *margin* followed by the *plot*. Are the two class correctly classified with about the same reliability? If so, why might a physician want to know that? If not, why might a physician want to know that?
6. The votes are stored as part of the random forests object. Construct a histogram of the votes separately for each of the two outcome classes. How do votes differ from margins?
7. Now imagine that a physician did not have the results of the diabetes test but wanted to start treatment immediately, if appropriate. Each of the predictors are known for that patient but not the diagnosis. Using the predictor values for that

patient, a random forests forecast is made. What should the physician use to measure the reliability of that forecast? Given some examples of high and low reliability.

Endnotes

[1] One might think weighting trees by some measure of generalization error would help. Better performing trees would be given more weight in the averaging. So far at least, the gains are at best small (Winham et al. 2103). Because better performing trees tend to have more variation over terminal node fitted values, a form of self-weighting is in play.

[2] Geurts and his colleagues (2006) have proposed another method for selecting predictors that can decrease dependence across trees and further open up the predictor competition. They do not build each tree from a bootstrap sample of the data. Rather, for each random sample of predictors, they select splits for each predictor at random (with equal probability), subject to some minimum number of observations in the smaller of the two partitions. Then, as in random forests, the predictor that reduces heterogeneity the most is chosen to define the two subsets of observations. They claim that this approach will reduce the overall heterogeneity at least as much as other ensemble procedures without a substantial increase in bias. However, this conclusion would seem to depend on how good the predictors really are.

[3] In practice, there will be some tuning if for no other reason than to closely approximate the target cost ratio. The pristine nature of the out-of-bag data will be compromised at least a bit. In practice, the consequences for proper inferences are usually not serious. But if one has concerns, the option of real hold-out test data is still available. One would be most concerned if the sample size is small (e.g., < 200) and large number of fitting attempts is large (e.g., >20).

[4] All of the other procedures tried performed even more poorly.

[5] R code is not provided because it is too early in the exposition. Lots of R code is provided later.

[6] It might seem strange that the classification accuracy of one outcome is not 1 minus the classification accuracy of the other. If a case is not classified as DV, it must be classified as a DV case. But one is conditioning on the actual outcome, and the denominators of the classification errors differ. Accuracy depends in part on the base.

[7] The notation is a little confusing. Something like $\mathbf{X}_i$ might be better.

[8] The concept of training data gets fuzzy at this point. The training data for a given tree is the random sample drawn with replacement from the dataset on hand. But for the random forest the entire dataset is the training data.

[9] There are other implementations for random forests in R that are briefly discussed later.

[10] For example, if there is a tiny random forest of 3 trees (more like very small stand), and the ith observation has 3 weights of 0.2, 0.3, and 0.1, the average weight over the 3 trees is 0.2. This assumes that each all three cases are OOB.

[11] The package *quantregForest* is authored by Nicolai Meinshausen and Lukas Schiesser.

[12] Using the procedure *randomForest* in R written by Leo Breiman and Ann Culter, and later ported to R by Andy Liaw and Matthew Wiener, the stratified sampling argument was *sampsize=c(100,100)*. The order of the two sample sizes depends on the order of the response variable categories. They are ordered alphabetically or numerically low to high depending on how the outcome variable is coded. For classification procedures in R, it is a good idea to always construct the outcome variable as a factor. The procedure *randomForest* will automatically know that the task is classification. If a binary response variable is defined as numeric with a value of 0 and a value of 1, and if the type of procedure within *randomForest* is not identified as classification, *randomForest* will proceed with regression. This is a common error.

[13] Sometimes Granger-cause is called predictive cause.

[14] For example, if getting a job is coded 1 and not getting a job is coded 0, the mean of the 1s and 0s is the proportion p that got a job. The logit is $\log[p/(1 - p)]$.

[15] $e^{[2(-0.693)]}/(1 + (e^{[2(-0.693)]}) = 0.20$.

[16] The term "centered" is used because mean of the K logged proportions is the reference.

[17] The bars use the value of zero as the base and move away from 0.0 upwards or downwards. This is consistent with the mean logit centering.

[18] They are not literally reduced forms results because there is no structural model.

[19] For the employment data (N = 6723), doing the MDS using *cmdscale* on an iMac with an 3.4 GHz intel Core i7 and 32 GB of memory using took about 30 min.

[20] This is not to say that MDS is inappropriate in principle or that it will not work well for other kinds of applications.

[21] As is often the case with quantitative response variables, the defaults in *randomForest* worked well.

[22] The authors are Nicolai Meinshausen and Lukas Schiesser. The version used for these analyses (version 1.1) seems to have some bugs in the plotting routines, which is why the code shown in Fig. 5.16 is so lengthy and inelegant. The plots had to be constructed from more basic procedures.

[23] The procedure *randomForestSRC* is written by Udaya Kogalur and Hermant Ishwaran.

[24] Keep in mind that random forests does not provide fitted probabilities for outcome classes and the votes over trees address a different question. As discussed in the chapter on CART, conformal inferential approaches for forecasted classes do not correspond to the uncertainty questions usually asked about those classes. But, recall that the bootstrap can address the uncertainty in useful ways.

[25] *Rborist* wins the award for the cutest name.

[26] Currently, up to 53 classes are allowed for any given categorical input in *randomForest*.

[27] Wu et al. (2007) define a "pinball prior" for tree generation. The pinball prior and Fig. 5.17 have broadly similar intent, but the details are vastly different.

[28] Convolutional neural networks, discussed in a later chapter, commonly is used to analyze image and speech data for which it is uniquely suited. For these kinds of data, random forests is at least far less effective and arguably inappropriate.

References

Berk, R. A. (2003). *Regression analysis: A constructive critique*. Newbury Park, CA.: SAGE.

Berk, R. A., Kriegler, B., & Ylvisaker, D. (2008). Counting the Homeless in Los Angeles County. In D. Nolan & Speed, S. (Eds.). *Probability and statistics: Essays in honor of David A. Freedman*. Monograph Series for the Institute of Mathematical Statistics.

Biau, G. (2012). Analysis of a random forests model. *Journal of Machine Learning Research, 13*, 1063–1095.

Biau, G., & Devroye, L. (2010). On the layered nearest neighbor estimate, the bagged nearest neighbor estimate and the random forest method in regression and classification. *Journal Multivariate Analysis, 101*, 2499–2518.

Biau, G., Devroye, L., & Lugosi, G. (2008). Consistency of random forests and other averaging classifiers. *Journal of Machine Learning Research, 9*, 2015–2033.

Breiman, L. (2001a). Random forests. *Machine Learning, 45*, 5–32.

Breiman, L., Friedman, J. H., Olshen, R. A., & Stone, C. J. (1984). *Classification and regression trees*. Monterey, CA: Wadsworth Press.

Chaudhuri, P., & Loh, W.-Y. (2002). Nonparametric estimation of conditional quantiles using quantile regression trees. *Bernoulli, 8*(5), 561–576.

Chipman, H. A., George, E. I., & McCulloch, R. E. (2010). BART: Bayesian additive regression trees. *Annals of Applied Statistics, 4*(1), 266–298.

de Leeuw, J., & Mair, P. (2009). Multidimensional scaling using majorization: SMACOF in R. *Journal of Statistical Software, 31*(3), 11557–11587.

Friedman, J. H. (2001). Greedy function approximation: A gradient boosting machine. *The Annals of Statistics, 29* 1189–1232

Geurts, P., Ernst, D., & Wehenkel, L. (2006). Extremely randomized trees. *Machine Learning, 63*(1), 3–42.

Granger, C. W. J., & Newbold, P. (1986). *Forecasting economic time series*. New York: Academic Press.

Hastie, T., Tibshirani, R., & Friedman, J. (2009). *The elements of statistical learning* (2nd edn.). New York: Springer.

Ishwaran, H. (2015). The effect of splitting on random forests. *Machine Learning, 99*, 75–118.

Ishwaran, H., Kogalur, U. B., Blackstone, E. H., & Lauer, T. S. (2008). Random survival forests. *The Annals of Applied Statistics, 2*(3), 841–860.

Ishwaran, H., Gerds, T. A., Kogalur, U. B., Moore, R. D., Gange, S. J., & Lau, B. M. (2014). Random survival forests for competing risks. *Biostatistics, 15*(4), 757–773.

Ishwaran H., & Lu, M. (2019) Standard errors and confidence intervals for variable importance in random forest regression, classification, and survival. *Statistics in Medicine, 38*(4), 558–582.

Kapelner, A., & Bleich, J. (2014). bartMachine: Machine learning for Bayesian additive regression trees. asXiv:1312.2171v3 [stat.ML].

Lin, Y., & Jeon, Y. (2006). Random forests and adaptive nearest neighbors. *Journal of the American Statistical Association, 101*, 578–590.

Loh, W.-L. (2014). Fifty years of classification and regression trees (with discussion). *International Statistical Review, 82*(3), 329–348.

Mathlourthi, W., Fredette, M., & Larocque, D. (2015). Regression trees and forests for non-homogeneous Poisson processes. *Statistics and Probability Letters, 96*, 204–211.

Meinshausen, N. (2006). Quantile regression forests. *Journal of Machine Learning Research, 7*, 983–999.

Mentch, L., & Hooker, G. (2015). Quantifying uncertainty in random forests via confidence intervals and hypothesis tests. Cornell University Library, arXiv:1404.6473v2 [stat.ML].

Scornet, E., Biau, G., & Vert, J.-P. (2015). Consistency of random forest methods. *The Annals of Statistics, 43*(4), 1716–1741.

Schwarz, D. F., König, I. R., & Ziegler, A. (2010). On safari to random jungle: A fast implementation of random forests for high-dimensional data. *Bioinformatics, 26*(14), 1752–1758.

Seligman, M. (2015). Rborist: Extensible, parallelizable implementation of the random forest algorithm. R package version 0.1–0. http://cran.r-project.org/package=Rborist.

Thompson, S. K. (2002). *Sampling* (2nd edn). New York: Wiley.

Wager, S. (2014). Asymptotic theory for random forests (2014). Working Paper arXiv:1405.0352v1.

Wager, S., & Walther, G. (2015). Uniform convergence of random forests via adaptive concentration. Working Paper arXiv:1503.06388v1.

Wager, E., Hastie, T., & Efron, B. (2014). Confidence intervals for random forests: The Jackknife and infinitesimal Jackknife. *Journal of Machine Learning Research, 15*, 1625–1651.

Winham, S. J., Freimuth, R. R., & Beirnacka, J. M. (2103). A weighted random forests approach to improve predictive performance. *Statitical Analysis and Data Mining, 6*(6): 496–505.

Wright, M. N., & Ziegler, A. (2017). Ranger: A fast implementation of random forests for high dimensional data in C++ and R. *Journal of Statistical Software, 77*(1), 7671–7688.

Wu, Y., Tjelmeland, H., & West, M. (2007). Bayesian CART: Prior specification and posterior simulation. *Journal of Computational and Graphical Statistics, 16*(1), 44–66.

Wyner, A. J., Olson, M., Bleich, J., & Mease, D. (2017), Explaining the Success of AdaBoost and Random Forests as Interpolating Classifiers, *Journal of Machine Learning Research, 18*, 1–33.

Xu, B., Huang, J. Z., Williams, G., Wang, Q., & Ye, Y. (2012). Classifying very high dimensional data with random forests build from small subspaces. *International Journal of Data Warehousing and Mining, 8*(2), 44–63.

Zhang, H., Wang, M., & Chen, X. (2009). Willows: A memory efficient tree and forest construction package. *BMC Bioinformatics, 10*(1), 130–136.

Ziegler, A., & König, I. R. (2014). Mining data with random forests: Current options for real world applications. *Wiley Interdisciplinary Reviews: Data Mining and Knowledge Discovery, 4*(1), 55–63.

Chapter 6
Boosting

Summary In this chapter we continue the use of fitting ensembles. We focus on boosting with an emphasis on classifiers. The unifying idea is that the statistical learning procedure makes many passes through the data and constructs fitted values for each. However, with each pass, observations that were fit more poorly on the last pass are given more weight. In that way, the algorithm works more diligently to fit the hard-to-fit observations. In the end, each set of fitted values is combined in an averaging process that serves as a regularizer. Boosting can be a very effective statistical learning procedure.

6.1 Introduction

As already discussed, one of the reasons why random forests is so effective for a complex $f(\mathbf{X})$ is that it capitalizes interpolation. As a result, it can respond to highly local features of the data in a robust manner. Such flexibility is desirable because it can substantially reduce the bias in fitted values. But the flexibility usually comes at a price: the risk of overfitting. Random forests consciously addresses overfitting using OOB observations to construct the fitted values and measures of fit, and by averaging over trees. The former provides ready-made test data, while the latter is a form of regularization. Experience to date suggests that this two-part strategy can be highly effective.

But the two-part strategy, broadly conceived, can be implemented in other ways. An alternative method to accommodate highly local features of the data is to give the observations responsible for poor statistical performance more weight in the fitting process. When in the binary case, for example, a fitting function misclassifies certain observations, that function can be applied again, but with extra weight given to the misclassified observations. Then, after a large number of fitting attempts, each with difficult-to-classify observations given relatively more weight, overfitting

© Springer Nature Switzerland AG 2020   297
R. A. Berk, *Statistical Learning from a Regression Perspective*,
Springer Texts in Statistics, https://doi.org/10.1007/978-3-030-40189-4_6

can be reduced if the fitted values from the different fitting attempts are averaged in a sensible fashion. Ideas such as these lead to very powerful statistical learning procedures that compare favorably to random forests. These procedures are called "boosting."

Boosting as originally conceived gets its name from its ability to take a "weak learning algorithm," which performs just a bit better than random guessing, and "boosting" it into an arbitrarily "strong" learning algorithm (Schapire 1999: 1). It "combines the outputs from many weak classifiers to produce a powerful committee" (Hastie et al. 2009: 337). Like random forests, it constructs and combines an ensemble of learners.

But, boosting as initially formulated differs from random forests in at least five important ways. First, in traditional boosting, there are no chance elements introduced. At each iteration, boosting works with the full training sample and all of the predictors. Some more recent developments in boosting exploit random samples from the training data, but these developments are enhancements that are not fundamental to the usual boosting algorithms. Second, with each iteration, the observations that are misclassified, or otherwise poorly fitted, are given more relative weight. No such weighting is used in random forests. Third, the ultimate fitted values are a linear combination over a large set of earlier fitting attempts. But the combination is not a simple average as in random forests. The fitted values are weighted in a manner to be described shortly. Fourth, the fitted values and measures of fit quality are usually constructed from the data in-sample. There are no out-of-bag observations, although some recent developments make that an option. Finally, although small trees can be used as weak learners, boosting is not limited to an ensemble of classification or regression trees.

To appreciate how these pieces can fit together, we turn to AdaBoost.M1 (Freund and Schapire 1996, 1997), which is perhaps the earliest and the most widely known boosting procedure. For reasons we soon examine, the "ada" in AdaBoost stands for "adaptive" (Schapire 1999: 2). AdaBoost illustrates well boosting's key features and despite a host of more recent boosting procedures is still among the best classifiers available (Mease and Wyner 2008).

6.2   AdaBoost

We will treat AdaBoost.M1 as the poster child for boosting in part because it provides such a useful introduction to the method. It was designed originally for classification problems, which once again are discussed first.

Consider a binary response Y coded as 1 or -1. AdaBoost.M1 then has the following general structure. The pseudocode that follows is basically a reproduction of what (Hastie et al. 2009) show on their page 339.[1]

1. Initialize the observation weights $w_i = 1/N, i = 1, 2, \ldots, N$ observations.
2. For $m = 1$ to M passes over the data:

(a) Fit a classifier $G_m(x)$ to the training data using the weights w_i.

(b) Compute: $err_m = \frac{\sum_{i=1}^{N} w_i I(y_i \neq G_m(x_i))}{\sum_{i=1}^{n} w_i}$.

(c) Compute $\alpha_m = \log[(1 - err_m)/err_m]$.

(d) Set $w_i \leftarrow w_i \cdot \exp[\alpha_m \cdot I(y_i \neq G_m(x_i))], i = 1, 2, \ldots, N$.

3. Output $G(x) = \text{sign}\left[\sum_{m=1}^{M} \alpha_m G_m(x)\right]$.

There are N cases and M iterations. $G_m(x)$ is a classifier for pass m over the data x. It is the source of the fitted values used in the algorithm. Any number of procedures might be used to build a classifier, but highly truncated trees (called "stumps") are common. The operator I is an indicator variable equal to 1 if the logical relationship is true, and 0 otherwise. Because the binary response is coded 1 and -1, the sign defines the outcome.

Classification error for pass m over the data is denoted by err_m; it is essentially the proportion of cases misclassified. In the next step, err_m is in the denominator and $(1 - err_m)$ is in the numerator before the log is taken. A larger value of α_m means a better fit.

The new weights, one for each case, are then computed, The value of w_i is unchanged if the ith case is correctly classified. If the ith case is incorrectly classified, it is "upweighted" by e^{α_m}. AdaBoost.M1 will pay relatively more attention in the next iteration to the cases that were misclassified. In some expositions of AdaBoost (Freund and Schapire 1999), α_m is defined as $\frac{1}{2}\log(1-err_m/err_m)$. Then, incorrectly classified cases are upweighted by e^{α_m} and correctly classified cases are downweighted by $e^{-\alpha_m}$.

In the final step, classification is determined by a sum of fitted values over the M classifiers G_m, with each set of fitted values weighted by α_m. This is in much the same spirit as the last step in the random forest algorithm; there is again a linear combination of fitted values. But for AdaBoost, the contributions from classifiers that fit the data are better and are given more weight, and the class assigned depends on the sign of the sum.

It is important to distinguish between the role of w_i and the role of α_m. The weights w_i are used solely to alter the relative importance of cases when the classifier is applied to the data in step 2a. Each case i has its own weight, which depends on its actual class and its fitted class. In steps 2b, 2c, and 2d, new weights are constructed for the next pass through the data. The weights play no role when the M sets of fitted values are linearly combined. The fit measure α_m is needed to compute the next set of weights, and in step 3, for the linear combination of the M sets of fitted values.

If AdaBoost results are used for forecasting, the actual outcome class is not known. Consequently, one cannot compute new weights w_i. But that does not matter. One has stored the M sets of fitted values and the associated predictor values for each fitted value in each set. One has also stored all of the α_m. The predictor values for any new case whose outcome class needs to be forecasted are assigned the fitted values for each of the M earlier passes through the data depending on the predictor values for that case. Step 3 is then repeated for the new case.

To summarize, AdaBoost combines a large number of fitting attempts of the data. Each fitting attempt is undertaken by a classifier using weighted observations. The observation weights are a function of how poorly an observation was fitted in the previous iteration. The fitted values from each iteration are then combined as a weighted sum. There is one weight for each fitting attempt, applied to all of the fitted values, which is a function of the overall classification error of that fitting attempt. The observation weights and the iteration weights both are a function of the classification error, but their forms and purposes are quite different.

6.2.1 A Toy Numerical Example of AdaBoost.M1

To help fix these ideas, it is useful to go through a numerical illustration with very simple data. There are five observations with response variable values for $i = 1, 2, 3, 4, 5$ of $1, 1, 1, -1, -1$, respectively.

1. Initialize the observations with each weight $w_i = 1/5$.
2. For the first iteration using the equal weights, suppose the fitted values from some classifier for observations $i = 1, 2, 3, 4, 5$ are, respectively, $1, 1, 1, 1, 1$. The first three are correct and the last two are incorrect. Therefore, the error for this first iteration is

$$err_1 = \frac{(0.20 \times 0) + (0.20 \times 0) + (0.20 \times 0) + (0.20 \times 1) + (0.20 \times 1)}{1} = 0.40.$$

3. The weight to be given to this iteration is then

$$\alpha_1 = \log \frac{(1 - 0.40)}{0.40} = \log(0.60/0.40) = \log(1.5) = 0.41.$$

4. The new weights are

$$w_1 = 0.20 \times e^{(0.41 \times 0)} = 0.20$$

$$w_2 = 0.20 \times e^{(0.41 \times 0)} = 0.20$$

$$w_3 = 0.20 \times e^{(0.41 \times 0)} = 0.20$$

$$w_4 = 0.20 \times e^{(0.41 \times 1)} = 0.30$$

$$w_5 = 0.20 \times e^{(0.41 \times 1)} = 0.30.$$

5. Now we begin the second iteration. We fit the classifier again and for $i = 1, 2, 3, 4, 5$ get, respectively, $1, 1, 1, 1, -1$. The first three and the fifth are correct. The fourth is incorrect. The error for the second iteration is

$$err_2 = \frac{[(0.20 \times 0) + (0.20 \times 0) + (0.20 \times 0) + (0.30 \times 1) + (0.30 \times 0)]}{1.2} = 0.25.$$

6. The weight to be given to this iteration is

$$\alpha_2 = \log\frac{(1-25)}{0.25} = \log(0.75/0.25) = 1.1.$$

7. We would normally continue iterating, beginning with the calculation of a third set of weights. But suppose we are done. The classes assigned are

$$\hat{y}_1 = \text{sign}[(1 \times 0.41) + (1 \times 1.1)] > 0 \Rightarrow 1$$
$$\hat{y}_2 = \text{sign}[(1 \times 0.41) + (1 \times 1.1)] > 0 \Rightarrow 1$$
$$\hat{y}_3 = \text{sign}[(1 \times 0.41) + (1 \times 1.1)] > 0 \Rightarrow 1$$
$$\hat{y}_4 = \text{sign}[(1 \times 0.41) + (1 \times 1.1)] > 0 \Rightarrow 1$$
$$\hat{y}_5 = \text{sign}[(1 \times 0.41) + (-1 \times 1.1)] < 0 \Rightarrow -1.$$

One can see in this toy example how in the second iteration the misclassified observations are given relatively more weight. One can also see that the class assigned (i.e., +1 or −1) is just a weighted sum of the classes assigned at each iteration. The second iteration had fewer wrong (one out of five rather than two out of five) and so was given more weight in the ultimate averaging. These principles would apply even for very large datasets and thousands of iterations. The key point, however, is that operationally, there is nothing very mysterious going on.

6.2.2 Why Does Boosting Work so Well for Classification?

Despite the operational simplicity of boosting, there is no consensus on why it works so well. At present, there seem to be three complementary perspectives. All three are interesting, and each has some useful implications for practice.

6.2.2.1 Boosting as a Margin Maximizer

The first perspective comes from computer science and the boosting pioneers. The basic idea is that boosting is a margin maximizer (Schapire et al. 1998; Schapire and Freund 2012). From AdaBoost, the margin for any given case i is defined as

$$mg^* = \sum_{y=G_m} \alpha_m - \sum_{y \neq G_m} \alpha_m, \tag{6.1}$$

where the sums are over the number of passes through the data for correct classifications or incorrect classifications, respectively. This expression is different from Breiman's margin (mr) but in the same spirit. In words, for any given case i, the margin is the difference between the sum of the iteration weights when the classification is correct and the sum of the iteration weights when the classification is incorrect.[2]

Looking back at the toy example, the classifier is two for two for the first three observations, one for two for the last observation, and zero for two for the fourth observation. In practice, there would be hundreds of passes (or more) over the data, but one can nevertheless appreciate that the classifications are most convincing for the first three observations and least convincing for the fourth observation. The fifth observation is in between. Equation (6.1) is just an extension of this idea.

The sum of the correct or incorrect classifications becomes the sum of the weights when the classification is correct or the sum of the weights when the classification is incorrect, with the weights equal to α_m. For the first three cases in the toy example, the margin $(0.41 + 1.1) - 0 = 1.51$. The margin for the fourth case is $0 - (0.41 + 1.1) = -1.51$. The margin for the fifth case is $1.1 - 0.41 = 0.69$. The evidence for the first three cases is the highest. The evidence for the fourth case is the lowest, and the evidence for the fifth case is in between.

And now the punch line. "Boosting is particularly good at finding classifiers with large margins in that it concentrates on those examples whose margins are small (or negative) and forces the base learning algorithm to generate good classifications for those examples" (Schapire et al. 1998: 1656).[3] Indeed, as the number of passes through the data increase, the margins over observations generally increase, although whether they are maximized depends on the base classifier. For instance, the margins are generally not maximized using stump classification trees but one often can do better with large classification trees. The issues are subtle.

Improvements in the margin over passes through the data reformulate the overfitting problem. It is possible in principle to fit the training data perfectly. One would ordinarily halt the boosting well before that point because of concerns about overfitting. But with a perfect fit of the data, generalization error in test data can be surprisingly good because the weighed averaging works in a manner much like the averaging in bagging or random forests. (Look again at the final step in the AdaBoost.M1 algorithm.) Moreover, boosting *past* a perfect fit of the data can further reduce generalization error because the margins are getting larger. In short, concerns about overfitting for boosting seem to have been somewhat overstated.

There is one exception in which overfitting has actually been understated. When a classifier is also used to compute the probabilities associated with each class, boosting to minimize generalization error pushes the conditional proportions/probabilities for each observation toward 0.0 or 1.0 (Mease et al. 2007; Buja et al. 2007). With the goal of accurately assigning classes to observations, fitted probabilities are just scores that serve as a means to the end of accurate classification. There is no need for the probability interpretation. The more that such scores can differ for different outcome classes, the smaller the generalization error. Distinctions between outcome classes are more definitive.

In summary, one reason why boosting works so well as a classifier is that it can in practice approximate a margin maximizer. An important implication for using classifiers such as AdaBoost.M1 is that overfitting often is not be a serious problem. One can even boost past the point at which the fit in the training data is perfect. Another important implication for practice is that if classification trees are used as the classifier, large trees are desirable. And if large trees are desirable, so are large samples.

6.2.2.2 Boosting as a Statistical Optimizer

The second perspective sees AdaBoost as a stagewise additive model using basis functions in much the same spirit as CART and random forests. Consider again the final step in the algorithm for AdaBoost.M1

$$G(x) = \text{sign} \left[\sum_{m=1}^{M} \alpha_m G_m(x) \right]. \tag{6.2}$$

Each pass through the data involves the application of a classifier $G_m(x)$, the culmination of which is a stage. The results of M stages are combined in an additive fashion with the M values of α_m as the computed weights. This means that each $G_m(x)$ relies on a linear basis expansion of X, much as discussed in Chap. 1.

If boosting can be formulated as a stagewise additive model, an important question is what loss function is being used. From Friedman and his colleagues (2000), AdaBoost.M1 iterations are implicitly targeting

$$f(X) = \frac{1}{2} \log \frac{P(Y = 1|X)}{P(Y = -1|X)}. \tag{6.3}$$

This is just one-half of the usual log-odds (logit) function for $P(Y = 1|X)$. The $1/2$ results from using the sign to determine the class. This is the "population minimizer" for an exponential loss function $e^{-yf(x)}$. More formally,

$$\arg \min_{f(x)} \text{E}_{Y|x}(e^{-Yf(x)}) = \frac{1}{2}(\log) \frac{P(Y = 1|x)}{P(Y = -1|x)}. \tag{6.4}$$

AdaBoost.M1 is attempting to minimize exponential loss with the observed class and the fitted class as its arguments. The focus on exponential loss raises at least two important issues for practice.

First, emphasizing the mathematical relationship between the exponential loss function and conditional probabilities can paper over a key point in practice. Although at each stage, the true conditional probability is indeed the minimizer, over stages there can be gross overfitting of the estimated probabilities. In other words, the margin maximizing feature of boosting can trump the loss function optimizing feature of boosting.

Second, a focus on the exponential loss function naturally raises the question of whether there are other loss functions that might perform better. Hastie and his colleagues (2009: 345–346) show that minimizing the negative binomial log-likelihood (i.e., the deviance) is also (as in AdaBoost) in service of finding the true conditional probabilities, or the within-sample conditional proportions (i.e., a Level II or Level I analysis, respectively). Might this loss function, implemented as "LogitBoost," be preferred? On the matter of overfitting conditional probabilities, the answer is no. The same overfitting problems surface (Mease et al. 2007).

With respect to estimating class membership, the answer is maybe. Hastie et al. (2009: 346–349) show that the LogitBoost loss function is somewhat more robust to outliers than the AdaBoost loss function. They argue that, therefore, LogitBoost may be preferred if a significant number of the observed classes of the response variable are likely to be systematically wrong or noisy. There are other boosting options as well (Friedman et al. 2000). But, it is not clear how the various competitors fare in practice and for our purposes at the moment, that is beside the point. The loss function optimization explanation, whatever the proposed loss function, is at best a partial explanation for the success of boosting.

6.2.2.3 Boosting as an Interpolator

The third perspective has already been introduced. One key to the success of random forests is that it is an interpolator that is then locally robust. Another key is the averaging over a large number of trees. Although the details certainly differ, these attributes also apply to boosting (Wyner et al. 2017). As the margins are increased, the fitted values better approximate an interpolation of the data. Then, the weighted average of fitted values provides much the same stability as the vote over trees provides for random forests. For classifiers, "... the additional iterations in boosting way beyond the point at which perfect classification in the training data (i.e., interpolation) has occurred has the effect of smoothing out the effects of noise rather than leading to more and more overfitting" (Wyner et al. 2017: 24).

All three perspectives help explain why boosting performs so well as a classifier. From a statistical perspective, boosting is a stagewise optimizer targeting the same kinds of conditional probabilities that are the target for logistic regression. One of the several different loss functions can be used depending on the details of the data. This framework places boosting squarely within statistical traditions. But boosting is far more than a round-about way to do logistic regression. The margin maximization perspective helps to explain why and dramatically reduces concerns about overfitting, at least for classification. When the classifiers are trees, large trees perform better, which suggests that in general, complex base classifiers are to be preferred. Finally, the interpolation perspective links boosting to random forests and shows that boosting classifiers have many of the same beneficial properties. In so doing, there is a deeper understanding about why maximizing margins can be so helpful, although it is not nearly the whole story. In the end, interpolation may be the key.

The boosting implications for classification in practice are fourfold:

1. complex base learners (e.g., large classification trees) help;
2. boosting beyond a perfect fit in the training data can help;
3. a large number of observations can help; and
4. a rich set of predictors can help (subject to the usual caveats such as very high multicollinearity).

6.3   Stochastic Gradient Boosting

At present, there are many different kinds of boosting that all but boosting mavens will find overwhelming. Moreover, there is very little guidance about which form of boosting should be used in which circumstances. For practitioners, therefore, stochastic gradient boosting is a major advance (Friedman 2001, 2002). It is not quite a one-size-fits-all boosting procedure, but within a single statistical framework provides a rich menu of options. As such, it follows directly from the statistical perspective on boosting.

Suppose that the response variable in the training data is binary and coded numerically as 1 or 0. The procedure is initialized with some constant such as the overall proportion of 1s. This constant serves as the fitted values from which residuals are obtained by subtraction in the usual way. The residuals are then appended to the training data as a new variable. Next, a random sample of the data is drawn without replacement. One might, for example, sample half the data. A regression tree, not a classification tree, is applied to the sample with the residuals as the response. Another set of fitted values is obtained for all of the data. From these, a new set of residuals is obtained and appended. Another random sample is taken from the training data and the fitting process is repeated. The entire cycle is repeated many times: (1) fitted values, (2) residuals, (3) sampling, (4) a regression tree. In the end, the fitted values from each pass through the data are combined in a linear fashion. For classification, these can be interpreted as proportions or probabilities depending on whether the analysis is at Level I or level II, respectively. Commonly, observations with $\hat{y}_i > 0.5$ are assigned a 1, and observations with $\hat{y}_i \leq 0.5$ are assigned a 0. Numeric response variables also are permitted, and the steps are largely the same.[4]

The weighting so central to boosting occurs implicitly through the residuals from each pass. Larger positive or negative residuals imply that for those observations, the fitted values are less successful. As each regression tree attempts to maximize the quality of the fit, it responds more to the observations with larger positive or negative residuals.

6.3.1 Gradient Boosting More Formally

Consider now somewhat more formally the sources of the term "gradient" in gradient boosting. The discussion that follows draws heavily on Ridgeway (1999) and on Hastie et al. (2009: sections 10.9–10.10).

A *given* tree can be represented as

$$T(x; \Theta) = \sum_{j=1}^{J} \gamma_j I(x \in R_j), \tag{6.5}$$

with the tree parameters $\Theta = \{R_j, \gamma_j\}$, where j is an index for the terminal node, $j, \ldots, J$, R_j a predictor-space region defined by the jth terminal node, and γ_j is the value assigned to each observation in the jth terminal node. The goal is to construct values for the unknown parameters Θ_m so that the loss function is minimized.[5] At this point, no particular loss L is specified, and we seek a single tree such that

$$\hat{\Theta} = \arg\min_{\Theta} \sum_{j=1}^{J} \sum_{x_i \in R_j} L(y_i, \gamma_j). \tag{6.6}$$

As noted earlier, minimizing the loss function for a single tree is challenging. For stochastic gradient boosting, the challenge is even greater because of the need to minimize the loss over a collection of trees. In response, the algorithm proceeds in a stagewise fashion so that at iteration m,

$$\hat{\Theta}_m = \arg\min_{\Theta_m} \sum_{i=1}^{N} L(y_i, f_{m-1}(x_i) + T(x_i; \Theta_m)), \tag{6.7}$$

where $f_{m-1}(x_i)$ now is fixed, and $T(x_i; \Theta_m)$ is a new tree; the intent is to reduce the loss as much as possible incorporating the fitted values from a new tree. This can be accomplished through an astute determination of $\hat{\Theta}_m = [R_{jm}, \gamma_{jm}]$ for $j = 1, 2, \ldots, J_m$. In other words, Eq. (6.7) expresses the aspiration of updating the fitted values in an optimal manner through $T(x_i; \Theta_m)$.

Equation (6.7) can be reformulated as a numerical optimization task. For the ith observation on iteration m, g_{im} is the partial derivative of the loss with respect to the fitted value. Thus,

$$g_{im} = -\left[\frac{\partial L(y_i, f(x_i))}{\partial f(x_i)} \right]_{f(x_i)=f_{m-1}(x_i)}. \tag{6.8}$$

Equation (6.8) represents for each observation i the potential reduction in the loss as its fitting value $f(x_i)$ is altered. The larger the value of g_{im}, the greater is the reduction in the loss as $f(x_i)$ changes. So, an effective fitting function should respond more to the larger absolute values of g_{im} than small ones.[6] The connections to Eqs. (6.5) through (6.7) are made through Θ, which determines the $f(x_i)$.

The g_{im} will generally vary across observations. A way must be found to exploit the g_{im} so that over all of the observations, the loss is reduced the most it can be. One approach is to use a numerical method called "steepest descent," in which a "step length" ρ_m is found so that

$$\rho_m = \arg \min_{\rho} L(\mathbf{f}_{m-1} - \rho \mathbf{g}_m). \tag{6.9}$$

In other words, a scalar ρ_m is determined for iteration m so that when it multiplies the full set of partial derivatives, the new loss is minimized.[7] Then, the current fitted values are updated by

$$\mathbf{f}_m = \mathbf{f}_{m-1} - \rho \mathbf{g}_m. \tag{6.10}$$

This exercise is repeated for the next iteration in a stagewise, greedy fashion. Because $\mathbf{g}_m$ depends on the fitted values that, in turn, depend on Θ_m, the algorithm finds the values of Θ that reduce the loss the most.

The updating process is very aggressive because $-\mathbf{g}_m$, sometimes called the "directional derivative," is the updating direction that reduces the loss by the greatest amount. Subsequent iterations follow in the same manner until no further reduction in the loss can be obtained. The fitted values are as good as they can be.

To get a better sense of what is meant by "direction," Fig. 6.1 illustrates in cartoon fashion the basics of the process when there are only two fitted values ($N = 2$). These are on the horizontal axis. The loss is on the vertical axis. In this case, the loss function is convex. The minimized loss is represented by the red filled circle.

As represented in Eqs. (6.9) and (6.10), the algorithm starts at some arbitrary point and proceeds one step at a time determined by the direction and step length for which the loss is reduced the most, subject to a constraint on the length of the step. The direction of each step is dictated by the sizes of the components of the directional gradient. In two dimensions, for example, Fig. 6.2 shows how the step will be pulled in the direction of the larger partial derivative because in that direction the loss is reduced more. The step vector in blue is the sum of the components of the gradient in vector form. Typically, there will be many observations, but the ideas represented in Fig. 6.1 directly generalize.

For all of these steps to play through, the values of the partial derivatives must be obtained at each iteration. For gradient boosting, one can use regression tree residuals r_{im} as empirical proxies for the gradients. These are sometimes called "pseudo-residuals." Friedman (2002) shows that there is, then, a least squares solution to finding effective parameter values for the fitting function at each iteration. For iteration m, one fits a regression tree to the negative gradients. That is,

$$\tilde{\Theta}_m = \arg \min_{\Theta} \sum_{i=1}^{N} (-g_{im} - T(x_i; \Theta))^2. \tag{6.11}$$

Fig. 6.1 An illustration of steepest descent looking down into a convex loss function (The two sets of fitted values are on the horizontal axes. Loss is represented on the vertical axis.)

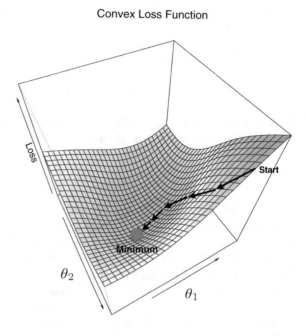

Convex Loss Function

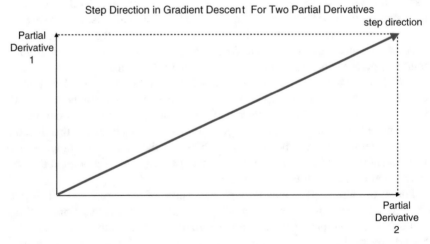

Step Direction in Gradient Descent For Two Partial Derivatives

Fig. 6.2 The step direction is the sum of two partial derivatives in vector form (A longer vector indicates a steeper partial derivative)

In practice, one fits successive regression trees by least squares. This is not a heavy computational burden and depending on how the r_{im} are constructed, a variety of sensible loss functions can be defined. These different loss functions result in boosting variants for the generalized linear model and more.

6.3.2 Stochastic Gradient Boosting in Practice

We turn, then, to stochastic gradient boosting, implemented in R as *gbm*, that is an explicit generalization of Friedman's original gradient boosting. Among the differences are the use of sampling in the spirit of bagging and a form of shrinkage.[8]

Consider a training dataset with N observations and p predictors x, and the response y.

1. Initialize $f_0(x)$ so that the constant κ minimizes the loss function: $f_0(x) = \arg\min_\kappa \sum_{i=1}^{N} L(y_i, \kappa)$.[9]
2. For m in $1, \ldots, M$, do steps a–e.

   (a) For $i = 1, 2, \ldots, N$ compute the negative gradient approximation as the working response

   $$r_{im} = -\left[\frac{\partial L(y_i, f(x_i))}{\partial f(x_i)} \right]_{f=f_{m-1}}.$$

   (b) Randomly select without replacement W cases from the dataset, where W is less than the total number of observations. This is a simple random sample, not a bootstrap sample, which seems to improve performance. How large W should be is discussed shortly.

   (c) Using the randomly selected observations, each with their own r_{im}, fit a regression tree with J_m terminal nodes to the r_{im}, giving regions R_{jm} for each terminal node $j = 1, 2, \ldots, J_m$.

   (d) For $j = 1, 2, \ldots, J_m$, compute the optimal terminal node prediction as

   $$\gamma_{jm} = \arg\min_\gamma \sum_{x_i \in R_{jm}} L(y_i, f_{m-1}(x_i) + \gamma),$$

   where region R_{jm} denotes the set of x-values that define the terminal node j for iteration m.

   (e) Drop all of the cases down the tree grown from the sample, and update $f_m(x)$ as

   $$f_m(x) = f_{m-1}(x) + \nu \cdot \sum_{j=1}^{J_m} \gamma_{jm} I(x \in R_{jm}),$$

   where ν is a "shrinkage" parameter that determines the learning rate. The importance of ν is discussed shortly.

3. Output $\hat{f}(x) = f_M(x)$.

Ridgeway (1999) has shown that using this algorithmic structure, all of the procedures within the generalized linear model, plus several extensions of it, can properly be boosted by the stochastic gradient method. Stochastic gradient boosting relies on an empirical approximation of the true gradient (Hastie et al. 2009: section 10.10) for which the trick is determining the right r_i for each special case; the "residuals" need to be defined. Among the current definitions of r_i are the following, each associated with a particular kind of regression mean function: linear regression, logistic regression, robust regression, Poisson regression, quantile regression, and others.

1. Gaussian: $y_i - f(x_i)$: the usual regression residual.
2. Bernoulli: $y_i - \frac{1}{1+e^{-f(x_i)}}$: the difference between the binary outcome coded 1 or 0 and the fitted proportion for the conventional logit link function for logistic regression.
3. Poisson: $y_i - e^{f(x_i)}$: the difference between the observed count and the fitted count for the conventional log link function as in Poisson regression.
4. Laplace: $\text{sign}[y_i - f(x_i)]$: the sign of the difference between the values of the response variable and the fitted medians, a form of robust regression.
5. AdaBoost: $-(2y_i - 1)e^{-(2y_i-1)f(x_i)}$: based on exponential loss and closely related to logistic regression.
6. Quantile: $\alpha(I(y > f(x_i)) - (1 - \alpha)I(y_i \leq f(x_i))$: for quantile regression the weighted difference between two indicator variables is equal to 1 or 0 depending on whether residual is positive or negative with the weights α or $(1 - \alpha)$, and α as the percentile target.

There are several other options built into *gbm*, which does stochastic gradient boosting in R.[10] Hastie and his colleagues (2009: 321) derive the gradient for a Huber robust regression. Ridgeway (2012) offers boosted proportional hazard regression. No doubt there will be additional distributions added in the future.

Stochastic gradient boosting also can be linked to various kinds of penalized regression of the general form discussed in earlier chapters. One insight is that the sequence of results that is produced with each pass over the data can be seen as a regularization process akin to shrinkage (Bühlmann and Yu 2004; Friedman et al. 2004).

In short, with stochastic gradient boosting, each tree is constructed much as a conventional regression tree. The difference is how the "target" for the fitting is defined. Using disparities defined in particular ways, a wide range of fitting procedures can be boosted. It is with good reason that "gbm" stands for "generalized boosted regression models."

6.3.3 Tuning Parameters

Stochastic gradient boosting has a substantial number of tuning parameters, many of which affect the results in similar ways. There is no analytical way to arrive at an optimal tuning parameter values in part because how they perform is so dependent on the data (Buja et al. 2007). An algorithmic search over values might be helpful in principle, but would be computationally demanding, and there would likely be many sets of tuning parameter values leading to nearly the same performance. Fortunately, the results from stochastic gradient boosting are often relatively robust to sensible variation in the tuning parameters, and common defaults usually work quite well.

The most important tuning parameters provided by *gbm* are as follows:

1. Number of Iterations—The number of passes through the data is typically the most important tuning parameter and is in practice empirically determined. Because there is no convergence and no clear stopping rule, the usual procedure is to run a large number of iterations and inspect a graph of the fitting error (e.g., residual deviance) plotted against the number of iterations. The error should decline rapidly at first and then level off. If after leveling, there is an inflection point at which the fitting error begins to increase, the number of iterations can be stopped shortly before that point. If there is no inflection point, the number of iterations can be determined by when reductions in the error effectively cease. There is a relatively large margin for error because plus or minus 50–100 iterations rarely lead to meaningful performance differences.

2. Subsample Size—A page is taken from bagging with the use of random sampling in step 2b to help control overfitting. The sampling is done without replacement, but as noted earlier, there can be an effective equivalence between sampling with and without replacement, at least for conventional bagging (Buja and Stuetzle 2006). When sampling without replacement, the sample size is a tuning parameter, and the issues are rather like those that arise when one works with split samples. Sampling about half the data is a common choice.

3. Learning Rate—A slow rate at which the updating occurs can be very useful. Setting the tuning parameter v to be less than 1.0 is standard practice. A value of 0.001 often seems to work reasonably well, but values larger and smaller by up to a factor of 10 are sometimes worth trying as well. By slowing down the rate at which the algorithm learns, a larger number of basis functions can be computed. Flexibility in the fitting process is increased, and the small steps increase shrinkage, which improves stability. A cost is a larger number of passes through the data. Fortunately, one can usually slow the learning process down substantially without a prohibitive increase in computing.

4. Interaction Depth—Another tuning parameter that affects the flexibility of the fitting function is the "depth" of the interaction. This name is a little misleading because it does not directly control the order of the interactions allowed. Rather it controls the number of splits allowed. If the interaction depth is 1, there is only a split of the root node data. If the interaction depth is 2, the two resulting data partitions of the root node data are split. If the interaction depth is 3, the four resulting partitions are split. And on it goes. Interaction depth is a way to limit the size of the regression trees, and values from 1 to 10 are used in practice. As such, the interaction depth determines the *maximum* order of any interactions, but the order of the interactions can be less than the interaction depth. For example, an interaction depth of 2 may result in four partitions defined by a single predictor at

different break points. There are no interaction effects because interaction effects are commonly defined as the product of two or more predictors. If interaction depth is set to 2, the largest possible interaction effect is two (i.e., a two-way interaction involving two predictors).

5. Terminal Node Size—Yet another tuning parameter that affects fitting function flexibility is the minimum number of observations in each tree's terminal node. For a given sample size, smaller node sizes imply larger trees and a more flexible fitting function. But smaller nodes also lead to less stability for whatever is computed in each terminal node. Minimum terminal node sizes of between 5 and 15 seem to work reasonably well in many settings, but a lot depends on the loss function that is being used. By the interpolation thinking introduced earlier, some argue for terminal node sizes of 1 for binary response variables.

In practice, the tuning parameters can interact. For example, terminal node size may be set too high for the interaction depth specified to be fully implemented. Also, more than one tuning parameter can be set in service of the same goal. The growth of larger trees, for instance, can be encouraged by small terminal node sizes and by greater interaction depth. In short, sometimes tuning parameters compete with one another and sometimes tuning parameters complement one another.

A major obstacle to effective tuning is the need for test data. Even with the sampling built into stochastic gradient boosting, there is no provision for retaining the unsampled data for performance evaluation. The out-of-bag data may be used only to help determine the number of iterations.[11] Common tuning advice, therefore, is limited to in-sample performance. But recall that for classification, one can have a perfect fit to the data and still reduce generalization error with more iterations. For classification and regression, using the test data for honest performance evaluation seems like a good idea.

6.3.4 Output

The key output from stochastic gradient boosting is much the same as the key output from random forests. However, unlike random forests, there are not the usual out-of-bag observations that can be used as test data. Consequently, confusion tables depend on resubstituted data; the data used to grow the trees are also used to evaluate their performance. The same applies to fitted values for numerical response variables. Consequently, overfitting can be a complication. Ideally, this problem should be addressed with test data.

Just as for random forests, the use of multiple trees means that it is impractical to examine tree diagrams to learn how individual predictors perform. The solutions currently available are much like those implemented for random forests. There are variable importance measures and partial dependence plots that are similar to those used in random forests.

The partial dependence plots must be treated cautiously when the outcome variable is binary.[12] Recall that in an effort to classify well, boosting can push the fitted probabilities away from 0.50 toward 0.0 and 1.0. For *gbm*, partial dependence plots with binary response variables use either a probability or logit scale (i.e., $\log [p_i /(1 - p_i)]$) on the vertical axis. Both are vulnerable if measures of classification performance are used to tune and if the number passes through the data is large. If tuning is done through measures of fit such as the deviance, one has no more than the usual concerns about overfitting. But, in that case, classification accuracy (should one care) will perhaps be sacrificed.[13]

The exact form taken by the variable importance measures depends on options in the software. One common choice is reductions of the loss function that can be attributed to each predictor. The software sums for each tree how much the loss decreases when any predictor defines a data partition. For example, if for a given tree a particular predictor is chosen three times to define data partitions, the three reductions in the loss function are summed as a measure of that predictor's contribution to the fit for that tree. Such sums are averaged over trees to provide the contribution that each predictor makes to the overall fit. The contributions can be reported in raw form or as percentages of the overall reduction in loss.

In *gbm*, there is on a somewhat experimental basis a random shuffling approach to importance based on classification accuracy. To date, however, out-of-bag observations are not used so that true forecasting accuracy is not represented. Recall that for random forests, importance is defined by contributions to classification accuracy in the out-of-bag data. One option is to use test data properly to determine classification accuracy overall. It is then easy to write a function that will shuffle one predictor at a time and compute the reduction in classification accuracy. Another option is to use the procedure *caret*, which provides several useful ways to work with *gbm* output.[14]

6.4 Asymmetric Costs

All of the available loss functions for categorical outcomes use symmetric costs. False positives count the same as false negatives. For stochastic gradient boosting, there are two ways to easily introduce asymmetric costs. For binary outcomes, the first is to place a threshold on the fitted values that differs from 0.5 (or on the logit scale that differs from 0.0). This option was discussed earlier for several other procedures. For example, if a positive is coded 1 and a negative is coded 0, placing the threshold at 0.25 means false negatives can be 3 times most costly than false positives. The problems with this approach were also discussed. All other boosting output is still based on symmetric costs. One has boosted to the wrong approximation.

Moreover, there can be operational difficulties if the distribution of the fitted values is either very dense or very sparse in the neighborhood of the threshold. If very dense, small changes in the threshold that make no material difference can alter classification performance dramatically. At the very least, this may be counterintuitive and will likely increase instability for the classes assigned. If very sparse, it can be difficult set the threshold so that the desired cost ratio in a confusion table is produced. The distribution is too lumpy.

The second alternative is also for binary outcomes: use weights. This is much like altering the prior for CART. And like with CART, some trial and error is involved before the classification table with the desired cost ratio is produced. One can then think of the weights as tuning parameters for the cost ratio in a confusion table; one tunes toward the target cost ratio. The intent is to upweight the outcome for which classification errors are more costly relative to the outcome for which classification error is less costly. An example is provided below.[15]

For numerical response variables, the options are to date rather limited. The only loss function for which asymmetric costs are naturally available is the quantile regression loss function. By choosing the appropriate quantile, underestimates can be given different costs from overestimates. For example, if one estimates the 75th percentile, underestimates are three times more costly than overestimates. Looking back at the quantile regression residual expression shown earlier when the algorithm for stochastic gradient boosting was introduced, the value of α is set to the target percentile and is the weight given to all positive residuals. The value of $(1 - \alpha)$ is the weight given to all negative residuals. Positive residuals are underestimates, and negative residuals are overestimates.

Figure 6.3 shows the shape of the loss function when the quantile is greater than 0.50. As illustrated by the red line, the loss grows more rapidly for underestimates (i.e., positive residuals) than for overestimates (i.e., negative residuals). For quantiles less than 0.50, the reverse is true. For a quantile of 0.50, the red and blue line have the same rate of growth.

Fig. 6.3 Asymmetric loss function for the Quantile loss function with the Quantile set at 0.75

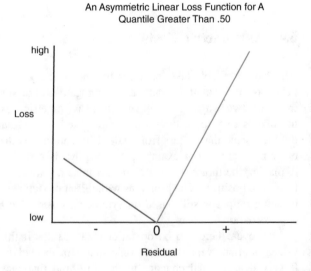

6.5   Boosting, Estimation, and Consistency

The most important output from boosting is the fitted values. For a Level I analysis, these are just statistics computed for the data on hand. But, often there is an interest in using the values as estimates of the fitted values in the joint probability distribution responsible for the data. This is a Level II analysis. Just as for random forests, no claims are made that boosting will provide accurate estimates of the true response surface. At best, one can get a consistent estimate of generalization error for a given sample size, boosting specification and set of tuning parameters values (Jiang 2004, Zhang and Yu 2005, Bartlett and Traskin 2007). But existing proofs either impose artificial conditions or are limited to a few of the "easier" loss functions such as exponential loss and quadratic loss. And even then, the implications for practice are not clear. There can be a Goldilocks stopping strategy for a given number of observations at which the number of iterations is neither too few nor too many. But how to find that sweet spot for a given analysis is not explained.

The best one can do in practice is apply some empirical heuristic and hope for the best. As already noted, that heuristic can be the point at which the decrease in the loss function levels off as the number of iterations increases. Some measure of fit between the observed response values and the fitted values can then be used as a rough proxy for generalization error for that sample size, stopping decision, specification, and associated tuning parameter settings. Conventionally, this is an in-sample estimate. A more honest estimate of generalization error can be obtained from a test sample and as described earlier, one can use the nonparametric bootstrap to approximate the variability in that estimate. This is essentially the same approach to a Level II analysis as used for random forests.

6.6   A Binomial Example

We return to the Titanic data for some applications of stochastic boosting as implemented in *gbm* for a Level I analysis. Recall that the response is whether a passenger survived. It is coded here numerically as 1 for survived and 0 for perished.[16] The predictors we use are gender ("sex"), age, class of cabin ("pclass"), number of siblings/spouses aboard ("sibsp"), and the number of parents/children aboard ("parch"). The code used for the analysis with Bernoulli loss is provided in Fig. 6.4. At the top, the data are loaded, and a new dataset is constructed. A weighting variable is constructed for later use. All NA entries removed. Removing NAs in advance is required when a procedure does not discard them automatically.

Consistent with our earlier discussion, the minimum terminal node size is set to 1, and the interaction depth set to three. Setting it to a larger value (e.g., 8) led to fewer iterations but essentially the same results. Setting it to a smaller value (e.g., 1) led to more iterations, but also essentially same results. The number of iterations

```
# Load and Clean Up Data
library(PASWR)
data("titanic3")
attach(titanic3)
wts<-ifelse(survived==1,1,3) # for asymmetric costs if needed
Titanic3<-na.omit(data.frame(fare,survived,pclass,
                             sex,age,sibsp,parch,wts))

# Boosted Binomial Regression
library(gbm)
out2<-gbm(survived~pclass+sex+age+sibsp+parch,
        data=Titanic3,n.trees=4000,interaction.depth=3,
        n.minobsinnode = 1,shrinkage=.001,bag.fraction=0.5,
        n.cores=1,distribution = "bernoulli")

# Output
gbm.perf(out2,oobag.curve=T,method="OOB",overlay=F) # 3245
summary(out2,n.trees=3245,method=permutation.test.gbm,
        normalize=T)
plot(out2,"sex",3245,type="response")
plot(out2,"pclass",3245,type="response")
plot(out2,"age",3245,type="response")
plot(out2,"sibsp",3245,type="response")
plot(out2,"parch",3245,type="response")
plot(out2,c("sibsp","parch"),3245,type="response") # Interaction

# Fitted Values
preds2<-predict(out2,newdata=Titanic3,n.trees=3245,
                type="response")
table(Titanic3$survived,preds2>.5)
```

Fig. 6.4 R code for Bernoulli regression boosting

was set to 4000 anticipating that 4000 should be plenty. If not, the number could be increased. All else were the defaults, except that the number of cores available was one. Even with only one core, the fitting took about a second in real time.[17]

Figure 6.5 shows standard *gbm* performance output. On the horizontal axis is the number of iterations. On the vertical axis is the change in the Bernoulli deviance based on the OOB observations. The OOB observations provide a more honest assessment than could be obtained in-sample. However, they introduce sampling error so that the changes in the loss bounce around a bit. The reductions in the deviance decline as the number of iterations grows and becomes effectively 0.0 shortly after the 3000th pass through the data. Any of the iterations between 3000 and 4000 lead to about the same fit of the data, but the software selects iteration 3245

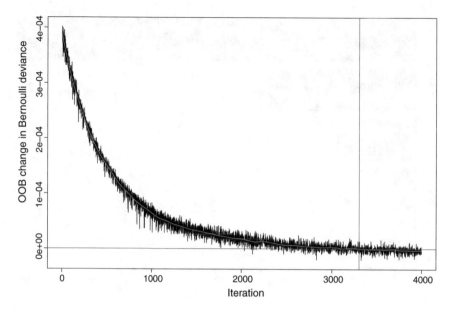

Fig. 6.5 Changes in Bernoulli deviance in OOB data with Iteration 3245 as the stopping point (N=1045)

as the stopping point. Consequently, the first 3245 trees are used in all subsequent calculations.[18]

Figure 6.6 is a variable importance plot shown in the standard *gbm* format. Importance is measured by the contribution to the fit. The shuffling option is chosen, with the reductions in fit contributions averaged over the entire training dataset, not for the OOB data. Also, the contribution of each input is standardized as its percentage contribution to the total contributions across all predictors. For example, gender is the most important predictor with a relative performance of 60 (i.e., 60%). The class of passage is the next most important input with a relative performance score of about 25, followed by age with a relative performance score of about 12. If you believe the accounts of the Titanic's sinking, these contributions make sense. But just as with random forests, each contribution includes any interaction effects with other variables unless the tree depth is equal to 1 (i.e., *interaction.depth=1*). So, the contributions in Fig. 6.6 cannot be attributed to each input by itself. Equally important, contributions to the fit are not regression coefficients and or contributions to forecasting accuracy. It may not be clear, therefore, how to use them when real decisions have to be made.

Figure 6.7 presents two partial dependence plots with the fitted proportion on the vertical axis. One has the option of reporting the results as proportions or logits. One can see that class of passage really matters. Survival drops from a little over 0.6 to a little under 0.30 from first class to second class to third class. Survival is also strongly related to age. The survival drops from about 0.70 to about 0.40 as age

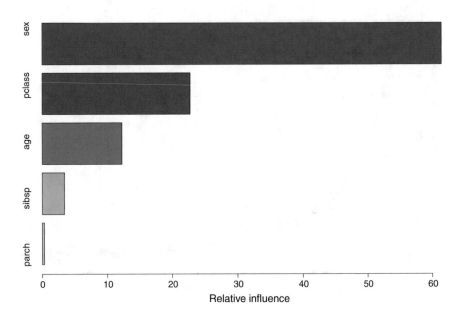

Fig. 6.6 Titanic data variable importance plot for survival using binomial regression boosting (N=1045)

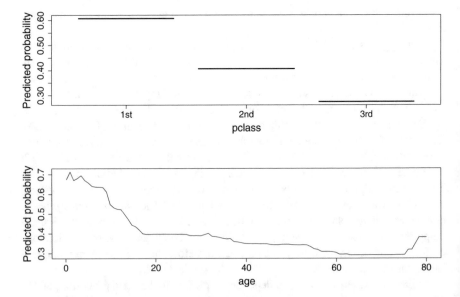

Fig. 6.7 Titanic data partial dependence plots showing survival proportions for class of passage and age using binomial regression boosting (N=1045)

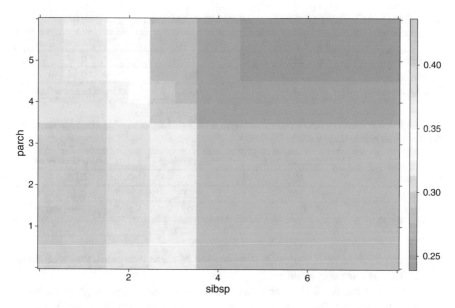

Fig. 6.8 Interaction partial dependence plot: survival proportions for the number of Siblings/Spouses aboard and the number of parents/children aboard using binomial regression boosting (N=1045)

increases from about 1 year to about 18. There is another substantial drop around age 55 and an increase around age 75. But there are very few passengers older than 65, so the apparent increase could be the results of instability.[19]

Figure 6.8 is a partial dependence plot designed to show two-way interaction effects. The two inputs are the number of siblings/spouses aboard and the number of parents/children aboard, which are displayed as a generalization of a mosaic plot. The inputs are shown on the vertical and horizontal axes. The color scale is shown on the far right. A combination of sibsp >5 and parch >4 has the smallest chances of survival; about a quarter survived. A combination of sibsp <2 and parch <3 has the largest chances of survival; a little less than half survived.[20] In this instance, there does not seem to be important interaction effects. The differences in the colors from top to bottom are about the same regardless of the value for sibsp. For example, when sibsp is 6, the proportion surviving changes from top to bottom from about 0.25 to about 0.30. The difference is −0.05. When sibsp is 1, the proportion surviving changes from top to bottom from about 0.35 to about 0.40. The difference is again around −0.05. Hence, the association between sibsp and survival is approximately the same for both values of sibsp.

It is difficult to read the color scale for Fig. 6.8 at the necessary level of precision. One might reach different conclusions if numerical values were examined. But the principle just illustrated is valid for how interaction effects are represented. And it is still true for these two predictors that a combination of many siblings/spouses and

Table 6.1 Confusion table for titanic passengers with default 1 to 1 weights (N=1045)

	Fitted perished	FittedSurvived	Classification error
Perished	561	57	0.09
Survived	126	301	0.29
Prediction error	0.18	0.16	Overall error = 0.18

Table 6.2 Confusion table for titanic passengers with 3–1 weights making classification errors for those who perished more costly (N=1045)

	Fitted perished	Fitted survived	Classification error
Perished	601	17	0.03
Survived	195	232	0.46
Prediction error	0.24	0.08	Overall error = 0.21

many parents/children is the worst combination of these two predictors whether or not their effects are only additive.

Table 6.1 is the confusion table that results when each case is given the same weight. This is the default. The empirical cost ratio in the confusion table is about 2.2 to 1 with misclassification errors for those who perished about twice as costly as misclassification errors for those who survived. Whether that is acceptable depends on how the results would be used. In this instance, there are probably no decisions to be made based on the classes assigned, so the cost ratio is probably of little interest.

Stochastic gradient boosting does a good job distinguishing those who perished from those who survived. Only 9% of those who perished were misclassified, and only 29% of those who survived were misclassified. The prediction errors of 18% and 16% are also quite good although it is hard to imagine how these results would be used for forecasting.

Table 6.2 repeats the prior analysis but with survivor observations weighted as 3 times more than the observations for those who perished. Because there are no decisions to be made based on the analysis, there is no grounded way to set the weights. The point is just to illustrate that weighting can make a big difference in the results that, in turn, affect the empirical cost ratio of a confusion table. That cost ratio is now 11.5 so that misclassifications of those who perished are now over 11 times more costly than misclassifications of those who survived. Consequently, the proportion misclassified for those who perished drops to 3%, and the proportion misclassified for those who survived increases to 46%. Whether these are more useful results than the results shown in Table 6.1 depends on how the results would be used.[21]

Should one report the results in proportions or probabilities? For these data, proportions seem more appropriate. As already noted, the Titanic sinking is probably best viewed as a one time event that has already happened, which implies there may be no good answer to the question "probability of what?" Passengers either perished or survived, and treating such an historically specific event as one of many identical, independent trials seems a stretch. This is best seen as a Level I analysis.

6.7 Boosting for Statistical Inference and Forecasting

When one can make the case that the dataset is comprised of IID realizations from a relevant joint probability distribution, the stage is set for proper statistical inference, including statistical tests and confidence intervals. Attention centers on the boosting fitted values. Just as for bagging and random forests, uncertainty in the fitted values, as well as various summary statistics of the fitted values, can be usefully addressed employing test data combined with the nonparametric bootstrap.

Test data are used as new, input data in the R *predict* function, once the boosting algorithmic structure has been determined with training data. The boosting algorithm is *not* applied to the test data; just like CART, bagging, and random forests, boosting engages in automated data snooping and the need for empirical tuning.

6.7.1 An Imputation Example

Sometimes the boosting results can be productively used in imputation or forecasting, and here too, uncertainty properly can be addressed asymptotically. Consider the *Pima.te* dataset in the *MASS* library. From the documentation in R, "A population of women who were at least 21 years old, of Pima Indian heritage and living near Phoenix, Arizona, was tested for diabetes according to World Health Organization criteria. The data were collected by the US National Institute of Diabetes and Digestive and Kidney Diseases. We used the 532 complete records after dropping the (mainly missing) data on serum insulin."

It might be productive to consider the genetic, biomedical, and social process that predispose people to get diabetes, perhaps conditional on having a Pima Indian heritage. Those processes might be usefully summarized with a joint probability distribution characterizing relevant variables. Depending on how the data were actually collected, it might also be reasonable to treat each observation as an IID realization from that joint probability distribution. But one would need extensive information on exactly how the data were collected. The data would not be IID realizations, for example, if study subjects were recruited from a single, local clinic or through referrals from family and friends.

For didactic purposes, assume the data can be treated as IID. There is an outcome variable coded "1" if an individual had diabetes and "0" otherwise. There also are variables thought to be related to diabetes that might be used as predictors. A conventional fitting exercise could then be undertaken with stochastic gradient boosting. To what end? A physician might be able to use the results as a diagnostic

```
library(MASS)
data("Pima.te")
summary(Pima.te)
Diab<-ifelse(Pima.te[,"type"]=="Yes",1,0) # Make response numeric
dta<-data.frame(Pima.te[,1:7],Diab)

# Split data
index<-sample(1:332,166,replace=F) # For split
train<-dta[index,] # Split 1
test<-dta[-index,] # Split 2

# Apply stochastic gradient boosting
library(gbm)
gbm1<-gbm(Diab~.,data=train,distribution = "bernoulli",
          interaction.depth=3, cv.folds=5,
          n.minobsinnode = 1) # Fit gbm
best.iter<-gbm.perf(gbm1,method="cv") # get number of trees

# Compute Ordered Residuals and the value of k
Yhat<-predict(gbm1,newdata=test,ntrees=best.iter,
              type="response") # Honest fitted values
resids<-sort(abs(Yhat-test[,8])) # Sorted honest residuals
k<-ceiling(((nrow(test)/2)+1)*.95) # Computer constant for CI
wiggle<-resids[k] # kth sorted residual

# Compute confidence interval for new patient
newd<-data.frame(npreg=10,glu=119,bp=80,skin=35,
                              bmi=29,ped=0.263,age=29)
Y.hat<-predict(gbm1,newdata = newd,n.trees=best.iter,
             type="response") # Forecast
CIlow<-Y.hat-wiggle # Lower boundary
CIhigh<-Y.hat+wiggle # Upper boundary
data.frame(Lower=CIlow, Forecast=Y.hat,Upper=CIhigh) # 95% CI
```

Fig. 6.9 Illustrative R code for split sample conformal prediction interval

aid. What are the chances that a given patient actually has diabetes that heretofore had not be diagnosed? This is an imputation task.

The code for such an analysis is shown in Fig. 6.9. Readers seeking more information about the nature of each predictor should consult the R documentation. The example shows for a single patient how one can use *gbm* and split sample, conformal prediction intervals to construct a 95% around the probability of having diabetes. For the patient with the input values shown, the probability of having diabetes is 0.34. The 95% interval ranges from 0.12 to 0.57. The diagnosing physician would need to provide a medical interpretation of the results, but perhaps the risk is large enough to at least undertake more extensive tests and plan for frequent follow-up evaluations.[22]

6.8   A Quantile Regression Example

For the Titanic data, the fare paid in dollars becomes the response variable, and the other predictors are just as before. With a few very large fares, there might be concerns about how well boosted normal regression would perform. Recall that boosted quantile regression is robust with respect to response variable outliers or a highly skewed distribution and also provides a way to build in relative costs for fitting errors. Figure 6.10 shows the code for a boosted quantile regression fitting the conditional 75th percentile.

There are two significant changes in the tuning parameters. First, the distribution is now "quantile" with alpha as the conditional quantile to be estimated. We begin by estimating the conditional 75th percentile. Underestimates are taken to be 3 times more costly than overestimates. Second, we also require an increase in the number of iterations. Figure 6.11 shows that a much large number of iterations is needed than for boosted binomial regression. For the conditional 75th percentile, only a little over 4000 iterations are needed. But we will see shortly that for other conditional percentiles at least 12,000 iterations are needed. There is a very small computational penalty for 12,000 iterations for these data.[23]

Figure 6.12 is the same kind of importance plot as earlier except that importance is now represented by the average improvement over trees in fit for the quantile loss function as each tree is grown. This is an in-sample measure.[24] Nevertheless, the plot is interpreted essentially in the same fashion. Fare is substantially associated with the class of passage, just as one would expect. The number of siblings/spouses is the second more important predictor, which also makes sense. With so few predictors, and such clear differences in their contributions, an OOB approach and the in-sample approach will lead to about the same substantive contributions.

Figure 6.13 shows for illustrative purposes two partial response plots. The upper plot reveals that the fitted 75th percentile is about $46 for females and a little less than $36 for males with the other predictors held constant. It is difficult to know what this means, because class of passage is being held constant and performs just as one would expect (graph not shown). One possible explanation is that there is variation in amenities within class of passage, and females are prepared to pay more for them. The lower plot shows that variation in fare with respect to age is at most around $3 and is probably mostly noise, given all else that is being held constant.

Figure 6.14 is an example of an interaction partial plot. The format now shows a categorical predictor (i.e., class of passage) and a numerical predictor (i.e., age). There are apparently interaction effects. Fare declines with age for a first class passage but not for a second or third class passage. Perhaps older first class passengers are better able to pay for additional amenities. Perhaps, there is only one fare available for second and third class passage.[25]

```
# Load Data and Clean Up Data
library(PASWR)
data("titanic3")
attach(titanic3)
Titanic3<-na.omit(data.frame(fare,pclass,
                             sex,age,sibsp,parch))

# Boosted Quantile Regression
library(gbm)
out1<-gbm(fare~pclass+sex+age+sibsp+parch,data=Titanic3,
          n.trees=12000,interaction.depth=3,
          n.minobsinnode = 10,shrinkage=.001,bag.fraction=0.5,
          n.cores=1, distribution = list(name="quantile",
          alpha=0.75))

#Output
gbm.perf(out1,oobag.curve=T) # 4387
summary(out1,n.trees=4387,method=relative.influence)
par(mfrow=c(2,1))
plot(out1,"sex",4387,type="link")
plot(out1,"age",4387,type="link")
plot(out1,"sibsp",4387,type="link")
plot(out1,"parch",4387,type="link")
plot(out1,c("pclass","age"),4448,type="link") # Interaction

# Fitted Values
preds1<-predict(out1,newdata=Titanic3,n.trees=4387,type="link")
plot(preds1,Titanic3$fare,col="blue",pch=19,
     xlab="Predicted Fare", ylab="Actual Fare",
     main="Results from Boosted Quantile Regression
     with 1 to 1 line Overlaid: (alpha=.75)")
     abline(0,1,col="red",lwd=2)
```

Fig. 6.10 R code for quantile regression boosting

Figure 6.15 is a plot of the actual fare against the fitted fare for the 75th percentile. Underestimates are treated as 3 times more costly than overestimates (i.e., $0.75/0.25 = 3$). Overlaid is a 1-to-1 line that provides a point of reference. Most of the fitted values fall below the 1-to-1 line, as they should be given the conditional percentile being fitted. Still, four very large fares are grossly underestimated. The full set of fitted values range from near \$0 to over \$200, but there are several actual fares over \$500. Roughly speaking, the fitted 75th percentile increases linearly with the actual fares. The correlation between the two is over 0.70. In short, performance seems reasonable overall if one can overlook the few very large underestimates.

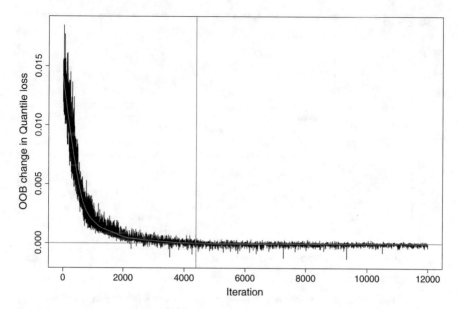

Fig. 6.11 Changes in the quantile loss function with OOB titanic data and with iteration 4387 as the stopping point (N= 1045)

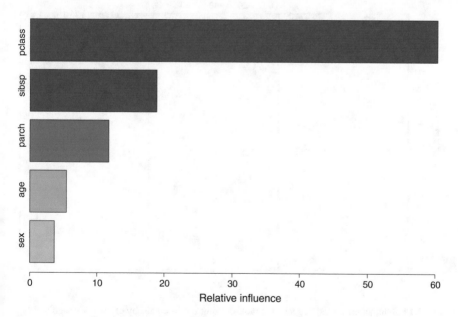

Fig. 6.12 Variable importance plot for the fare paid using quantile regression boosting with the 75th percentile (N=1045)

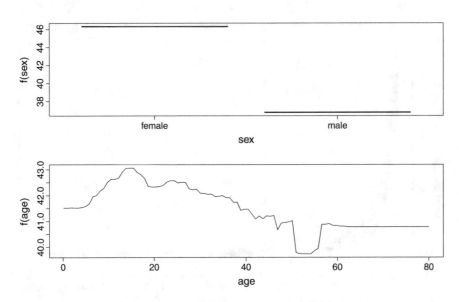

Fig. 6.13 Two partial dependence plots showing the fare paid as a function of sex or age using quantile regression boosting fitting the 75th percentile (N=1045)

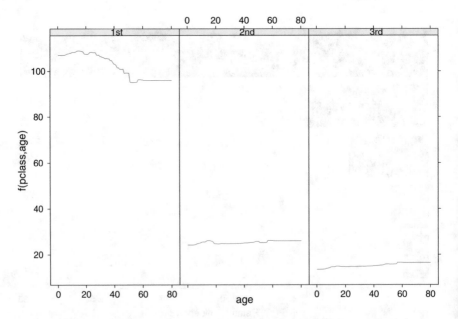

Fig. 6.14 Interaction partial dependence plot showing the fare paid by class of passage and age using quantile regression boosting fitting the 75th percentile (N=1045)

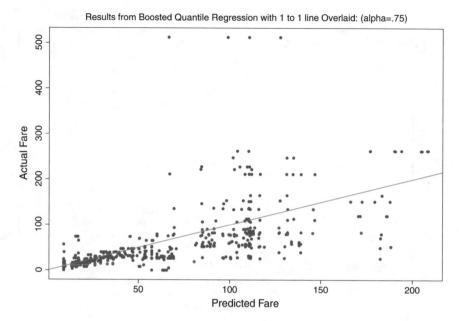

Fig. 6.15 Actual fare against fitted fare for a boosted quantile regression analysis of the titanic data with a 1-to-1 line overlaid (alpha = 0.75, N=1045)

Figure 6.16 is a plot of the actual fare against the fitted fare for the 25th percentile. Overestimates now are taken to be three times more costly than underestimates (i.e.,$0.25/0.75 = 1/3$). Overlaid again is a 1-to-1 line that provides a point of reference. Most of the actual fares fall above the 1-to-1 line. This too is just as it should be. The fitted values range from a little over $0 to about $75. Overall, the fit still looks to be roughly linear, and the correlation is little changed.[26]

Without knowing how the results from a boosted quantile regression are to be used, it is difficult to decide which quantiles should be fitted. If robustness is the major concern, using the 50th percentile is a sensible default rather than conditional means. But there are many applications where for subject-matter or policy reasons other percentiles can be desirable. As discussed earlier, for example, if one were estimating the number of homeless in a census tract (Berk et al. 2008), stakeholders might be very unhappy with underestimates because social services would not be made available where they were most needed. Fitting the 90th percentile could be a better choice. Or, stakeholders might on policy grounds be interested in the 10th percentile if in a classroom setting, there are special concerns about students who are performing poorly. It is the performance of kids who struggle that needs to be anticipated.

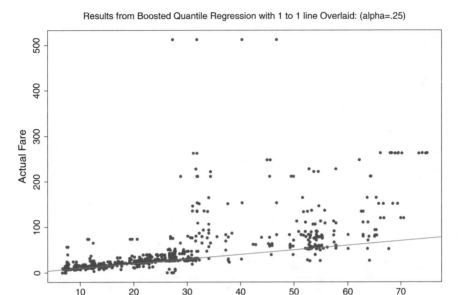

Results from Boosted Quantile Regression with 1 to 1 line Overlaid: (alpha=.25)

Fig. 6.16 Actual fare against fitted fare for a boosted quantile regression analysis of the titanic data with a 1-to-1 line overlaid (alpha = 0.25, N=1045)

6.9 Boosting in Service of Causal Inference in Observational Studies

When one is trying with observational data to estimate the causal effect of some intervention, a Level III analysis is being undertaken. It is well known that covariates associated with the intervention and the outcome produce confounding. Unless something is done to adjust properly for the confounding, estimates the true causal effect will be biased.[27]

We considered the main issues in Chapter 1. A conventional regression solution to confounding takes the form $Y = f(T, \mathbf{X}) + \varepsilon$, where T is the intervention (often binary), $\mathbf{X}$ is a set of covariates thought to be responsible for the confounding, and ε is the usual regression disturbance term.[28] The $f(T, \mathbf{X})$ is assumed to be linear. As discussed earlier, adjusting for confounding with linear regression has been correctly and widely criticized for the untestable assumptions required for the usual first order and second order conditions to be met. The same criticisms apply to nonlinear parametric regressions.

When there is a single intervention of interest and a set of "nuisance" covariates, the estimation challenge can be broken down into two components:

1. the manner in which the intervention is related to the covariates; and
2. the manner in which the response variable is related to the covariates.

When there is random assignment, the treatment assigned is on the average unrelated to the covariates; there is on the average no confounding. Furthermore, the means by which the intervention is assigned are known in the sense that the probability of any study unit receiving the intervention is determined by the research design.[29] That probability is commonly called a "propensity score" (Rosenbaum and Rubin 1983).

In observational studies (i.e., studies lacking random assignment to interventions), propensity scores can be estimated by a statistical model. Logistic regression is a popular choice. If the first and second order conditions of the propensity score model are met, one can condition on, or weight by, the estimated propensity scores and proceed as if one has random assignment. Nature has conducted the equivalent of a randomized experiment using the propensity scores as the assignment probabilities. Unbiased estimates of the average treatment effect (ATE) can be the reward.[30]

Alternatively, if one can correctly model how the treatment and the covariates are related to the response variable, unbiased estimates of an average treatment effect can be computed, even if the propensity score model is misspecified. One must meet a different set of the first and second order conditions. In short, getting *either* estimation exercise right leads to an unbiased estimate of the ATE (Scharfstein et al., 1994; Tchetgen Tchetgen et al., 2010). One has "double robustness."

An important concern for double robustness is the functional forms assumed. Linear relationships between the outcome variable and all of the included predictors is the standard supposition. Linearity also is the standard supposition for relationships between the treatment indicator and the other predictors.[31] Can one do better? Maybe. Some recent work suggests that machine learning can help (Chernozhukov et al. 2017). In effect, one unpacks the automatic, residualizing steps in linear regression and allows machine learning to find nonlinear relationships if they exist.

One begins in Equations 6.12 and 6.13 by removing systematic associations between T and $\mathbf{X}$. Ideally, all systematic variation – whether linear or nonlinear – is eliminated. Likewise, in a second operation shown in Equations 6.14 and 6.15, one removes systematic associations between Y and $\mathbf{X}$. How complete both residualizations are depends on $g(\mathbf{X})$ and $h(\mathbf{X})$. Both functions can be estimated with a form of statistical learning that can capture nonlinear associations. Stochastic gradient boosting is well suited for this task.

The result is two sets of residuals: ζ_i as the residualized T and υ_i as the residualized Y. One cannot prove that in either case all sources of confounding are gone, but the nonlinear approximations of $g(\mathbf{X})$ and $h(\mathbf{X})$ should do better than linear approximations, or at least not worse.

$$T_i = g(\mathbf{X}_i) + \zeta_i \tag{6.12}$$

$$\zeta_i = T_i - g(\mathbf{X}_i) \tag{6.13}$$

$$Y_i = h(\mathbf{X}_i) + \upsilon_i \tag{6.14}$$

$$\upsilon_i = Y_i - h(\mathbf{X})_i \tag{6.15}$$

Using Equation 6.16, it a simple matter to regress υ_i on ζ_i, where β_1 is the estimated average treatment effect, and ξ_i is another disturbance term. One can also directly compute the difference between means $\bar{\upsilon}$ and $\bar{\zeta}$.

$$\upsilon_i = \beta_0 + \beta_1 \zeta_i + \xi_i \tag{6.16}$$

Estimates $\hat{g}(\mathbf{X})$ and $\hat{h}(\mathbf{X})$ obtained from data are best seen as approximations of the true population functionals. One hopes that the asymptotic bias in $\hat{\beta}_1$ is small or at least smaller than the bias when linear relationships are assumed.

Just as in so much of statistical learning, statistical inference is challenging because of data snooping built into procedures like stochastic gradient boosting. We have discussed the problem extensively in past chapters. Once again, one can rely on test data. Equations 6.12 and 6.14 are implemented with the training data subject to data snooping. Equations 6.13, 6.15, and 6.16 are implemented with test data, which are not tainted from the fitting process in Equations 6.12 and 6.14. Asymptotic statistical inference using the bootstrap or sandwich standard errors properly can follow. One has an asymptotically unbiased estimate of the ATE, but only for a population *approximation*.

As in earlier chapters, the training data and fitted boosting structure are treated as fixed. One is not considering uncertainty that would result from initiating the study again using new training data from which a new fitted boosting structure would be constructed. One might think that wrapping the entire procedure in a bootstrap would save the day. However, data snooping internal to the algorithm likely would jeopardize the entire enterprise.

Another major weakness of this approach is that splitting the data into a training sample and a test sample reduces the number of observations for each compared to the full dataset. A clever solution, at least for Equation 6.16, is to reuse the data. In a first pass through the data, the training data are used for fitting, and the test data are used to construct the residuals. In a second pass through the data, the roles are reversed. The test data are used for fitting, and the training data are used to construct the residuals.

One now has two vectors for ζ and two vectors for υ. Each pair can be concatenated so that one has the full number of observations for each. The two vectors that result are then used in Equation 6.16. Estimation and statistical inference follows as before, but with a much larger number of observations. The downside is that each fitting exercise is still undertaken with each of the two sample splits. The upside is that with a sufficiently large number of observations, the fitting process will work well nevertheless. A few hundred observations for each split will often be adequate.

One might wonder what legitimately can be learned about an ATE from an acknowledged approximation. For example, how should one proceed when the null hypothesis that the ATE = 0 is rejected? For observational studies, biased causal effect estimates are ubiquitous. One is almost always working with approximations. The introduction of statistical learning into the doubly robust form of analysis, arguably is a way to obtain better approximations, but all of the usual interpretive challenges remain. Yet, when randomized experiments are not an option, strong observational studies are probably the best one can do (Rosenbaum 2010: chapter 1).

6.10   Summary and Conclusions

Boosting is a very rich approach to statistical learning. The underlying concepts are interesting and the use to date creative. Boosting has also stimulated very productive interactions among researchers in statistics, applied mathematics, and computer science. Perhaps most important, boosting has been shown to be very effective for many kinds of data analysis.

However, there are important limitations to keep in mind. First, boosting is designed to improve the performance of weak learners. Trying to boost learners that are already strong is not likely to be productive. Whether a set of learners is weak or strong is a judgment call that will vary over academic disciplines and policy areas. If the list of variables includes all the predictors known to be important, if these predictors are well measured, and if the functional forms with the response variables are largely understood, conventional regression will then perform well and provide outputs that are much easier to interpret.

Second, if the goal is to fit conditional probabilities, boosting can be a risky way to proceed. There is an inherent tension between reasonable estimates of conditional probabilities and classification accuracy. Classification with the greatest margins is likely to be coupled with estimated conditional probabilities that are pushed toward the bounds of 0 or 1.

Third, boosting is not alchemy. Boosting can improve the performance of many weak learners, but the improvements may fall far short of the performance needed. Boosting cannot overcome variables that are measured poorly or important predictors that have been overlooked. The moral is that (even) boosting cannot overcome a seriously flawed measurement and badly executed data collection. The same applies to all of the statistical learning procedures discussed in this book.

Finally, when compared to other statistical learning procedures, especially random forests, boosting will allow for a much wider range of applications, and for the same kinds of applications, perform competitively. In addition, its clear links to common and well-understood statistical procedures can help make boosting understandable.

Exercises

Problem Set 1

Generate the following data. The systematic component of the response variable is quadratic.

```
x1=rnorm(1000)
x12=x1^2
ysys=1+(-5*x12)
y=ysys+(5*rnorm(1000))
dta=data.frame(y,x1,x12)
```

1. Plot the systematic part of y against the predictor $x1$. Smooth it using *scatter.smooth*. The smooth can be a useful approximation of the $f(x)$ you are trying to recover. Plot y against $x1$. This represents the data to be analyzed. Why do they look different?
2. Apply *gbm* to the data. There are a lot of tuning parameters and parameters that need to be set for later output so, here is some bare-bones code to get you started. But feel free to experiment. For example,

```
out<-gbm(y~x1,distribution="gaussian",n.trees=10000,
    data=dta)
gbm.perf(out,method="OOB").
```

   Construct the partial dependence plot using

```
plot(out,n.trees=???),
```

   where the ??? is the number of trees, which is the same as the number of iterations. Make five plots, one each of the following number of iterations: 100, 500, 1000, 5000, 10,000 and the number recommended by the out-of-bag method in the second step above. Study the sequence of plots and compare them to the plot of the true $f(X)$. What happens to the plots as the number of iterations approaches the recommended number and beyond? Why does this happen?
3. Repeat the analysis with the interaction.depth=3 (or larger). What in the performance of the procedure has changed? What has not changed (or at least not changed much)? Explain what you think is going on. (Along with n.trees, interaction.depth can make an important difference in performance. Otherwise, the defaults usually seem adequate.)

Problem Set 2

From the *car* library load the data "Leinhardt." Analyze the data using *gbm*. The response variable is infant mortality.

1. Plot the performance of *gbm*. What is the recommended number of iterations?

2. Construct a graph of the importance of the predictors. Which variables seem to affect the fit substantially and which do not? Make sure your interpretations take the units of importance into account.
3. Construct the partial dependence plot for each predictor. Interpret each plot.
4. Construct all of the two-variable plots. Interpret each plot. Look for interaction effects. (There are examples in the *gbm* documentation that can be accessed with *help*.)
5. Construct the three-variable plot. (There are examples in the *gbm* documentation that can be accessed with *help*.) Interpret the plot.
6. Consider the quality of the fit. How large is the improvement compared to when no predictors are used? You will need to compute measures of fit. There is none in *gbm.object*.
7. Write a paragraph or so, on what the analysis of these data has revealed about correlates of infant mortality at a national level.
8. Repeat the analysis using random forests. How do the results compare to the results from stochastic gradient boosting? Would you have arrived at substantially different conclusions depending on whether you used random forests or stochastic gradient boosting?
9. Repeat the analysis using the quantile loss function. Try values for α of 0.25, 0.50, and 0.75, which represent different relative costs for underestimates compared to overestimates. How do the results differ in the number of iterations, variable importance, partial dependence plots, and fit? How do the results compare to your early analysis using stochastic gradient boosting?

Problem Set 3

The point of this problem set is to compare the performance of several different procedures when the outcome is binary and decide which work better and which work worse for the data being analyzed. You also need to think about why the performance can differ and what general lessons there may be.

From the *MASS* library, analyze the dataset called Pima.tr. The outcome is binary: diabetes or not (coded as "Yes" and "No" for the variable "type"). Assume that the costs of failing to identify someone who has diabetes are three times higher than the costs of falsely identifying someone who has diabetes. The predictors are all of the other variables in the dataset.

The statistical procedures to compare are logistic regression, the generalized additive model, random forests, and stochastic gradient boosting. For each, you will need to determine how to introduce asymmetric costs. (Hint: for some you will need to weight the data by outcome class.) You will also need to take into account the data format each procedure is expecting (e.g., can missing data be tolerated?). Also feel free to try several different versions of each procedure (e.g., "AdaBoost" v. "Bernoulli" for stochastic gradient boosting). The intent is to work across material from several earlier chapters.

1. Construct confusion tables for each model. Be alert to whether the fitted values are for "resubstituted" data or not. Do some procedures fit the data better than others? Why or why not?
2. Cross-tabulate the fitted values for each model against the fitted values for each other model. How do the sets of fitted values compare?
3. Compare the "importance" assigned to each predictor. This is tricky. The units and computational methods differ. For example, how can sensible comparisons be made between the output of a logistic regression and the output of random forests?
4. Compare partial response functions. This too is tricky. For example, what can you do with logistic regression?
5. If you had to make a choice to use one of these procedures, which would you select? Why?

Endnotes

[1] Even though the response is binary, it is treated as a numeric. The reason will be clear later.

[2] A more general definition is provided by Schapire and his colleagues (1998: 1697). A wonderfully rich and more recent discussion about the central role of margins in boosting can be found in Schapire and Freund (2012). The book is a remarkable mix from a computer science perspective of the formal mathematics and very accessible discussions of what the mathematics means.

[3] In computer science parlance, an "example" is an observation or case.

[4] The response is represented by y_i because it is a numeric residual regardless of whether the original response was numeric or categorical. Categorical response variables are coded as a numeric 1 or 0 so that arithmetic operators can be applied.

[5] Θ here does not represent random integers used in random forests.

[6] Naming conventions get a little confusing at this point. Formally, a gradient is a set (vector) of partial derivatives. But it also is common to speak of those partial derivatives as gradients.

[7] The response variable is no longer shown because it does not change in the minimization process.

[8] For very large datasets, there is a scalable version of tree boosting called *XGBoost* (Chen and Guestrin 2016) that can provide noticeable speed improvements but has yet to include the range of useful loss functions found in *gbm*. There is also the need to configure the data in particular ways that differ from data frames. But for large datasets, it is worth the trouble. More will be said about *XGBoost* when "deep learning" is briefly considered in Chap. 8.

[9] Other initializations such as least squares regression could be used, depending on loss function (e.g., for a quantitative response variable).

[10] The original gbm was written by Greg Ridgeway. The current and substantially revised gbm is written by Brandon Greenwell, Bradley Boehmke, and Jay Cunningham, who build on Ridgeway's original code.

[11] For gbm, the data not selected for each tree are called "out-of-bag" data although that is not fully consistent with the usual definition because in *gbm* the sampling is without replacement.

[12] The partial dependence plots as part of *gbm* work well. One can also use the partial dependence plots in the library *pdp*, written by Brandon Greenwell, that come with more options.

[13] A useful indication of whether there are too many passes through the data is if the distribution of the fitted proportions/probabilities starts to look bimodal. There is no formal reason why a bimodal distribution is necessarily problematic, but with large trees, the distribution should not

be terribly lumpy. A lumpy distribution is far less of a potential problem if there is no interest in interpreting the fitted proportions/probabilities.

[14]The *caret* library is written by Max Kuhn. There are also procedures to automate *gbm* tuning, but like all automated tuning, subject-matter expertise plays no role. Considerable caution is warranted.

[15]The R procedure *XGBoost* allows for categorical response variables with more than two categories. Weighting can still be used to tune the results. Usually, more trial and error is required than for the binary case.

[16]Because *gbm* depends on regression trees even for binary outcome variables, outcome variables need to be numeric.

[17]For these analyses, the work was done on an iMac with a single core. The processor was a 3.4 Ghz Intel Core i7.

[18]If forecasting were on the table, it might have been useful to try a much larger number of iterations to reduce estimates of out-of-sample error.

[19]The plots are shown just as *gbm* builds them, and there are very few options provided. But just as with random forests, the underlying data can be stored and then used to construct new plots more responsive to the preferences of data analysts. One also has the prospect of doing the plotting in *pdp*.

[20]Because both inputs are integers, the transition from one value to the next is the midpoint between the two.

[21]It is not appropriate to compare the overall error rate in the two tables (0.18–0.21) because the errors are not weighted by costs. In Table 6.2, classification errors for those who perished are about 5 times more costly than in Table 6.1.

[22]Ideally, there would be far more data and a much more narrow 95% confidence interval. If a reader runs the code shown again, slightly different results are almost certain because of a new random split of the data. It also is possible to get an upper or lower bound outside of the 0.0–1.0 range. Negative values should be treated as values of 0.0. Positive values larger than 1.0 should be treated as values of 1.0. Valid coverage remains.

[23]Only order matters so compared to estimates of conditional means, a lot of information is discarded. Working with very high or very low quantiles can exacerbate the problem, because the data are usually less dense toward the tails.

[24]The out-of-bag approach was not available in *gbm* for boosted quantile regression.

[25]The library *pdp* constructs partial dependence plots for a variety of machine learning methods offering a wide range of useful options including access to the *ICEbox* library. *ICEbox* is written by Alex Goldstein, Adam Kapelner, and Justin Bleich, and *pdp* is written by Brandon Greenwell.

[26]The size of the correlation is being substantially determined by actual fares over $200. They are still being fit badly, but not a great deal worse.

[27] Causality is *not* a feature of the data itself. It is an interpretive overlay that depends on how the data were generated (i.e., an experiment in which the intervention is manipulated) and/or subject-matter theory (e.g, force equals mass times acceleration). Discussions about the nature of causality have a very long history. The current view, and the one taken here, is widely, if not universally, accepted. Imbens and Rubin (2015) provide an excellent and accessible treatment.

[28] *T* can also be numeric, most commonly conceptualized as a "dose" of some intervention. For purposes of this discussion, we need not consider numeric interventions.

[29]Whether in practice the intervention assigned is actually delivered is another matter that is beyond the scope of this discussion. Randomized experiments often are jeopardized when the intervention assigned is not delivered.

[30] The average treatment effect (ATE) is for a binary treatment *defined* as the difference between the response variable's mean or proportion under one study condition and the response variable's mean or proportion under the other study condition. One imagines the average outcome when all of the study subjects receive the treatment compared to the average outcome when all study subjects do not receive the treatment. A randomized experiment properly implemented provides and unbiased *estimate*. These ideas easily can be extended to cover studies with more than two study conditions.

[31] Regression diagnostics can help, but then what? You may learn that linearity is not plausible, but what functional forms are? What if the apparent nonlinearities are really caused by omitted variables not in the data?

References

Bartlett, P. L., & M. Traskin (2007). AdaBoost is Consistent. *Journal of Machine Learning Research, 8*, 23472368.

Berk, R. A., Kriegler, B., & Ylvisaker, D. (2008). Counting the homeless in Los Angeles county. In D. Nolan & S. Speed (Eds.), *Probability and statistics: Essays in honor of David A. Freedman*. Monograph series for the institute of mathematical statistics.

Bühlmann, P., & Yu, B. (2004). Discussion. *The Annals of Statistics, 32*, 96–107.

Buja, A., & Stuetzle, W. (2006). Observations on bagging. *Statistica Sinica, 16*(2), 323–352.

Buja, A., Mease, D., & Wyner, A. J. (2007). Boosting Algorithms: Regularization, Prediction and Model Fitting. *Statistical Science, 22*(4), 506–512.

Chen, T., & Guestrin, C. (2016). XGBoost: A scalable tree boosting system. arXiv:1603.02754v1 [cs.LG].

Chernozhukov, V., Chetverikov, D., Demirer, M., Esther Duflo, E., Hansen, C., & Newey, W. (2017). Double/Debiased/Neyman machine learning of treatment effects. arXiv:1701.08687v1 [stat.ML].

Freund, Y., & Schapire, R. (1996). Experiments with a new boosting algorithm. In *Machine learning: Proceedings for the thirteenth international conference* (pp. 148–156). San Francisco: Morgan Kaufmann.

Freund, Y., & Schapire, R. E. (1997). A decision-theoretic generalization of online learning and an application to boosting. *Journal of Computer and System Sciences, 55*, 119–139.

Freund, Y., & Schapire, R. E. (1999). A short introduction to boosting. *Journal of the Japanese Society for Artificial Intelligence, 14*, 771–780.

Friedman, J. H. (2001). Greedy function approximation: A gradient boosting machine. *The Annals of Statistics, 29*, 1189–1232

Friedman, J. H. (2002). Stochastic gradient boosting. *Computational Statistics and Data Analysis, 38*, 367–378.

Friedman, J. H., Hastie, T., & Tibshirani, R. (2000). Additive logistic regression: A statistical view of boosting (with discussion). *Annals of Statistics, 28*, 337–407.

Friedman, J. H., Hastie, T., Rosset S., Tibshirani, R., & Zhu, J. (2004). Discussion of boosting papers. *Annals of Statistics, 32*, 102–107.

Hastie, T., Tibshirani, R., & Friedman, J. (2009). *The elements of statistical learning* (2nd edn.). New York: Springer.

Imbens, G., & Rubin, D. B. (2015) *Causal inference for statistics, social, and biomedical sciences: An introduction*. Cambridge: Cambridge University.

Jiang, W. (2004). Process consistency for AdaBoost. *Annals of Statistics, 32*, 13–29.

Mease, D., & Wyner, A. J. (2008). Evidence contrary to the statistical view of boosting (with discussion). *Journal of Machine Learning, 9*, 1–26.

Mease, D., Wyner, A. J., & Buja, A. (2007). Boosted classification trees and class Probability/Quantile estimation. *Journal of Machine Learning, 8*, 409–439.

Ridgeway, G. (1999). The state of boosting. *Computing Science and Statistics, 31*, 172–181.

Ridgeway, G. (2012). Generalized boosted models: A guide to the gbm Package. Available at from *gbm* documentation in R.

Rosenbaum, P. R. (2010). *Design of observational studies*. New York: Springer.

Rosenbaum, P. R., & Rubin, D. B. (1983). The central role of the propensity score in observational studies for causal effects. *Biometrika, 70*(1), 41–55.

Schapire, R. E. (1999). A brief introduction to boosting. In *Proceedings of the sixteenth international joint conference on artificial intelligence.*

Schapire, R. E., & Freund, Y. (2012) *Boosting.* Cambridge: MIT Press.

Schapire, R. E., Freund, Y., Bartlett, P, & Lee, W.-S. (1998). Boosting the margin: A new explanation for the effectiveness of voting methods. *The Annals of Statistics, 26*(5), 1651–1686.

Scharfstein, D.O. Rotnitzky, A. and J.M. Robins (1994) "Adjusting for Non-Ignorable Drop-Out Using Semipara-Metric Non-Response Models." *Journal of the American Statistical Association* 94:1096–1120.

Tchetgen Tchetgen, E. J., Robins, J. M., & Rotnitzky, A. (2010). On doubly robust estimation in a semiparametric odds ratio model. *Biometrika, 97*(1), 171–180.

Wyner, A. J., Olson, M., Bleich, J, & Mease, D. (2017). Explaining the success of AdaBoost and random forests as interpolating classifiers. *Journal of Machine Learning Research, 18*, 1–33.

Zhang, T., & Yu, B. (2005). Boosting with early stopping: Convergence and consistency. *Annals of Statistics, 33*(4), 1538–1579.

Chapter 7
Support Vector Machines

Summary Support vector machines perhaps has the best mathematical pedigree of any statistical learning procedure. It was originally developed as a classifier that maximizes a somewhat different definition of a margin, which leads to a novel "hinge" loss function. Also distinctive is the use of kernels in place of the usual design matrix. The kernels allow for very complicated linear basis expansions derived from the full set of predictors. Support vector machines competes well with other statistical learning classifiers, but because kernels are $N \times N$, support vector machines does not scale well. That can be a major problem in the era of big data.

7.1 Introduction

Support vector machines (SVM) was developed as a type of classifier, largely in computer science, with its own set of research questions, conceptual frameworks, technical language, and culture. A substantial amount of the initial interest in support vector machines stemmed from the important theoretical work surrounding it (Vapnick 1996). For many, that remains very attractive.

The early applications of SVM were not especially compelling. But, over the past decade, the applications to which support vector machines have been applied have broadened (Christianini and Shawe-Taylor 2000; Moguerza and Munõz 2006; Ma and Gao 2014), available software has responded (Joachims 1998; Chen et al. 2004; Hsu et al. 2010; Karatzoglou et al. 2015), and relationships between support vector machines and other forms of statistical learning have become better understood (Bishop 2006: chapters 6 and 7; Hastie et al. 2009: 417–437). SVM has joined a mainstream of many machine/statistical learning procedures. It incorporates some unique features to be sure, but many familiar features as well. In practice, SVM can be seen as a worthy classification competitor to random forests and stochastic gradient boosting.

© Springer Nature Switzerland AG 2020

R. A. Berk, *Statistical Learning from a Regression Perspective*,
Springer Texts in Statistics, https://doi.org/10.1007/978-3-030-40189-4_7

This chapter will draw heavily on material covered in earlier chapters. In particular, regression kernels, discussed in Chap. 2, will make an important encore appearance. Much of the earlier material addressing why boosting works so well also will carry over, at least in broad brush strokes. Support vector machines (SVM) can be understood in part as a special kind of margin maximizer and in part as a loss function optimizer with an unusual loss function.

Different expositions of support vector machines often use rather different notation. In particular, the notational practices of computer science and statistics rarely correspond. For example, the excellent treatment of support vector machines by Bishop (2006: Chapter 7) and the equally excellent treatment of support vector machines by Hastie et al. (2009: Chapter 12) are difficult to compare without first being able to map one notional scheme on to the other. In this chapter, the notation of Hastie and colleagues will be used, by and large, because it corresponds better to the notation employed in earlier chapters.

7.2 Support Vector Machines in Pictures

Support vector machines has more demanding mathematical underpinnings than boosting or random forests. In some ways, it is another form of penalized regression. But before we get to a technical discussion, let us take a look at several figures that will make the key ideas accessible.

7.2.1 The Support Vector Classifier

Suppose there is a binary response variable coded, as is often done in boosting, as 1 and -1. There is also a $f(x)$, where x is a vector of one or more predictors. The function can be written in a familiar linear manner using vector notation as

$$f(x) = \beta_0 + x^T \beta. \tag{7.1}$$

Equation 7.1 is essentially a linear regression with a binary outcome of 1 or -1 and no restrictions in practice on what numeric values the function yields. The $f(x)$ might be 0.6 for one observation, -1.2 for another observation, 2.1 for another observation, and so on. We are *not* fitting logits, proportions, or probabilities. This is a fundamental difference compared to, say, logistic regression.

How are classes assigned? If $f(x)$ is a positive number, the label 1 is assigned to an observation. If $f(x)$ is a negative number, the label -1 is assigned to an observation. One can then compare the 1s and -1s from the function to the 1s and -1s of the response variable. The problem to be tackled in the pages ahead is how to make the two sets of 1s and -1s correspond as much as possible, not just in the data on hand, but in new realizations of the data. The task is to produce accurate

Fig. 7.1 A support vector
classifier with two predictors
X and Z and two linearly
separable classes shown as
red or blue

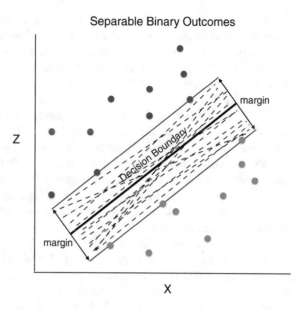

classifications, which has been a major theme of past chapters. But the way SVM
goes about this is novel. We begin with the support vector classifier.[1]

Figure 7.1 shows a three-dimensional scatter plot much like those used in earlier
chapters. As before, there are two predictors (X and Z) and a binary response that
can take on values of red or blue. Red might represent dropping out of school,
and blue might represent graduating. (Blue could be coded as 1, and red could be
coded as -1.) The two predictors might be reading grade level and the number of
truancies per semester. In this figure, the blue circles and red circles are each located
in quite different parts of the two-dimensional space defined by the predictors. In
fact, there is substantial daylight between the two groups, and a linear decision
boundary easily could be drawn to produce perfect homogeneity. In SVM language,
a linear separating hyperplane could be drawn to produce separation between the
two classes. More such SVM language will be introduced as we proceed.

In Fig. 7.1, there is a limitless number of linear decision boundaries producing
separation. These are represented by the dashed lines in Fig. 7.1. Ideally, there is a
way to find the best linear decision boundary.

Enter the support vector classifier. When there is separation, the support vector
classifier solves the problem of which line to overlay by constructing two parallel
lines on either side of, and the same distance from, the decision boundary. The two
lines are placed as far apart as possible without including any observations within
the space between them. One can think of the two lines as fences defining a buffer
zone. In other words, the support vector classifier seeks two parallel fences that
maximize their perpendicular distance from the decision boundary. There can be
only one such straight line parallel to the fences and midway between them. That
decision boundary is shown with the solid black line.

Observations can fall right on either fence but not on their wrong sides. Here, there are no blue circles below the upper fence and no red circles above the lower fence. Observations that fall on top of the fences are called "support vectors" because they directly determine where the fences will be located and hence, the optimal decision boundary. In Fig. 7.1, there are two blue support vectors and three red support vectors.

In Fig. 7.1, the total width of the buffer zone is shown with the two double-headed arrows. The distance between the decision boundary and either fence is called the "margin," although some define the margin as the distance between the two fences (which amounts to the same thing). The wider the margin, the greater the separation between the two classes. Although formally, the margin for a support vector classifier differs from the margins used by boosting and random forests, larger margins remain desirable because generalization error usually will be smaller. The separation is more definitive.

Classification follows directly. Cases that fall on one side of the decision boundary are labeled as one class. Cases that fall on the other side of the decision boundary are labeled as the other class. Subsequently, any new cases for which the outcome class is not known will be assigned the class determined by the side of the decision boundary on which they fall. And that location will be a function of X and Z. The classification rule that follows from the decision boundary is called "hard thresholding," and the decision boundary is often called the "separating hyperplane." Sometimes the two fences are called the "margin boundary."

The data shown in Fig. 7.1 are very cooperative, and such cooperation is in practice rare. Figure 7.2 shows a plot that is much like Fig. 7.1, but the two sets of values are no longer linearly separable. Three blue circles and the two red circles

Fig. 7.2 A support vector classifier with predictors X and Z when there are two classes that are not linearly separable

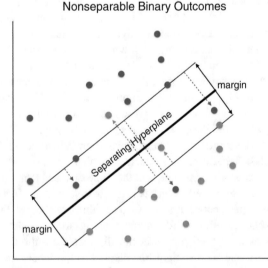

violate their margin boundaries. They are on the wrong side of their respective buffer zone fences with each distance represented by an arrow. Moreover, there is no way to relocate and/or narrow the buffer zone so that there is a linear separating hyperplane able to partition the space into two perfectly homogeneous regions. There is no longer any linear solution to the classification problem.

One possible response is to permit violations of the buffer zone. One can specify some number of the observations that would be allowed to fall on the wrong side of their margin boundary. These are called "slack variables." One can try to live with a result that looks a lot like Fig. 7.2. The idea might be to maximize the width of the buffer zone conditional on the slack variables.

But that is not quite enough. Some slack variables fall just across their margin boundary, and some fall far away. In response, the distance between the relevant fence and the location of the slack variable can be taken into account. The sum of such distances can be viewed as a measure of how permissive one has been when the margin is maximized. If one is more permissive by allowing for a larger sum, it may be possible to locate a linear, separating hyperplane within a larger margin. Again, larger margins are good. More stable classifications can follow. But more permissive solutions imply more bias because misclassifications will be introduced. A form of the bias–variance tradeoff reappears. It follows that the sum of the distances can be a tuning parameter when a support vector classifier is applied to data. Fitting the support vector classifier with slack variables is sometimes called "soft thresholding."

7.2.2 Support Vector Machines

There is a complementary solution to classification problems when the classes are not linearly separable. One can allow for a nonlinear decision boundary in the existing predictor space by fitting a separating hyperplane in higher dimensions. We introduced this idea in Chap. 1 when linear basis expansions were discussed, and we elaborated on it in Chap. 2 when regression kernels were considered in some depth. Support vector classifiers become support vector machines when a kernel replaces a conventional set of predictors. However, the use of kernels is not straightforward. As already noted, there can be several kernel candidates with no formal guidance on which one to choose. In addition, kernels come with tuning parameters whose values usually have to be determined empirically. Finally, recall that kernel results are scale dependent (and normalizing papers over the problem) with categorical predictors a major complication.

In summary, support vector machines estimates the coefficients in Eq. 7.1 by finding a separating hyperplane producing the maximum margin, subject to a constraint on the sum of the slack variable distances. With those estimates in hand, fitted values are produced. Positive fitted values are assigned a class of 1, and negative fitted values are assigned a class of -1.

7.3   Support Vector Machines More Formally

With the main conceptual foundations of support vector machines addressed, we turn briefly to a somewhat more formal approach. To read the literature about support vector machines, some familiarity for the underlying mathematics and notation is important. What follows draws heavily on Hastie et al. (2009: 417–438) and on Bishop (2006: Chapters 6 and 7).

7.3.1   The Support Vector Classifier Again: The Separable Case

There are N observations in the training data. Each observation has a value for each of p predictors and a value for the response. A response is coded 1 or -1. The separating hyperplane is defined by a conventional linear combination of a vector of predictors as

$$f(x) = \beta_0 + x^T \beta = 0. \tag{7.2}$$

Notice that the value of 0 is half way between -1 and 1. If you know the sign of $f(x)$, you know the class assigned. That is, classification is then undertaken by the following rule:

$$G(x) = \text{sign}(\beta_0 + x^T \beta). \tag{7.3}$$

A lot of information can be extracted from the two equations. One can determine for any i whether $y_i f(x_i) > 0$ and, therefore, whether it is correctly classified.[2] $\beta_0 + x^T \beta$ can be used to compute the signed distance of any fitted point in the predictor space from the separating hyperplane. Hence, one can determine whether a fitted point is on the wrong side of its fence and if so, how far.

For the separable case, the trick is to find values β and β_0, to maximize the margin. Let M be the distance from the separating hyperplane to the margin boundary. The goal is

$$\max_{\beta, \beta_0, \|\beta\|=1} M, \tag{7.4}$$

subject to

$$y_i(\beta_0 + x_i^T \beta) \geq M, \quad i = 1, \ldots, N, \tag{7.5}$$

where for mathematical convenience the regression coefficients are standardized to have a unit length.[3] In words, our job is to find values for β and β_0 so that M is as large as possible for observations that are correctly classified. Some define the margin as $2M$.

The left-hand side of Eq. 7.5 in parentheses is the distance between the separating hyperplane and a fitted point. Because M is a distance centered on the separating hyperplane, Eq. 7.5 identifies correctly classified observations on or beyond their margin boundary. No cases are inside their fences. Thus, M is sometimes characterized as producing a "hard boundary" because it is statistically impermeable. That is basically the whole story for the support vector classifier when the outcomes are linearly separable.

It can be mathematically easier, if less intuitive, to work with an equivalent formulation:[4]

$$\min_{\beta,\beta_0} \|\beta\| \tag{7.6}$$

subject to

$$y_i(\beta_0 + x_i^T \beta) \geq 1, \quad i = 1, \ldots, N. \tag{7.7}$$

Because $M = 1/\|\beta\|$, Eqs. 7.6 and 7.7 now seek to *minimize the norm* of the coefficients through a proper choice of the coefficient values (Hastie et al. 2009: section 4.5.2). Equation 7.7 defines a linear constraint and requires that the points closest to the separating hyperplane are at a distance of 1.0, and that all other observations are farther away (i.e., distance >1). Equations 7.6 and 7.7 do not change the underlying optimization problem and lead to a more direct, easily understood solution (Bishop 2006: 327–328).

7.3.2 The Nonseparable Case

We return for the moment to Eqs. 7.4 and 7.5, but for the nonseparable case, some encroachments of the buffer zone have to be tolerated. Suppose one defines a set of "slack" variables $\xi = (\xi_1, \xi_2, \ldots, \xi_N)$, $\xi_i \geq 0$, that measure how far observations are on the wrong side of their fence. We let $\xi_i = 0$ for observations that are on the proper side of their fence or right on top of it; they are correctly classified and not in the buffer zone. The farther an observation moves across its fence into or through the buffer zone, the larger is the value of the slack variable.

The slack variables lead to a revision of Eq. 7.5 so that for case i

$$y_i(\beta_0 + x_i^T \beta) \geq M(1 - \xi_i) \tag{7.8}$$

for all $\xi_i \geq 0$, and $\sum_{i=1}^{N} \xi_i \leq W$, with W as some constant quantifying how tolerant of misclassifications one is prepared to be.

The right-hand side of Eq. 7.8 equals M when an observation falls on top of its margin. For observations that fall on the wrong side of their margin, ξ_i is positive. As the value of ξ_i becomes larger, the margin-based threshold becomes smaller and more lenient as long as the sum of the ξ_i is less than W (Bishop 2006: 331–332). Equation 7.8 changes a hard thresholding as a function M into a soft thresholding as a function of $M(1 - \xi_i)$. The fence is no longer statistically impermeable.

There is again an equivalent and more mathematically convenient formulation, much like the one provided earlier as Eqs. 7.6 and 7.7 (Hastie et al. 2009: 373):

$$\min_{\beta, \beta_0} \|\beta\| \qquad (7.9)$$

subject to

$$y_i(\beta_0 + x_i^T \beta) \geq 1 - \xi_i, \quad i = 1, \dots, N, \qquad (7.10)$$

for all $\xi_i \geq 0$, and $\sum_{i=1}^{N} \xi_i \leq W$, with W as some constant. As before the goal is to minimize the norm of the coefficients but with special allowances for slack variables. For larger ξ_i's, the linear constraint is more lenient. Once again, there is soft thresholding. In expositions from computer science traditions, Eqs. 7.9 and 7.10 sometimes are considered "canonical."

Figure 7.3 is a small revision of Fig. 7.2 showing some important mathematical expressions. Observations for which $\xi_i > 1$ lie on the wrong side of the separating hyperplane and are misclassified. Observations for which $0 < \xi_i \leq 1$ lie in the buffer zone but on the correct side of the separating hyperplane. Observations for which $\xi_i = 0$ are correctly classified and on the margin boundary. The circles with borders are support vectors.

Equations 7.9 and 7.10 constitute a quadratic function with linear constraints whose quadratic programming solution can be found using Lagrange multipliers (Hastie et al. 2009: section 12.2.1). Figure 7.4 shows a toy example in which there

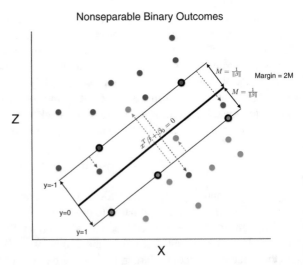

Fig. 7.3 A support vector classifier with some important mathematical expressions for predictors X and Z when there are two classes that are not separable (support vectors are circled.)

Fig. 7.4 Finding the minimum of a quadratic function with a linear constraint

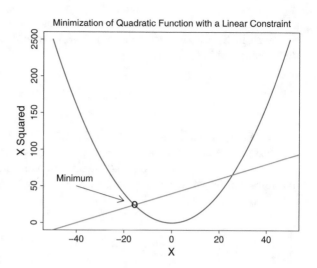

is single variable (i.e., x), a quadratic function of that variable in blue, and a linear constraint in red. The minimum when the constraint is imposed is larger than the minimum when the linear constraint is not imposed. The quadratic programming challenge presented by the support vector classifier is that the single x is replaced by the coefficients in Eq. 7.9, and the simple linear constraint is replaced by the N linear constraints in Eq. 7.10.

In the notation of Hastie et al. (2009: 421), the solution has

$$\hat{\beta} = \sum_{i=1}^{N} \hat{\alpha}_i y_i x_i, \tag{7.11}$$

where $\hat{\alpha}_i$ represents a new coefficient for each i whose value needs to be estimated from the data. All of the N values for $\hat{\alpha}_i$ are equal to 0 except for the support vectors that locate the separating hyperplane. The value of $\hat{\beta}_0$ is estimated separately. With all of the coefficients in hand, classification is undertaken with Eq. 7.3: $\hat{G}(x) = \text{sign}(\hat{\beta}_0 + x^T \hat{\beta})$.

7.3.3 Support Vector Machines

We now turn from the support vector classifier to the support vector machine. The transition is relatively simple because support vector machines is essentially a support vector classifier that uses kernels as predictors. Kernels were considered at some length in Chap. 2 and will not be reconsidered here. But as we proceed, it is important to recall that (1) the choice of kernel is largely a matter of craft lore and can make a big difference, (2) factors are formally not appropriate when kernels are constructed, and (3) there can be several important tuning parameters.

The Lagrangian is defined as before except that in place of the predictors contained in **X**, support vector machines works with their linear basis expansions $\Phi(\mathbf{X})$ contained in **K**. The result is

$$\hat{f}(x) = \hat{\beta}_0 + \sum_{i=1}^{N} \hat{\alpha}_i y_i K(x, x_i), \tag{7.12}$$

where $K(x, x_i)$ is the kernel (Hastie et al. 2009: 424; Bishop 2006: 329). All else follows in the same manner as for support vector classifiers.

For $f(x) = h(x)^T \beta + \beta_0$, the optimization undertaken for support vector machines can be written in regularized regression-like form (Hastie et al. 2009: 426; Bishop 2006: 293):

$$\min_{\beta_0, \beta} \sum_{i=1}^{N} [1 - y_i f(x_i)]_+ + \frac{\lambda}{2} \|\beta\|^2, \tag{7.13}$$

where the + next to the right bracket indicates that only the positive values are used. The product $y_i f(x_i)$ is negative when there is a misclassification. Therefore, the term in brackets is positive unless a case is classified correctly and is on the correct side of its fence. The term in brackets is also linear in $y_i f(x_i)$ before becoming 0.0 for values that are not positive. $\|\beta\|^2$ is the squared norm of the regression coefficients, and λ determines how much weight is given to the sum of the slack variables. This is much like the way ridge regression penalizes a fit. A smaller value of λ makes the sum of slack variables less important and moves the optimization closer to the separable case. There will be a smaller margin, but the separating hyperplane can be more complex (Bishop 2006: 332).[5]

Equation 7.13 naturally raises questions about the loss function for support vector machines (Hastie et al. 2009: section 12.3.2; Bishop 2006: 337–338). Figure 7.5 shows with a blue line the "hinge" SVM loss function. The broken magenta line is a binomial deviance loss of the sort used for logistic regression. The binomial deviance has been rescaled to facilitate a comparison.

Some refer to the support vector loss function as a "hockey stick." The thick vertical line in red represents the separating hyperplane. Values of $yf(x)$ to the left indicate observations that are misclassified. Values of $yf(x)$ to the right indicate observations that are properly classified. The product of y and $f(x)$ will be ≥ 1 if a correctly classified observation is on the proper side of its fence.

Consider the region defined by $yf(x) < 1$. Moving from left to right, both loss functions decline. At $yf(x) = 0$, the hinge loss is equal to 1.0, and an observation is a support vector. Moving toward $yf(x) = 1$, both loss functions continue to decline. The hinge loss is equal to 0 at $yf(x) = 1$. The binomial deviance is greater than 0. For $yf(x) > 1$, the hinge loss remains 0, but the binomial deviance continues to decline, with values greater than 0.

One can argue that the two loss functions are not dramatically different. Both can be seen as an approximation of misclassification error. The misclassification

Fig. 7.5 Binomial and hinge loss as a function of the product of the true values and the fitted values

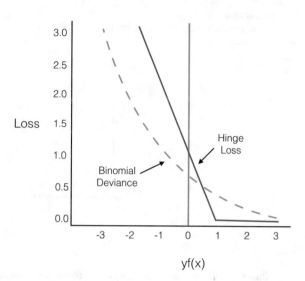

loss function would be a step function equal to 1.0 to the left $yf(x) = 0$ and equal to 0.0 at or to the right of $yf(x) = 0$. It is not clear in general when the hinge loss or the binomial deviance should be preferred although it would seem that the hinge loss would be somewhat less affected by outliers.

7.3.4 SVM for Regression

Support vector machines can be altered to apply to quantitative response variables. One common approach is to ignore in the fitting process residuals smaller in absolute value than some constant (called ϵ-insensitive regression). For the other residuals, a linear loss function is applied. Figure 7.6 provides an illustration.

The result is a robustified kind of regression. Any relative advantage in practice from support vector machine regression compared to any of several forms of robust regression is not clear, especially with what we have called kernelized regression in the mix. But readers interested in regression applications will find what they need in the *kernlab* or *e1071* libraries.

7.3.5 Statistical Inference for Support Vector Machines

To this point, the discussion of support vector machines has been presented as a Level I problem. But a Level II analysis can be on the table. Equation 7.13 makes

Fig. 7.6 An example of an
ϵ-insensitive loss function
that ignores small residuals
and applies symmetric linear
loss to the rest

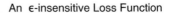

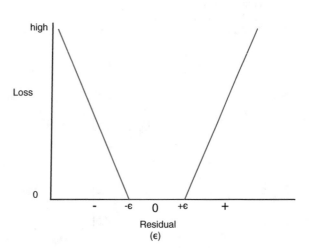

clear that support vector machines is a form of penalized regression. In particular, it is essentially kernelized ridge regression with a hinge loss function. But just as for a ridge regression, there is tuning that becomes a data snooping issue.

Therefore, the discussion of statistical inference undertaken in Chap. 2 applies. A clear and credible account of an appropriate data generation process is essential. A proper estimation target must be articulated. And then, having legitimate test data can be very important, or at least an ability to construct sufficiently large split samples. However, the results of support vector machines are sample size dependent because a kernel matrix is $N \times N$. This affects how the estimation target is defined. For example, kernels from split samples will necessarily be smaller than $N \times N$, which alters the estimation target. The estimation target is now a support vector machine for a kernel matrix based on fewer than N observations. In effect, the number of predictors in $\mathbf{K}$ is reduced. Using a split sample each with $N/2$ observations, one would have a new SVM formulation and a new SVM estimand that could be estimated with test data as usual. Whether this is a sensible approach would need to be addressed on a case-by-case basis.

7.4   A Classification Example

Support vector machines performs much like random forests and stochastic gradient boosting. However, there can be much more to tune. We undertake here a relatively simple analysis using the Mroz dataset from the *car* library in R. Getting fitted values with a more extensive set of inputs is not a problem. The problem is linking the inputs to outputs with graphical methods, as we will soon see.

The data come from a sample survey of 753 husband–wife households. The response variable is whether the wife is in the labor force. None of the categorical predictors can be used,[6] which leaves household income exclusive of the wife's income, the age of the wife, and the log of the wife's expected wage. For now, two predictors are selected: age and the log of expected wage. About 60% of the wives are employed, so the response variable is reasonably well balanced, and there seems to be nothing else in the data to make an analysis of labor force participation problematic.

'Figure 7.7 shows the code to be used. The recoding is undertaken to allow for more understandable variables and to code the response as a factor with values of 1 and −1. The numerical values make the graphical output examined later easier to interpret.

The first analysis is undertaken with a radial kernel, which has a reputation of working well in a variety of settings. There are two tuning parameters. C is the penalty parameter determining the importance of the sum of the slack variables in the Lagrangian formulation. A larger value forces the fit toward the separable solution. We use the default value of 1. The other tuning parameter is σ, which sits in the denominator of the radial kernel. We let its value be determined by an empirical procedure that "estimates the range of values for the sigma parameter which would return good results when used with a Support Vector Machine (*ksvm*). The estimation is based upon the 0.1 and 0.9 quantile of $\|x - x'\|^2$. Basically any value in between those two bounds will produce good results" (online documentation for *ksvm* in the library *kernlab*). A single measure of spread is being provided for the entire set of predictors. The squared norm is larger when cases are more dissimilar over the full set of predictors. Finally, a cross-validation measure of classification error is included to get a more honest measure of performance.

Table 7.1 shows an in-sample confusion table. There are no out-of-bag observations or test data; the table is constructed in-sample. But C was set before the analysis began, and σ was determined with very little data snooping. The proportion misclassified in the training data was 0.28, and the fivefold cross-validation figure was 0.29.[7] Because the two proportions are very similar, overfitting apparently is not an important problem for this analysis.

Table 7.1 is interpreted like all of the earlier confusion tables, although the sign of the fitted values determines the class assigned. The empirical cost ratio is little less than two (i.e., 139/72). Incorrectly classifying a wife as in the labor force is about two times more costly than incorrectly classifying a wife as not in the labor force. That cost ratio would need to be adjusted, should it be inconsistent with the preferences of stakeholders.

The results look quite good. Overall, the proportion misclassified is 0.28, although it should be cost weighted to be used properly as a performance measure. When a logistic regression was run on the same data with the same predictors, the proportion misclassified was 0.45. The large gap is an excellent example of the power of support vector machines compared to more conventional regression approaches. Classification error and prediction error also look good. For example,

```
#### SVM With Mroz Employment Data ####
library(car)
data(Mroz)
attach(Mroz)

# Recodes
Participate<-as.factor(ifelse(lfp=="yes",1,-1)) # For clarity
Age<-age
LogWage<-lwg
Income<-inc
mroz<-data.frame(Participate,Age,LogWage,Income)

### Radial kernel with defaults: kpar="automatic",type="C-svc"
library(kernlab)
svm1<-ksvm(Participate~Age+LogWage,data=mroz,kernel="rbfdot",
           cross=5)
preds1<-predict(svm1,newdata=mroz) # Fitted values
summary(preds1) # Standard output
table(mroz$Participate,preds1) # Confusion table
prop.table(table(mroz$Participate,preds1),1) # Percentage
plot(svm1,data=mroz) # Plot separating hyperplane

### ANOVA kernel
#Define Weights
wts<-table(Participate) #Connects levels to Counts
wts[1]=.47 # Replace count for -1 class
wts[2]=.53 # Replace count for 1 class

library(kernlab)
svm2<-ksvm(Participate~Age+LogWage+Income,data=mroz,
           kernel="anovadot",kpar=list(sigma=1,degree=1),
           C=5,cross=3,type="C-svc",class.weights=wts)
svm2 # Standard output
preds2<-predict(svm2,newdata=mroz) # Fitted classes
table(mroz$Participate,preds2) # Confusion table
prop.table(table(mroz$Participate,preds2),1) # Percentage
plot(svm2,data=mroz,slice=list(Income=17))# At median income
```

Fig. 7.7 R code for support vector machine analyses of labor force participation

when a wife is predicted to be in the labor force, that classification is correct about 80% of the time.

There are no variable importance plots or partial dependence plots available in *kernlab*.[8] However, one can plot the separating hyperplane for two predictors in the units of those predictors. Figure 7.8 is a contour plot showing the separating hyperplane for labor force participation in units of the fitted values. Positive fitted

Table 7.1 SVM Confusion table for forecasting labor force participation (radial kernel, default settings)

	Fitted Not labor force	Fitted Labor force	Classification error
Not labor force	253	72	0.22
Labor force	139	289	0.32
Use error	0.35	0.20	Overall error = 0.28

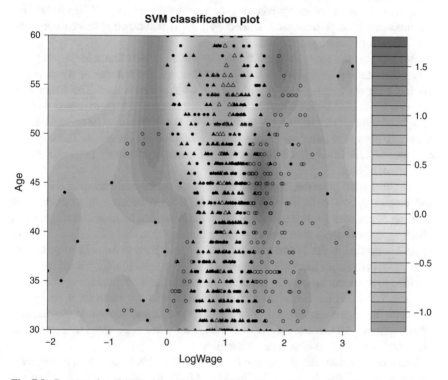

Fig. 7.8 Contour plot of SVM fitted values for labor force participation showing the separating hyperplane, observed values of the response, and support vectors (The circles are wives in the labor force. The triangles are wives not in the labor force. Filled circles or triangles are support vectors. A radial kernel with default settings was used.)

values in shades of blue mean that a wife was classified as in the labor force. Negative fitted values in shades of red mean that a wife was not classified as in the labor force. Age in years is on the vertical axis, and the log of expected wage is on the horizontal axis. Individuals in the labor force are shown with circles. Individuals not in the labor force are shown with triangles. Filled circles or triangles are support vectors.

The colors gradually shift from red to blue as the fitted values gradually shift from less than −1.0 to more than 1.5. The deeper the blue, the larger the positive fitted values. The deeper the red, the smaller the negative (i.e., more negative) fitted values. Deeper blues and deeper reds mean that an observation is farther from the separating hyperplane and more definitively classified. Consequently, the fitted values play a similar role to the vote proportions in random forests. Bigger is better because bigger implies more stability. If one were doing forecasting, the fitted value for each case could be used as a measure of the assigned class reliability.

The margin around the separating hyperplane is shown in white. Its shape and the location of the support vectors may seem strange. But recall that the separating hyperplane is estimated in a predictor space defined by a kernel. When the results are projected back into a space defined by the predictors, complicated nonlinear transformations have been applied.

But perhaps the story in Fig. 7.8 broadly makes sense. The middle pink area gets wider starting around age 50. At about that age, the number of wives not in the labor force increases over a wider range of expected wages. The larger blue areas on either side indicate that either a low expected or a high expected wage is associated with greater labor force participation. The former may be an indicator of economic need. The latter may be an indicator of good job prospects. There is little evidence of interaction effects because the pink area is effectively perpendicular to the horizontal axis.

For illustrative purposes, the same data can be reanalyzed changing the kernel and empirical cost ratio. An ANOVA kernel is used because in practice, it is often recommended for regression applications. Also, just as in stochastic gradient boosting, one can apply case weights to alter the empirical cost ratio. Here, a weight of 0.53 is applied to the 1s and a weight of 0.47 is applied to the -1s so that cases with wives in the labor force are given more relative weight. Finally, a third predictor is added to the mean function to illustrate later an interesting graphics option.

Table 7.2 shows the confusion table that results with the value for σ set to 1.0, the value for degree set to 1, the value for C set to 5.0, and household income as a third predictor. All three tuning values were determined after some trial and error using performance in confusion tables to judge.

The empirical cost ratio is now about 1 to 1 (i.e., 113/100), and classification error for being in the labor force has declined from 0.32 to 0.26. In trade, classification error for not being in the labor force has increased from 0.22 to 0.30. The overall proportion misclassified when *not weighted* by costs is effectively unchanged (i.e., 0.28). With so many alterations compared to the previous analysis, it is difficult

Table 7.2 SVM confusion table for forecasting labor force participation (ANOVA kernel, cost weighted, $\sigma = 1$, Degree $= 1, C = 5$)

	Fitted Not labor force	Fitted Labor force	Classification error
Not labor force	225	100	0.30
Labor force	113	315	0.26
Prediction error	0.33	0.24	Overall error $= 0.29$

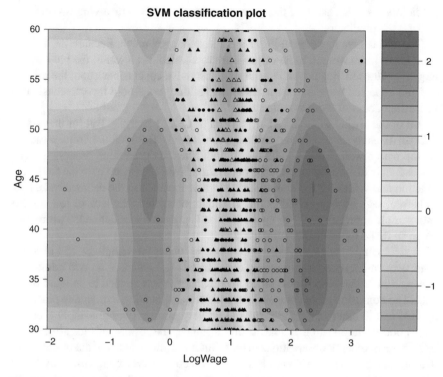

Fig. 7.9 Contour plot of SVM fitted values for labor force participation showing the separating hyperplane, observed values of the response, and support vectors (The circles are wives in the labor force. The triangles are wives not in the labor force. Filled circles or triangles are support vectors. An ANOVA kernel was used, cost weighted, with $\sigma = 1$, Degree $= 1$, $C = 5$, and household income values set to its median.)

to isolate the impact of each new feature of the analysis. However, it seems that including household income does not make a large difference.

Figure 7.9 shows the corresponding plot for the separating hyperplane. The layout is the same, but the content is different. Plots with two predictor dimensions mean that the roles of only two predictors can be displayed. Here, there are three predictors. In response, the plotting function (*ksvm.plot*) requires the predictors not displayed in the plot be set to some value. They are, in effect, held constant at that value. If any such predictors are not explicitly fixed at some value, the default has them fixed at 0.0. One can see from the last line of Fig. 7.7 that for all observations, the median of $17,000 is the assigned, fixed value.

This approach is less than ideal. It assumes that there are no interaction effects with the predictors whose values are fixed. An absence of interaction effects seems unlikely, so the issue is whether those interaction effects are large enough to matter. Perhaps the only practical way to get some sense is to examine a substantial number of plots like Fig. 7.9 with fixed values at other than the median. But even an exhaustive set of two-variable plots cannot be definitive unless there are only three predictors overall. That way, there are no interaction effects involving two or more of the fixed predictors.

The substantive message in Fig. 7.9 has not changed much. Because the 1s have been given more weight, more of them are forecasted. As a result, the blue area is larger, and the red area is smaller. But the substantive conclusions about the roles of age and expected wage are about the same. Holding household income constant at its median does not seem to matter much.

All of the results so far have been a form of Level I analysis. But for these data, a Level II analysis should be seriously considered. The data are from a sample survey with a well-defined, finite population. The data generation process is clear. A reasonable estimation target is the population SVM regression with the same loss function and values for the tuning parameters as specified in the data analysis. It is, as before, seen as an approximation. The main obstacle is the lack of test data. A split sample approach could be applied if one is prepared to redefine the estimation target so that it has a smaller sample size.

A split sample reanalysis was undertaken in which the sample of 753 observations was randomly split into nearly equal halves (i.e., there is an odd number of observations). The code for the radial kernel analysis was applied to one-half of the data. The confusion table code and the code for a separating hyperplane plot were applied to the other half. The results were very similar (within sampling error). An important implication is that in this instance, the results are not affected by cutting the number of observations in half. But it is difficult to know the mechanisms that are responsible. The kernel has been retuned and may compensate by better exploiting the smaller dimensions of the kernel. Also, with so few predictors, the need for a large kernel matrix may be effectively irrelevant. As in earlier chapters, a nonparametric bootstrap could be applied to the output from the second split of the data to provide useful information on the uncertainty of that output.

7.5 Summary and Conclusions

Support vector machines has some real strengths. SVM was developed initially for classification problems and performs well in a variety of real classification applications. As a form of robust regression, it may also prove to be useful when less weight needs to be given to more extreme residuals. And, the underlying fundamentals of support vector machines rest on well-considered and sensible principles.

Among academics, the adjective "interesting" is to damn with faint praise. But the applications discussed in Ma and Gao (2014) are genuinely interesting. They illustrate the rich set of data analysis problems to which support vector machines is being applied. They also document that a large number of talented researchers are working with and extending support vector machines.

In general, however, the comparative advantage of support vector machines, compared to random forests and stochastic gradient boosting, is not apparent. There is no evidence that it typically leads to smaller generalization error. Problems working with indicator predictor variables will often be a serious constraint. And choosing an appropriate kernel coupled with the required tuning can be a challenge. Finally, SVM may be overmatched by "big data."

Where support vector machines seems to shine is when the number of predictors and number of observations are modest. Then, kernels can have genuine assets that other machine learning procedures may not be able to match.

Exercises

Problem Set 1

Support vector machines begins with kernels. Review the section on kernels in Chap. 2 looking especially at the material on radial kernels. Load the R dataset *trees* and have a look at the three variables in the file. The code below will allow you to explore how the matrix derived from the radial kernel changes depending on the values assigned to σ. Try values of $0.01, 0.05, 0.1$, and 1. Consider how the standard deviation changes, excluding matrix elements equal to 1.0. Also have a look at the 3-D histograms depending on the value of σ. Describe what you see. How do the changes you see affect the complexity of the function that can be estimated?

```
library(kernlab) # you may need to install this
library(plot3D) # you may need to install this
X<-as.matrix(trees)
rfb<-rbfdot(sigma=.01) # radial kernel
K<-kernelMatrix(rfb,X)
sd(K[K<1]) # standard deviation with 1's excluded.
hist3D(z=K,ltheta=45,lphi=50,alpha=0.5,opaque.top=T,scale=F)
```

Problem Set 2

Construct a dataset as follows:

```
w<-rnorm(500)
z<-rnorm(500)
w2<-w^2
x<-(-1+3*w2-1*z)
p<-exp(x)/(1 + exp(x))
y<-as.factor(rbinom(500,1,p))
```

1. Regress y on w and z using logistic regression and construct a confusion table with the resubstituted data. You know that the model has been misspecified. Examine the regression output and the confusion table. Now regress y on $w2$ and

z using logistic regression and construct a confusion table with the resubstituted data. You know that the model is correct. Compare the two sets of regression coefficients, their hypothesis tests, and two confusion tables. How does the output from the two models differ? Why?

2. Can you do as well with SVM using w and z as when logistic regression is applied to the correct model? With w and z as predictors (not $w2$), use an ANOVA kernel in *ksvm* from the library *kernlab*. You will need to tune the ANOVA kernel using some trial and error. (Have a look at the material on the ANOVA kernel in Chap. 2.) Start with $sigma = 0.01$ and $degree = 1$. Increase both in several steps until $sigma = 10$ and $degree = 3$. Choose the values that give you the fewest classification errors. How does this confusion table from the well-tuned SVM compare to the confusion tables from the correct logistic regression? What is the general lesson?

3. Construct and interpret the SVM classification plot for the best SVM confusion table.

4. Repeat the SVM analysis, but with class weights. To construct the nominal weights with a ratio of, say 3 to 1, use

```
wts<-c(3,1) # specify weights
names(wts)<-c("0","1") #assign weights to classes
```

Insert these two lines of code before the call to *ksvm* and then include the argument *class.weights=wts* in *ksvm*. Try several different pair of nominal weights until you get a cost ratio in the confusion table such that the 1s are three times as costly as the 0s. How do the results differ?

Problem Set 3

1. From the *MASS* library, load the Pima.tr dataset. The variable "type" is the response. All other variables are predictors. Apply *ksvm* from the *kernlab* library and again use the ANOVA kernel and weights to address asymmetric costs. The doctor wants to be able to start treatment before the test results are in and thinks it is twice as costly to withhold treatment for a patient who needs it to compared to giving treatment to a patient does not need it. Apply SVM to the data so that the confusion table has a good approximation of the desired cost ratio and about as good performance as can be produced with these data. This will take some tuning of the ANOVA kernel and the tuning parameter C, which determines the weight given to the penalty in the penalized fit. (In Problem Set 2, C was fixed at the default value of 1.0.) A good strategy is to first set $C = 1$ and tune the ANOVA kernel. Then, see if you can do better altering the value of C.

2. Choose two predictors in which you think the doctor might be particularly interested and construct an SVM classification plot. Fix all other predictors at their means. Interpret the plot. Do you think there is any useful information in the plot to aid the physician. Why?

Endnotes

[1] In the SVM literature, the response variable is often called the "target variable," and the intercept in Eq. 7.1 is often called the "bias." Each observation is sometimes called an "example."

[2] Because y is coded as 1 and -1, products that are positive represent correctly classified cases. Because β and x are vectors, they should be in bold font. But Hastie et al. (2009) do not do that. Nevertheless, there should be no confusion.

[3] Because there is no intention to interpret the regression coefficients, nothing important is lost.

[4] There are several steps that require familiarity with matrix algebra. Interested readers should be able to find excellent treatments on the web. See, for example, lectures on support vector machines by Patrick H. Winston of MIT or by Yaser Abu-Mostafa of Caltech.

[5] λ is equal to the reciprocal of the weight given to the sum of the slack variables in the usual Lagrange expression (Hastie et al. 2009: 420, 426).

[6] How would you represent numerically a categorical variable with two categories, let alone more than two? Any decision would be arbitrary and affect the kernel calculations.

[7] Both are included as part of the regular *ksvm* output.

[8] The other popular support vector machines library in R is *e1071*. It works well, but has fewer kernel options than *kernlab* and many fewer features for working with kernels. It also lacks variable importance plots and partial dependence plots. The pdp library apparently can produce partial dependence plot from the procedure *ksm* in *kernlab* (Greenwald 2017: 424).

References

Bishop, C. M. (2006). *Pattern recognition and machine learning*. New York: Springer.

Chen, P., Lin, C., & Schölkopf, B. (2004). *A tutorial on v-support vector machines*. Department of Computer Science and Information Engineering, National Taiwan University, Taipei

Christianini, N., & Shawe-Taylor, J. (2000). *Support vector machines* (Vol. 93(443), pp. 935–948). Cambridge: Cambridge University Press.

Greenwald, B. M. (2017). pdp: An R package for constructing partial dependence plots. *The R Journal, 9*(1), 421–436.

Hastie, T., Tibshirani, R., & Friedman, J. (2009). *The elements of statistical learning* (2nd ed.). New York: Springer-Verlag.

Hsu, C., Chung, C., & Lin, C. (2010). *A practical guide to support vector classification*. Department of Computer Science and Information Engineering National Taiwan University, Taipei. http://www.csie.ntu.edu.tw/~cjlin/libsvm

Joachims, T. (1998). Making large-scale SVM learning practical. In B. Schölkopf, C. J. C. Burges, & A. J. Smola (Eds.), *Advances in Kernel Methods – Support Vector Learning*. Cambridge: MIT Press.

Karatzoglou, A., Smola, A., & Hornik, K. (2015). *kernlab – An S4 package for kernel methods in R*. https://cran.r-project.org/web/packages/kernlab/vignettes/kernlab.pdf

Ma, Y., & Gao, G. (2014). *Support vector machines applications*. New York: Springer.

Moguerza, J. M., & Munõz, A. (2006). Support vector machines with applications. *Statistical Science, 21*(3), 322–336.

Vapnick, V. (1996). *The nature of statistical learning theory*. New York: Springer-Verlag.

Chapter 8
Neural Networks

Summary Neural networks has its roots in the 1950s with the "perceptron." It is essentially sets of regression equations linked end to end in a manner that allows for nonlinear relationships. Neural networks performs no better than more recent statistical learning tools and typically, worse. However, about 10 years ago, computer scientists recognized that a special data management front end could make neural networks extremely effective in classifying images, translating languages and recognizing speech. Various elaborations and extensions of neural networks followed that some like to call "deep neural networks," or more broadly, "deep learning." These newer developments have generated both genuine excitement and some self-serving hype. In this chapter, we will begin with early neural networks and end with some of the impressive recent advances.

8.1 Introduction

Neural networks is actually a large collection of statistical learning procedures. The story begins in the 1950s with a technique called the "perceptron" (Rosenblatt 1958), based in part on early understandings of how brain neurons function. Advances that followed emphasized pattern recognition (Ripley 1996) for which a range of the formal properties were proved and better estimation procedures developed (Rumelhart et al. 1986). A popular application was to recognize each of the integers from 0 to 9 from handwritten examples. The result has been called "vanilla neural nets" by Hastie et al. (2009: 392). Until about a decade ago vanilla neural nets was effectively the entire neural networks enterprise, and it remains an important component of current practice. We start there. Consistent with one of the key storylines in this book, we are still focusing on the distribution of some response conditional on one or more predictors. The response can be numerical or categorical. Neural networks provides another way to arrive at some $f(\mathbf{X})$.

© Springer Nature Switzerland AG 2020

R. A. Berk, *Statistical Learning from a Regression Perspective*,
Springer Texts in Statistics, https://doi.org/10.1007/978-3-030-40189-4_8

361

8.2   Conventional (Vanilla) Neural Networks

From a statistical learning perspective, neural networks is a way to combine inputs in a nonlinear manner to arrive at outputs. Just as for random forests and boosting, a complicated $f(X)$ is approximated by an amalgamation of many, far more simple functions. There is also a regularization process by which the simple functions are combined. In the end, one has an interpolator (Olson et al. 2018). The foundational features of neural nets are no surprise, but for certain kinds of applications, additional steps are introduced into the analysis process and in this form, neural networks exploits some novel ideas.

For notational consistency, we build on Hastie et al. (2009: section 11.3). Figure 8.1 is a schematic of a very simple neural network. The p inputs are represented by $x_1, x_2, \ldots, x_p$. These are just the usual set of predictors. There is a single output, Y, although more complicated networks can have several different outputs. Y can be numerical or categorical and is just the usual response variable. In our notation, a categorical Y would be denoted by G. There is also in the simple example a single "hidden layer" $z_1, z_2, \ldots, z_M$ that can be understood as a set of M *unobserved*, latent variables. More typically, there are many hidden layers. All three components (i.e., inputs, output, and latent variables) are linked by associations that would be causal if one were trying to represent the actions of a collection of neurons. Figure 8.1 is called a "feedforward" neural network because there are no feedback loops. It is also called "fully connected" because going forward each input is linked to each latent variable and each latent variable is linked to the output.

It all starts with the inputs that are combined in a linear fashion for each latent variable. That is, each latent variable is a function of its own linear combination of the predictors. Each linear combination is sometimes called an "integration function." For the mth latent variable, one has

Fig. 8.1 A neural network with one response, one hidden layer, and no feedback

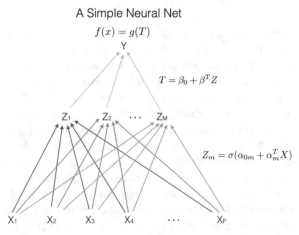

A Simple Neural Net

$$f(x) = g(T)$$

$$T = \beta_0 + \beta^T Z$$

$$Z_m = \sigma(\alpha_{0m} + \alpha_m^T X)$$

$$Z_m = \sigma(\alpha_{0m} + \alpha_m^T X), \tag{8.1}$$

where α_m^T is a vector of coefficients (also called "weights") that likely vary over the p inputs, α_{0m} is the intercept, called the "bias" in computer science, and σ is commonly a sigmoid "activation function." A key idea behind the S-shape is that a linear combination of inputs will more likely trigger an impulse as that linear combination of the inputs increases in value, but variation in the linear combination towards the middle of its range alters Z_m the most.[1] This is like logistic regression for which one also has a linear combination of inputs transformed by sigmoid link function. For neural networks, some of the possible link functions are not really sigmoid, but are still in that spirit. In the end, the transformed, linear combination of predictors serves as fitted values for the latent variables.

In the next step, a linear combination of the latent variable values is constructed as

$$T = \beta_0 + \beta^T Z, \tag{8.2}$$

where now the β^T is a vector of coefficients (also called "weights"), β_0 is the intercept/bias, and Z is the set of latent variables. One has a linear combination of the M latent variables that some also call an integration function. That linear combination can be subject to a transformation

$$f(x) = g(T), \tag{8.3}$$

where g is the transformation function. When Y is numerical, the transformation simply may be an identity function. When Y is categorical, the transformation may be logistic, much as in logistic regression.

There is no explicit representation of any disturbances, either for Z or Y, which is consistent with early machine learning traditions. The need to fit data with a neural network implies the existence of residuals, but they are not imbued with any formal, statistical properties. It is not apparent, therefore, how to get from a Level I analysis to a Level II analysis in the absence of the IID framework that has been deployed in earlier chapters. We revisit this issue later.

If one substituted the M versions of Eq. 8.1 into Eq. 8.2, each version of Eq. 8.1 would be multiplied by its corresponding value of β. Consequently, the relative impact of each set of linearly combined and then transformed inputs would be altered as a product of its β. When those results are inserted into Eq. 8.3, one has the option of applying another nonlinear transformation. In short, one has built a set of sequential, nonlinear transformations of the linearly combined inputs to arrive at the output; a series of simple linear combinations and transformations are used to approximate a complicated $f(X)$. In the process, there is new black box algorithm from which the associations between inputs and outputs are no longer apparent. Neural networks succeeds or fails by how well its fitted values for Y correspond to the actual values of Y. In that sense, there is nothing new.

Estimating the values of both sets of weights would be relatively straightforward if Z were observable. One would have something much like a conventional structural equation model in econometrics. But because Z is unobservable, estimation is undertaken in a more complicated fashion that capitalizes on the sequential structure of the neural network: from X to Z to Y.

As usual, a loss function associated with the response must be specified. For example, if the response is quantitative, quadratic loss would be a likely choice. Then, because of the sequential nature of Eqs. 8.1 through 8.3, the inputs are used to construct the values of the latent variable that, in turn, are combined to arrive at $\hat{Y}$. But one still needs values for both sets of the weights: the αs and the βs.

Consistent with many statistical learning algorithms discussed in earlier chapters, the weights first must be initialized. Values randomly drawn close to 0.0 are often a good choice because one starts out with something very close to a linear model; there is not much variation to transform by an activation function. Given the known values of X and an initialized weight for each α, fitted values for each Z_m follow directly. The initialized weight for each β then determine the fitted values for Y. From these, the loss is computed. The loss will almost always be unacceptably large given the initial weights.

By revising the weights, one hopes to reduce the loss overall. Suppose for simplicity that $g(T)$ is the identity function. Recall from the earlier discussion of gradient boosting that a gradient is essentially a set of partial derivatives. Consider first the βs. There are M βs, each having its own partial derivative: the partial derivative of the loss with respect to each β. As before, the partial derivatives determine how each β should be revised. A negative partial derivative, which implies a reduction in loss, leads to increases in the corresponding β. A positive partial derivative, which implies an increase in loss, leads to a reduction in the corresponding β. Over all partial derivatives, changes in the weights define a productive step down the face of the M dimensional loss function. More formally, largely using the notation of Hastie et al. (2009: 396)

$$\beta_{km}^{r+1} = \beta_{km}^r - \gamma_r \sum_{i=1}^{N} \frac{\partial L_i}{\partial \beta_{km}^r}, \tag{8.4}$$

where L_i is the loss for case i, r is the iteration, k is the response variable, m is a latent variable, and γ_r is the "learning rate," which discounts the impact of the partial derivative. Because of the learning rate, one is taking a smaller step down the face of the loss function to avoid advancing past better routes or past the minimum.

Things are a little more complicated for the αs because their impact on the loss passes through one or more of the partial derivatives for the βs. Look again at Fig. 8.1. To keep the discussion simple, suppose that σ is the identity function. The partial derivative of the loss with respect to each α_m is computed using the chain rule from calculus.[2] The partial derivative of the latent variable with respect to a given α is multiplied by the partial derivative of the loss with respect to a corresponding β. In the end, the revision of any α takes the same general form as the revision of any β. Thus,

$$\alpha_{kl}^{r+1} = \alpha_{kl}^{r} - \gamma_r \sum_{i=1}^{N} \frac{\partial L_i}{\partial \alpha_{kl}^{r}}, \tag{8.5}$$

where l is the predictor.[3]

This logic applies when $g(T)$ and σ are nonlinear transformations. The partial derivatives are just more complicated. Using the chain rule, one can work all the way back from the partial derivative of the loss with respect to each β to the partial derivative of the loss with respect to each α_m^T to compute all of the necessary partial derivatives. Each of the weights (i.e., the αs and the βs) can then be revised based on their partial derivatives with the loss. The weight revision process depends on this "backpropagation."

Despite the sequence from inputs to a hidden layer to an output, the fitting process is not stagewise. With each pass through the data, all of the weights are revised at once. In theory, this produces greater accuracy than had a stagewise approach been used. But there is a price: the tuning and fitting process can be far more demanding.

When there are several outcome variables, the same logic plays through. However, the loss function must now include a function of the errors for all of the outcome variables. For example, one might be interested in constructing a neural network for families in which the separate incomes from both partners are the fitting targets. Because these are not mutually exclusive outcomes, one has two different response variables.

Similar reasoning applies to categorical response variables, sometimes called a "multi-label" output. One does not have a single response variable with more than two mutually exclusive classes. Rather, there might be several categorical response variables for, say, arrested individuals who have different criminal charges that are not mutually exclusive (e.g., a property crime, a person crime, and a drug-related crime).

In the numeric or multi-label case, there is still a single loss function that is typically the sum of the losses across the different Ys or different Gs. With K numerical outcome variables, each error sum of squares is summed for $Y_1, Y_2, \ldots Y_K$. With K categorical outcomes variables for $G_1, G_2, \ldots G_K$, each cross-entropy is summed. Backpropagation works as before.

8.2.1 Implementation of Gradient Descent

For neural networks, implementation of gradient descent comes with several complications. First, start values can really matter because the loss functions typically are not convex. One can get stuck in a local minimum. A common approach is to repeat the fitting exercise several times with different sets of start values and then choose the result with the smallest loss. There are several clever tricks that can be applied as well. For example, one can capitalize on how fast the loss is dropping and allow that "momentum" to push the solution through a local minimum (Ghatak

2019: section 5.3.2). But even with the best current procedures and tools, one must always worry about being misled by a local solution.

Second, with so many weights, overfitting can be a serious problem. As a form of regularization, the integration functions help, but some additional forms of regularization are often needed.[4] Penalizing the fit in the spirit of ridge regression is one option. Others are discussed briefly later. In this context, evaluation data in addition to test data are very important.

Third, in part because the inputs can be highly correlated, some of the estimated weights can grow extremely large or approach zero over iterations. Such problems can be exacerbated by large values for some of the weight initializations and by strong associations between the weights themselves as the fitting proceds. Often the best one can do is to randomly reinitialize the weights and begin again. This can help break up some of the problematic dependence. Fancier options also exist such as randomly zeroing out some weights.

Fourth, the different units in which the inputs are measured can derail, or at least dramatically slow down, the convergence. Standardizing the inputs is usually helpful. There are several different kinds of standardization, including the common z-score transformation. Some argue that a min/max scaling is preferable for gradient descent. Thus, to get from the original variable to the transformed variable using maximum and minimum functions,

$$x_{new} = \frac{x_{old} - min(x_{old})}{max(x_{old}) - min(x_{old})}. \tag{8.6}$$

Standardization need not be limited to the inputs. One can also standardize the latent variables.[5]

Fifth, in Fig. 8.1, each input is connected to each latent variable, and each latent variable is connected to the response. The network is saturated (i.e., fully connected). No inputs are directly linked to the response, although that can be an option. In short, there can be in principle a large number of different network structures before the analysis begins.

Finally, the number of latent variables and hidden layers are tuning parameters typically arrived at through some combination of craft lore and performance in cross-validation. Sometimes hundreds of latent variables will be required. Tuning more generally is a major challenge in part because of the non-convex loss function. Lots of data snooping is required.

8.2.2   Statistical Inference with Neural Networks

Statistical inference for a neural network is no different fundamentally from statistical inference for random forests and boosting. One again treats the data as IID random realizations from a generative joint probability distribution. A plausible estimation target is, as before, an approximation of the true response surface. One imagines the neural network developed with the data is applied to the limitless number of observations that could be realized from the joint probability distribution. The fitted values constitute the approximation. The fitted values from test data constitute the estimate. From the test data fitted values, one can obtain an estimate of generalization error. Uncertainty in that estimate properly can be represented with a nonparametric bootstrap. Prediction intervals can be obtained with split conformal methods. As before, all of these inferential procedures assume that the training data and algorithm structure, once determined, are fixed. Important sources of uncertainty are unaddressed.

8.2.3 An Application

Neural networks can be used much like any of the stronger classifiers considered in earlier chapters. For this application, the data come from arraignments for marijuana possession in Toronto, Canada. The outcome is whether an offender is released. Predictors include the usual background variables and "Checks," which is the number of times an offender's name appears in criminal justice records. In the United States, this would fall under the rubric of prior record. The analysis code is shown in Fig. 8.2. Note the option of z-score standardizations rather than the min/max standardization provided for demonstration purposes.

There are several popular neural network programs that can be easily obtained, but their relative strengths and weaknesses are still to be well documented. Part of the challenge is that neural network procedures can be part of proprietary software whose performance and code are rarely disclosed in sufficient detail. Slick visuals and polished sales pitches do not qualify. The hype around "AI" has, if anything, made accurate assessment even more difficult.

Nevertheless, an important divide is between traditional neural networks and neural networks used as a component of what some call "deep learning." Here, we emphasize the former. The latter is addressed subsequently.

For this application, the R library *neuralnet* is used. Its syntax is by now familiar, and its performance can be quite good. However, like all neural network software, convergence is somewhat finicky. One can easily undertake a dozen or more attempts to arrive at acceptable tuning parameters for which there is convergence. Moreover, the fitting exercise usually needs to be repeated several times to help determine if the results are for a local or a global minimum. A very accessible discussion of the algorithm and how to proceed in practice is provided by Günther and Fritsch (2010). One important bit of advice is to start with a simple structure and complicate it gradually as needed (which is a form of model selection).

Figure 8.3 shows the estimated neural network. There are two hidden layers, each with two nodes. Error is in cross-entropy units. The algorithm implemented the usual alternating forward and backward process 43,454 times (i.e., "steps") to attain convergence. There is no definition of how many steps is too many, but if the

```
library(car)
data(Arrests)

# Scale in z-scores
attach(Arrests)
Released<-ifelse(released=="Yes",1,0)
Black<-scale(ifelse(colour=="Black",1,0))
Year<-scale(year)
Age<-scale(age)
Male<-scale(ifelse(sex=="Male",1,0))
Employed<-scale(ifelse(employed=="Yes",1,0))
Citizen<-scale(ifelse(citizen=="Yes",1,0))
Checks<-scale(checks)
detach(Arrests)
work1<-data.frame(Released,Black,Age,Year,Male,Employed,
                  Citizen,Checks)

# Split sample approach
index<-sample(1:5225,2000,replace=F)
Train<-work1[index,]
Test<-work1[-index,]

# Apply neuralnet
library(neuralnet)
nn1<-neuralnet(Released=="1"~., data=Train,hidden=c(2,2),
               linear.output = F, err.fct = "ce",
               threshold = 0.04, rep=1)
print(nn1)
plot(nn1)
preds<-predict(nn1,newdata=Test)
table(Test$Released,preds >.75) # confusion table

# Apply NeuralNetTools
library(NeuralNetTools)
olden(nn1) # importance plot

# Apply pdp
library(pdp)
partial(nn1,pred.var="Age",plot=T,chull=T, type="classification",
        which.class = 1,prob=T,smooth=T,rug=T)
```

Fig. 8.2 R code for neural networks application

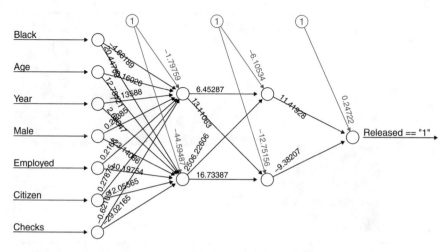

Fig. 8.3 Estimated neural network for release with seven inputs, two hidden layers with two neurons each, three "bias" neurons, and a single binary arraignment outcome ($N = 2000$)

algorithm fails to converge because the default number of steps has been reached (i.e., the default is *stepmax* $= 1e + 05$), there are several analysis options.

1. Run the procedure again from the beginning, which means that different random start values for the weights will be used.
2. Increase the number of steps allowed.
3. Make the convergence threshold more tolerant (e.g., use 0.05 rather than 0.01).
4. Simplify the neural network structure (e.g., reduce the number of hidden layers).

If some thought already has been given to options #2 through #4 before the algorithm was applied, option #1 is worth trying several times. And option #1 should be applied several times even if there is convergence to help determine if a local solution was produced. These steps can take hours.

A conventional confusion table was constructed but is not shown. There is apparently no way to alter the cost ratio by changing the prior or by weighting. As a fallback, a classifying threshold of 0.75 was used on the fitted proportions. The usual threshold of 0.50 led to all cases being classified as releases. Increasing the threshold set higher level of certainty for a case that was classified as a release. Incorrectly classifying a detention as a release was made far more costly. But as before, altering the threshold only affects the confusion table but not the neural network itself. Changing the threshold is not an ideal method for introducing asymmetric costs.

Importance plots can be produced using *olden* in the *NeuralNetTools* library. Figure 8.4 shows an importance plot that implements the "Olden" method (Olden et al. 2004). According to the documentation in R, the Olden method "calculates variable importance as the product of the raw input-hidden and hidden-output connection weights between each input and output neuron and sums the product across all hidden neurons." It is not clear exactly what to make of such in-

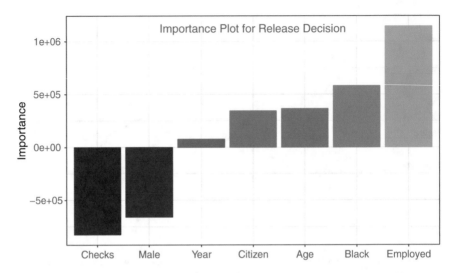

Fig. 8.4 Predictor importance measures for release at arraignment

sample values in part because one usually has standardized all of the predictors. The standardization affects the weight values. As noted several times earlier, standardization just papers over differences in the natural and interpretable units in which predictors are usually measured. Recall our discussion of the standardization of importance measures for random forests. For the Olden method, the most one learns is, *given the standardization*, the potential impact of each input in-sample on the fitted values. With a different form of standardization, the absolute and relative importance of each input can change substantially.

From Fig. 8.4 using the Olden method, employment appears to be the most important predictor associated with a release. Having a job is associated with an increase in the chances of release. The predictor Checks is a count (i.e., prior record) and is the second most important predictor. It is associated with a decrease in the chances of a release.

But such interpretations depend on the algorithm, how importance is defined, and how the algorithm performs with the training data available. The same analysis was undertaken using stochastic gradient boosting, and the predictor Checks was by far the most important variable. With each check, the fitted chances of a release declined. Employment was a distant second. Having a job increased only a bit the fitted chances of a release. One possible reason for the different results is that the required standardization for neural networks disadvantaged the Checks predictor by shrinking its variability relative to the binary employment variable.

Partial dependence plots are available using the *partial* procedure from the *pdp* library. It is not clear whether the *neuralnet* object is appropriate for *partial* but after a bit of fiddling, it ran with no error messages. Figure 8.5 shows the partial dependence plot for the predictor age. Note that age is in standard deviation units because of the earlier standardization of all predictors into z-scores. The vertical axis

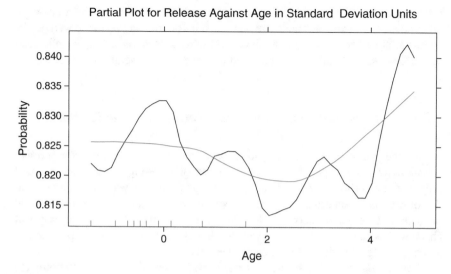

Fig. 8.5 Partial dependence plot for age

is in proportion/probability units. The black line is apparently an interpolation. The blue line is a loess smooth of the interpolation. One can see that age is not strongly associated with release, but that for those two standard deviations or more above the mean age, the chances of release increase slightly holding all other predictors constant.[6]

8.2.4 Some Recent Developments

There have been many recent enhancements in neural networks that are beyond the scope of this exposition, but two developments are worth a brief mention. First, with so many parameters, a form of regularization can be introduced by imposing a prior distribution on each. The result is "Bayesian neural nets" that for estimation relies on extensive preprocessing of the data and very sophisticated Markov Chain Monte Carlo (MCMC) methods (Neal and Zhang 2006). In practice, Bayesian neural nets seems to perform very well and can compete with the other statistical learning procedures discussed earlier.

However, the improved performance apparently has less to do with the formal Bayesian framework and more to do with enhancements discussed above: it becomes another form of regularization. Indeed, it seems likely that one can get similar improvement by bagging or boosting neural networks (Hastie et al. 2009: section 11.9.1).

Second, it is also sometimes possible to deploy a neural network in a manner that reduces computational burdens, ideally with no appreciable decline in accuracy. For example, one can fit the network by moving through hidden layers in a stagewise fashion. That is, the weights for the latent variables within one hidden layer are determined over many iterations and then fixed before moving on to the weights for latent variables for the next hidden layer.[7] Another strategy is to sample split, send the different splits to different GPUs, and then average the weights over splits.

8.2.5   Implications of Conventional Neural Nets for Practice

In the end, there does not seem to be any reason for deploying conventional neural networks compared to random forests or boosting, even with potential improvements using bagged or boosted neural nets. There is yet to be a compelling demonstration of superior performance especially when the expected dependence on data is taken into account. Moreover, there are the far greater operational challenges because of the non-convex loss function, the many tuning parameters, and overfitting from the large number of weights.

Nevertheless, there are special settings in which neural networks can dominate the competition. We turn to those now. We are still focused on the distribution of some response variable conditional on one or more predictors, although this overarching theme is obscured a bit by a host of new details.

8.3   Deep Learning with Neural Networks

These days, artificial intelligence (AI) is conflated with machine learning. Neither AI nor machine learning are well defined and, consequently, are routine components of sales pitches for software ranging from conventional statistics to the most advanced tools used for autonomous vehicles, facial recognition, and medical diagnoses. Complicating the definitions further is a renaming of many standard tools in statistics, often invented decades ago. For example, principal component analysis, invented by Karl Pearson in 1901, has been rebranded by computer scientists as unsupervised learning. Perhaps even more confusing, least squares regression, usually attributed to Karl Frederich Gauss and invented in the late eighteenth century, has been reborn as supervised learning.

Neural networks is a statistical learning procedure often included in the hype. Neural networks is actually a heterogeneous set of procedures, some pretty much ho-hum and some innovative and powerful. Traditional neural networks, just discussed, falls into the first category. Major extensions of traditional neural networks, such as convolutional neural networks, fall into the second category. The second category commonly goes by the name of "deep learning," which as a public relations gambit is nothing short of brilliant. Goodfellow et al. (2016) provide an excellent treatment that avoids most of the excesses. Still, one must be wary in general of performance claims that too often are limited to very particular applications and little more than "trust me" justifications.

There are many specialized tools under the rubric of deep learning, whose numbers seem to be growing almost daily. Formal proofs of actual performance in most cases lag far behind. Consequently, choices between different procedures and their tuning details are guided largely by craft lore.[8]

In practice, the tuning challenges briefly discussed for traditional neural networks can be orders of magnitude more difficult. Some claim that one needs a "neural net whisperer." In the deep learning setting, Chollet and Allaire (2018: 96) comment

> Unfortunately, there is no magical formula to determine the right number of layers or the right size of each layer. You must evaluate an array of different architectures (on your validation set, not your test set) in order to find the correct model size for your data. The general workflow is to find an appropriate model size to start with relatively few layers and parameters, and increase the size of the layers or add new layers until you see diminishing returns to validation loss.[9]

The same point can be made about all other characteristics of a neural network (e.g., activation functions) and its fitting process (e.g., learning rate, regularization), and we have yet to consider the new complications introduced by deep learning. Lapan (2018: 66) observes

> If you have ever tried to train a NN on your own, then you may know how painful and uncertain it can be. I am not talking about following the existing tutorials and demos, when all hyperparameters are already tuned for you, but about taking some data and creating something from scratch. Even with modern DL [deep learning] high-level toolkits, where all best practices such as proper weights initialization and optimizers' betas, gammas, and other options are set to sane defaults, and tons of other stuff hidden under the hood, there are still lots of decisions that you can make, hence lots of things can go wrong. As a result, your network almost never works from the first run and this is something that you should get used to.

Put another way, it usually takes a village to tune deep learning procedures on applications that matter (not just simple exercises). Otherwise, the tuning process will likely take far more time than a single practitioner has available. Tuning done within organizations that can allocate the necessary resources, including personnel, will have access to industrial-strength learning algorithms. But, even with superb software like *TensorFlow* and its growing collection of programming aids, deep learning requires far greater time investments than the statistical learning procedures discussed in earlier chapters. Solo data analysts take note.

8.3.1 Convolutional Neural Networks

Convolutional neural networks (CNN) is a major success story that illustrates well key features of deep learning. Viewed from 30,000 feet, CNN is a classifier. Its goal is to correctly assign an outcome class to an image. The algorithm trains on large number of images whose labels are determined in advance by humans. The algorithm learns how particular image features are associated with a given label. Subsequently, if an image has no label, the trained algorithm imputes it.

For example, training data might include many different images of trees or stop signs all labeled correctly. The algorithm learns how to distinguish between images of trees and images of stop signs by associating characteristics of an image with the appropriate label. Later, when presented with an unlabeled image of either a tree of a stop sign, a well-trained algorithm will usually assign the correct label.

There can be many image classes such as a tree, a stop sign, a pedestrian, or a bike rider. In medical applications, the visual objects could be brain damage from a stroke, plaque precursors of Alzheimer's, or thermal noise from an fMRI. For military applications, the visual objects might be a pickup truck carrying soldiers, a pickup truck carrying armaments, or a pickup truck carrying farm produce.

Each image is represented as a rectangular (usually) array of pixels. A pixel is as an input to the CNN, or in statistical language, a predictor. Each pixel can be characterized by several "channels." For example, one channel can be grayscale.[10] Other channels capture colors using one channel each for red, green, and blue. These primary colors are blended to construct virtually any color. Color saturation is yet another channel.

Ideally, each image is independently realized at random from an appropriate population of images on which the algorithm will be trained. A telling instance is the image recognition needed for autonomous vehicles. If the training data were assembled only from rural images, performance in cities could be problematic. One has moved from a population of rural images to a population of urban images that can differ in important ways. For example, there will likely be no trolly cars in rural locations.[11]

A key characteristic of pixelized images is that rows cannot be exchanged without altering the image to be detected. For example, if a stop sign is represented, exchanging the top five rows of pixels with the bottom five rows of pixels risks placing the face of the stop sign below the post on which it is attached. The same holds should any of the columns be exchanged. The word "stop" might be transformed into "opst." In contrast, most of the datasets used in earlier chapters allowed rows to be exchanged, or columns to be exchanged, leaving the analysis unaffected.

The rigidity of the row locations and the column locations is actually helpful. The location of each pixel in the image carries information. For example, pixels closer to one another may be more alike, and such information can be exploited. The red pixels in a red stop sign, for instance, will be in one location of the image. It is a bit like working with spatial data in which for observations characterized by longitude and latitude, proximity often matters. It is also a bit like working with temporal data when proximity in time can matter.

Convolutional neural networks faces the same tradeoffs discussed in earlier chapters. The complexity of the fitted values extracted plays into the bias–variance tradeoff. How one summarizes the information contained in the pixels must balance extracting fine details against the stability of those details. Computational demands are affected as well; trying to extract extensive detail can challenge even very large clusters of GPUs. Many of the creative advances built into convolutional neural networks speak to how effective tradeoffs can be made.

8.3.1.1 CNNs in More Detail

Consider for now a single image. Figure 8.6 shows an image that might be captured by a security camera, although actually taken from stock images in Keynote. To the human eye, the image contains a person, probably an adult male, dressed in a short jacket, standing erect and carrying a firearm that looks a lot a bit like an assault rifle with a pistol grip but no shoulder stock, and no banana clip. Suppose that assessment is correct. Would an algorithm be able to arrive at the same conclusion? Put in practical terms, from the set of very similar to very different images that might be captured by a security camera, can an algorithm be trained to correctly classify with high probability a heavily armed individual? For Fig. 8.6, that means learning from a large number of images that a security camera might produce, all correctly labeled.

For Fig. 8.6, the first step would be to "pixelate" the image. In Fig. 8.6, the pixels are represented by a set of rectangles shown with red vertical and horizontal lines. Each rectangle is an observational unit. There are 48 such pixels and, consequently, 48 observational units. Each is digitized to capture such things as color or brightness. For example, black and white images might be represented in grayscale values. The algorithm would use as inputs information about each pixel's content to learn the image.[12]

Figure 8.7 shows some of the subtleties images present. All five images contain that same armed man, but they differ in size, location in the frame, orientation, and color of the background. Literally, all of the images are different. Yet, the essence of an armed man must be extracted from each of the five images. Humans are able to do that easily. The major technical advance that often allows a computer to do

Fig. 8.6 An image with pixels outlined in red overlaid

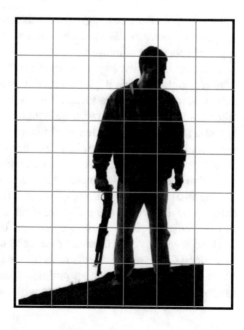

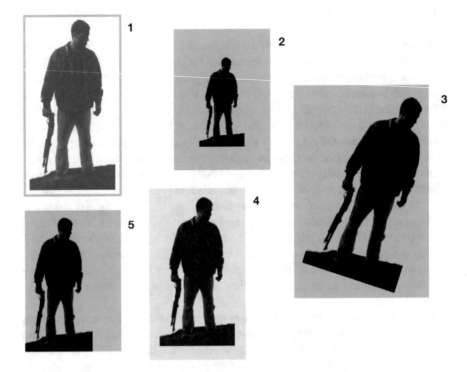

Fig. 8.7 An identical human image with different pixelated Information

the same is, in effect, to preprocess the data before a conventional neural network is applied. Some see this as a form of automated feature engineering. There are several types of operations employed.

Filtering is the first step. (Numerical details will follow shortly.) In Fig. 8.8, the blue rectangle contains a 3 by 3 set of 9 cells that together serve as a "filter." The filter is sometimes called a kernel; this is yet another kind of kernel. Each cell in the filter has a number to characterize a particular feature in the pixel beneath it. For example, each cell in the filter might contain the number 1. If the pixel overlaid is completely black that pixel might have been coded 1. A total of nine comparisons would be made, and the number of black pixels counted. The larger the sum, the more that "blackness" dominates the nine image pixels.[13]

The filter can be moved one pixel at a time left or right and/or one pixel at a time up or down until the entire figure is evaluated in 3 by 3 chunks. The filter always remains within the image, except for some tricks addressed briefly later. Each adjacent 3 by 3 set of image pixels are, in this example, summarized as to their blackness. One could learn where in the image the pixels gradually changed from black to white, from which an outline of the armed man might be approximated (although there are better ways, as we will soon see).

Fig. 8.8 Pixelized image
with a filter overlaid

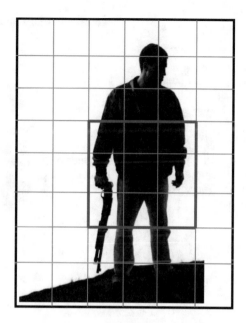

Equally important, the information from the nine image pixels will have been aggregated to provide a single number capturing their degree of blackness. A substantial data reduction has been accomplished; nine numbers have been replaced by a single number. One key benefit is that fewer parameters will need to be estimated, and a bias–variance tradeoff has been made.

The single numbers computed by the filtering are stored in a much smaller matrix that maintains the locations from which each filter's results were obtained. The filtering process is a "convolution" whose results are stored in a "feature map."[14]

For any image, many different filters are applied to extract different attributes of image. For example, one might want a filter for each of the primary colors. The results from each filtering operation are stored in its own feature map. If there are, for example, three filters, there are three feature maps.

Commonly, the output from filtering is transformed in a nonlinear fashion using an activation function, which helps to discard values that may not be informative. This can increase processing speed and help to sharpen the image. Some then call the image "rectified."

Each rectified feature map can be further reduced by "pooling." Several adjacent locations in a feature map are summarized with a single number. This is not usually thought of as filtering. For a 2 by 2 set of adjacent locations, for example, one might compute the largest previously filtered value. Not only can the size of a feature map be dramatically reduced, but a summary characterization akin to a summary statistic has been computed. Again there are tradeoffs between bias and variance, and typically reductions in computational demands.

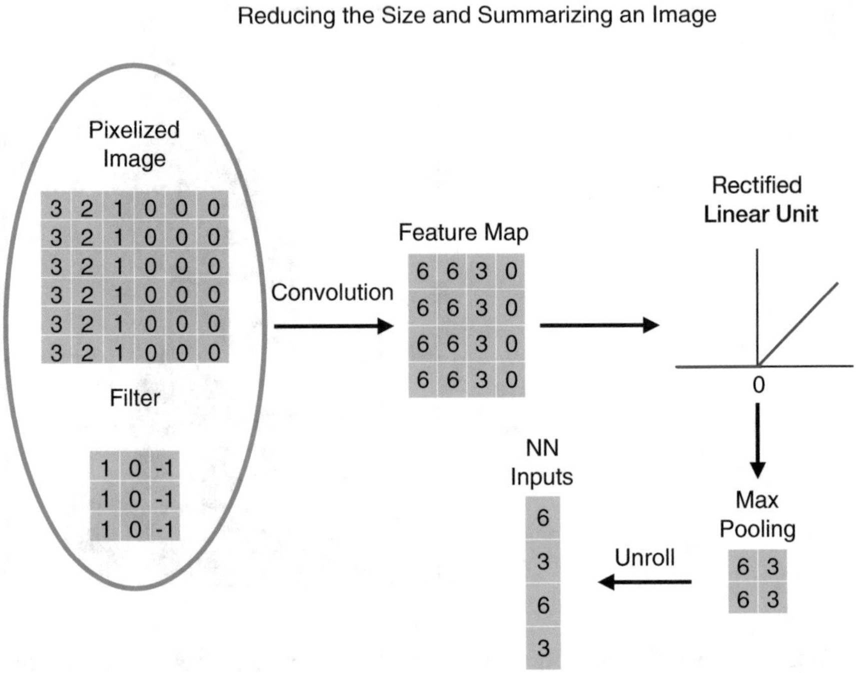

Reducing the Size and Summarizing an Image

Fig. 8.9 Learning an image by filtering and pooling

Greater numerical detail is provided in the following toy example based on a 6 by 6 image shown on the far left of Fig. 8.9. Suppose the pixel values are in grayscale units capturing variation from black to white. A value of 3 is black, a value of 0 is white, and values of 2 and 1 are consecutive shades of gray. The image is structured for didactic purposes so that one can easily see the transition from black to white moving from left to right. There is a clear vertical boundary between the white pixels and all other pixels. How might one find the vertical edge?

Below the 6 by 6 image is 3 by 3 filter. The values in those cells are designed to find a vertical edge. The filter begins in the upper left 3 by 3 set of pixels and produces a dot product of 6.[15]

The filter then moves one space to the right yielding a dot product of 6 once again. Shifting one pixel more to the right, the dot product is 3. And with one more shift to the right, the dot product is 0. These four values are stored in the top row of the feature map to the right. In a similar fashion, the filter can move one pixel lower, sweep over the image another time, and assemble the second row of the feature map—likewise for two more one pixel shifts downward.

In Fig. 8.9, the feature map retains the key information about the vertical edge. However, the values in each cell are no longer in the original grayscale units. The values are dot products (i.e., sums for cross products) of the image and the filter.

There is now a set of summary statistics, one for each 3 by 3 set of image pixels that ideally retains essential information about the image and discards distractions.

The size of the image analyzed and the nature of the filter are tuning parameters. In the first case, an image can be "padded" by including additional cells around the edge of the image with all pixel values set to 0. In Fig. 8.9, a padded image could append a single set of 0 cells around the periphery of image. The image would be 8 by 8: a new row at the top and bottom and a new column on the left edge and the right edge. The padding provides the original cells at the edges of the image an opportunity to be filtered more often, and one is not limited to padding with single new rows or columns.[16]

In the second case, there can be many filters, which may differ in dimensions, each designed to capture a particular feature of the image, such as different colors, textures, or edges. Each filter will have its own feature map. For example, one might employ a filter designed to capture horizontal edges or diagonal edges. Some filters are designed to move over the image horizontally or vertically one pixel at time, but others are designed to move two or more pixels at time. The number of pixels a filter moves is often called the "stride" of the filter, and it too is a tuning parameter.

In the next step, to the immediate right of the feature map in Fig. 8.9, each cell in a feature map is altered in a nonlinear fashion by an activation function. The "rectified linear unit" (ReLU) approach is perhaps the most popular. The ReLU function is piecewise linear with a knot at 0. Negative values become zeroes, and non-negative values are unaffected. One hopes to remove in a computationally efficient manner values that are effectively noise, and with the help of the nonlinear function, sharpen the image. In Fig. 8.9, all of the filtered values are non-negative, so the transformation has no effect.

The next operation is "pooling." In Fig. 8.9, each of the 2 by 2 sets of cells in the feature map is summarized by a single number that ideally measures the dominant characteristic of each disjoint set of 2 by 2 cells. Also, computational demands are further reduced. A common summary is simply the largest value in the four cells, called "max pooling." There are alternatives. For example, one can work with the mean value. The particular pooling method used is another tuning parameter. The same applies to the number of cells pooled. In Fig. 8.9, the max pooling results retain the information about the vertical edge.

To be consistent with the way inputs to a neural network are conventionally shown (e.g., Fig. 8.1), the pooled data in Fig. 8.9 are "unrolled" into a vector with a single column ready to be processed. One has a set of inputs distilled from the image.

The convolution processes, coupled with the pooling, are commonly repeated sequentially several times. For example, a matrix of pooled values can be subject to additional convolutions followed by more pooling. Also, pooling can be repeated several times on a given feature map. The number and ordering of such sequences are subject to tuning. In the end, an image of thousands of pixels is reduced to a matrix of much smaller dimensions that becomes input to a neural network. The cells in the matrix are unrolled so that they form a single vector just like the input for the neural network diagram shown in Fig. 8.1. It then becomes the job of a neural network to correctly classify images, in this case, as showing an armed person or not.

In practice, the steps in Fig. 8.9 can be rearranged and expanded in several different ways.

1. The values in each filter can be learned. They do not have to be specified in advance by the data analyst.
2. There often are several sets of filtering operations, each followed by pooling for a given image before the unrolling is done. In Fig. 8.9, the actions taken before unrolling can be implemented in the same sequence several times: filtering → pooling → filtering → pooling → filtering → pooling and so on.
3. There are different ways to structure the data file fed to a neural network. For example, if there are several feature maps, they can be stored in a three-dimensional tensor (i.e., a three-dimensional array). In Fig. 8.9, the width would be four pixels. The height would be four pixels, and the depth would be the number of feature maps, one for each filter.[17]
4. The convolutional neural networks trains on a large number of images, often thousands. Each image is a "sample" in statistical language or an "example" in computer science language.

The precise manner in which the unwound pixel information from a large number of images is processed by a neural network depends on many operational details, broadly the same as previously described. There is an initialization followed by a calculation of total loss over all images (i.e., the forward step). The backward step follows by which the weights are revised. The back and forth may be undertaken thousands of times.

The preprocessing adds many new complications in service of at least two major goals. The first is to reduce the amount of input a neural network needs to process. This is essential because each image is only a sample (i.e., "example") of one. In practice, there could be thousands of images, each with thousands of pixels.

The second goal is to extract the defining features of the image. In other language, one is seeking good "representations" of the important content in the image. When a human looks at an image, summary features are extracted and processed. The image is not examined and processed point by point. The convolutions and pooling are undertaken in the same spirit but depend on the filters and pooling to find and extract the essential features of the image. Looking back at Fig. 8.7, an effective extraction would not be distracted by the size, location, or orientation of the figure, or by the color of the background.

With all of the tuning and the very large number of weights, overfitting can be a serious problem for convolutional neural networks and deep neural networks in general. Several different regularization strategies are used.

1. Getting more data so that the overfitting is less pronounced.
2. Reducing the size and complexity of the neural network.
3. Reducing the amount of preprocessing.
4. Including a penalty function much as in ridge regression or the lasso.

5. At random, zeroing out some of the weights, which is the same as randomly dropping some of the paths between neurons.
6. Employing data augmentation, which means constructing new data from the data already on hand. For images, one alters the likeness a bit (e.g., rotating the image contents a small, random amount). The altered images are used along with the original image data.
7. Stopping the iterations early by making far fewer passes through the data. This is a well-understood regularization process in statistical learning more generally.

There do not seem to be any formal justifications for some forms of regularization over others. It is not even clear how to directly measure overfitting. In evaluation data, for instance, some differences are to be expected insofar as the evaluation data are also composed of IID observations. And even if sensible measures can be obtained, how much overfitting is too much? Once again, the guidelines depend on craft lore.

Currently, there is apparently not much interest in formal statistical inference for convolutional neural networks, at least among those who develop and deploy CNNs. Just as for conventional neural networks, the challenges are substantial. And just as with conventional neural networks, a partial solution can be obtained with test data. CNN presents no new problems except an even greater risk of serious data snooping and overfitting.

At the moment, there are several implementations of convolutional neural networks in R: *mxnet*, written in C++, but within an R wrapper; an R interface for *TensorFlow*; and two higher level interfaces for *TensorFlow*: *Keras* and *TF Estimators*. All have steep learning curves in part because of the many complexities just described (and more). Working with *Keras* perhaps has the best tradeoffs between flexibility and ease of use, and it is well exposited by Chollet and Allaire (2018). However, given the links from R to Python to *TensorFlow*, it can be difficult to understand how best to respond when there are error messages.[18]

There also are several popular forms of deep learning that are used for datasets that are not images. We will highlight recurrent neural networks (RNNs) and its most important variants because of the close parallels to forms of conventional regression analysis and because it is an option for data in which there is an important time dimension (as in conventional time series analysis).

8.3.2 Recurrent Neural Networks

The basic structure of a recurrent neural network (RNN) will be familiar to anyone who has worked with panel data. In its most generic form, RNN works with pooled cross-section time series observations. There is variation over time and variation over observational units. Such data long have been studied in econometrics (See Hsiao 1986, for an early review) and is now standard fare in any number of econometric text books (e.g., Greene 2003: Chapter 13). For example, one can have survey data in which a "panel" of respondents is re-interviewed every year for several years. The respondents are the cross-sectional units, and years are the temporal units.

For a panel data analysis, there often is a linear regression model such as

$$Y_t = \beta_0 + \beta_1 Y_{t-1} + \beta_2 X_{1,t} + \beta_3 X_{2,t} \ldots \beta_p X_{p-1,t} + \varepsilon_t, \tag{8.7}$$

where t is the subscript for temporal units, Y_t is some numeric response variable such as household income, β_0 through β_p are conventional coefficients for the intercept and $X_{1,t}$ through $X_{p-1,t}$, and ε_t is the usual disturbance term assumed to be realized independently with an expectation of zero and a constant variance σ^2. Allowance can be made for temporal dependence within the ε_t and for non-constant disturbance variances as well. The lagged Y_{t-1} is an autoregressive term explicitly capturing dependence over time in the response variable. Equation 8.7 can be altered to allow for some forms of the generalized linear and generalized additive models. For example, one is not limited to parametric functions of the right hand side variables. Random coefficient models also are available.

In most applications, Equation 8.7 is treated as a model in which the mechanisms by which the social social processes work are explicitly represented. Sometimes the regression coefficients are given causal interpretations; explanation is the top priority.

From an algorithmic perspective is which explanation is at best on a distant, back burner, one can formulate a structure for panel data within a recurrent neural network such that each temporal wave in the panel has its own conventional neural network. That is, each wave might have a neural network of the form shown in Figure 8.1. When there are no covatiates, Goodfellow and his colleagues (2016: section 10.1) write

$$\mathbf{s}^{(t)} = f(\mathbf{s}^{(t-1)}; \boldsymbol{\theta}), \tag{8.8}$$

where the vector $\mathbf{s}_t$ for our purposes can be the same as Y_t,[19] and the vector $\boldsymbol{\theta}$ is a set of weights, analogous to regression coefficients, that are generally fixed over time periods.[20] Note that here too, there is an autoregressive term. There is explicit dependence over time.

Within this notation, one can include an external input vector $\mathbf{x}^{(t)}$, which is the same as the usual covariates. Hence,

$$\mathbf{s}^{(t)} = f(\mathbf{s}^{(t-1)}, \mathbf{x}^{(t)}; \boldsymbol{\theta}). \tag{8.9}$$

One can use a similar formulation for a vector of hidden layers. For a hidden layer $\mathbf{h}^{(t)}$,

$$\mathbf{h}^{(t)} = f(\mathbf{h}^{(t-1)}, \mathbf{x}^{(t)}; \boldsymbol{\theta}). \tag{8.10}$$

An Internal Segment of a Recurrent Neural Network with Hidden Layers

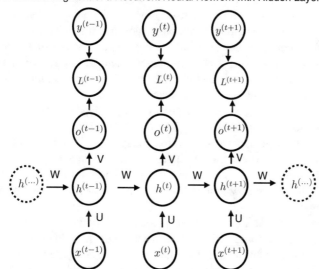

Fig. 8.10 A panel data recurrent neural network with $y^{(\cdot)}$ as the response variable, $x^{(\cdot)}$ as inputs, $h^{(\cdot)}$ the hidden layers, $o^{(\cdot)}$ the fitted values, $L^{(\cdot)}$ the loss, and U, V, and W as sets of weights

In other words, lagged information can be carried forward over time in the hidden layers. This is a key difference between the econometric approach and the statistical learning approach and is where nonlinearities can be captured.

None of the three equations represent causal models. They are meant to convey the existence of certain associations over time. There also is very little structure that would justify statistical inference. Uncertainty concerns seem at best an afterthought.

The components from Equations 8.8 through 8.10 can be assembled in many ways. Figure 8.10, taken from Goodfellow et al. (2016: 366), shows one example for an internal segment for panel data meant to represent how fitting is done. It is an example of a "vanilla" RNN. The external inputs and hidden layers are denoted as before and both are vectors, which means that in any time period, there can be many inputs and many nodes in the hidden layer. The neural network is recurrent because each vertical structure is a conventional neural network ordered from left to right in time. The conventional neural networks reoccur.

The vector, U, denotes the weights between the external vector of inputs and the nodes of the hidden layers. These weights do not change over time. The vector W denotes the weights linking the nodes in the hidden layer over time. These weights also do not change over time. The hidden layers produce outputs, $0^{(\cdot)}$, which are fitted values. Their vector of weights is shown by V, and they too do not change over time.

The response variable is represented by $y^{(\cdot)}$. It can be numeric or categorical. There is a loss $L^{(\cdot)}$ for each time period computed from the hidden layer output in that time period and the response variable values in that time period.

Figure 8.10 conveys that each hidden layer is a function of the immediately preceding hidden layer one time period earlier and the external inputs from the same time period. This allows the information from the external inputs to be carried forward in time in an autoregressive framework.

As a result, the response variable possesses time dependence, but only through time dependence of the hidden layers. To minimize the loss, the $o^{(\cdot)}$, which are products of the hidden layers, must be made to correspond well to the $y^{(\cdot)}$. These outputs are time dependent too because their hidden layers are time dependent. Readers are encouraged to study the far more complete discussion in Goodfellow et al. (2016: Chapter 10), including how gradients are computed such that appropriate weights can be obtained.

In the end, there is a complicated set of associations to account for the time dependence of the response variable. One is betting on the hidden layers to introduce useful nonlinear transformations that improve the fit compared to eq. 8.7. But, in an important sense, the two approaches are not comparable. Equation 8.7 takes uncertainty very seriously, which affects the form the model adopts. There are no such concerns in eq. 8.7. Likewise, because eq. 8.7 is usually treated as a model, in contrast to the algorithm represented in Figure 8.10, there can be important information about how the inputs are related to the response variable, and perhaps even causal interpretations.

Figure 8.10 can be easily reconfigured in a manner that transforms a vanilla RNN into a deep learning RNN. The usual approach is to introduce more hidden layers that can make the fitted values more complex. Drawing heavily on Pascanu and colleagues (2014), the RNN in Figure 8.11 at the top left is a reproduction of Figure 8.10 showing only the most essential components.

To its immediate right is a "deep output RNN" for which a new hidden layer in blue is interposed between each original hidden layer and the response. The asterisks are meant to indicate that the hidden layers differ, and there are no time-linked connections between the new hidden layers. Their job solely is to introduce greater complexity in the outputs from the original hidden layers. They add no additional time dependence.

At the lower left is a "deep transition RNN." Again, there is no additional time dependence introduce by the blue hidden layers. Allowance is made for greater complexity connecting the time dependent hidden layers. The temporal relationships can be more complex.

At the bottom right is a "stacked RNN." The new hidden layers in blue have the same architecture as the original hidden layers. A second source of time dependence is introduced for the possibility of more nonlinearity. Another source of complexity is introduced.

In short, what makes an RNN deep is including more hidden layers. Adding these layers can in principle improve the fit and reduce generalization error. But even the

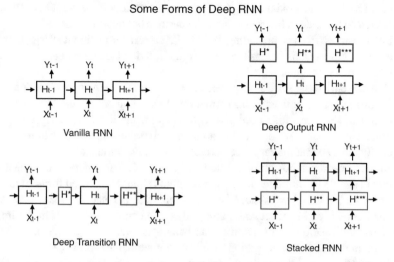

Fig. 8.11 Transforming vanilla RNNs into deep learning RNNs with the hidden layers in blue (The Y(.) are the response variable, the X(.) are the inputs, and the H(.) are the Hidden Layers. Asterisks are meant to show when hidden layers differ.)

craft lore on how best to proceed with what kinds of data is very skimpy, and adding hidden layers can make tuning still more challenging. As before, the structures in Figure 8.11 are *not* models. They are not a systematic response to subject matter theory. There is no help to be found there.

But there's more. Below is a very brief list of other kinds of RNN structures.

- Figure 8.10 has external inputs whose values change with each time period. Many kinds of inputs do not change with each time period (e.g., the year a company was founded, a person's genotype), and yet are related to the outputs through each hidden layer over time.
- Earlier values of the response variable can directly be related to later values of the response variable. That is, there can be associations even after conditioning on the external inputs. These associations over time for the response variable are not solely a function of the time dependent hidden layers.
- At least some of the weights can be allowed to change over time. This is much like approaches in econometrics for time varying parameters, which have been well studied for several decades (Pagan 1980; Robinson 1989; Tucci 1995).
- Hidden layers can be affected by hidden layers farther back in time than a single time period. The parallel in statistics is autoregressive models using several longer lags. This too has a rich history (Box et al. 1994).
- The impact of external inputs can affect the hidden layers through a set of longer lags. That is, hidden layers can be affected by earlier external inputs. This has been part of common practice for decades in regression analyses of longitudinal

data (Kedem and Fokianos 2002). One can also allow the external inputs to be related to the hidden layer in some time periods but not others.

- Fitted values from a preceding hidden layer can be an input along with the external inputs. This is feasible because the fitted values have been transformed in a nonlinear manner.
- One can enrich the relationships between between the sequence of hidden layers by introducing nonlinear transformations when combining the weights going from t to $t + 1$. An important goal is to keep the gradients from exploding over time. This is related to the need in autoregressive statistical models to restrict the coefficients so that the response variable has a finite variance.
- Hidden layers can be complemented by "gated cells" that determine which new inputs should be introduced, which past inputs should be passed forward in time, and which past inputs should be discarded. The balance between these three operations (i.e., introduce, pass along, discard) can be learned from the impact of the information on fit quality. One benefit is that consequential information from much earlier time periods can be "remembered," and recent, irrelevant information can be rapidly "forgotten." Such RNNs are called "long short-term memory" (LSTM) models, and have proved their worth in handwriting recognition and speech recognition.
- Recurrent neural networks can be restructured in a tree format called a "recursive neural network" (Goodfellow et al. 2016: section 10.6). There can be gains for computation efficiency, and for some applications, the tree format is more natural.
- RNNs can be configured for an analysis of a univariate time series. Given the very rich and powerful set of statistical tools available for time series analysis (e.g., Box et al. 1994), such an approach may be little more than a curiosity. Take a crack at the second exercise for this chapter.

8.3.2.1   Statistical Inference for RNNs

Even without the many variants of RNNs, statistical inference is a challenge. As usual, the first hurdle would be to make the case that the cross-sectional units are generated IID. Training and test data could be constructed by splitting the data pretty much as usual. A random subset of cases and all of their measures over time become the training data. The other cases and all of their measures over time become the test data.

When a single set of cases is selected at random and then followed over time, the case realizations could still be IID, and one would have a repeated measures design (Islam and Chowdhury 2017). Again, the nonparametric bootstrap could be adapted, but any statistical tests or confidence intervals would depend on how the outcome values were analyzed and from that, how to properly take into account any within case dependence.[21] Very similar considerations apply should the data be realized from a joint probability distribution consistent with a panel design or a repeated measures study. In practice, such premises would need to be persuasively argued based on subject-matter expertise and on how the data were collected.[22]

8.3.2.2 RNN Software

At the moment, there appear to be three viable RNN libraries in R. As before, *Keras* provides access to all of the current variants because of its dependence on *TensorFlow*, and the Chollet and Allaire volume (2018) explains the procedure well. As before, *Keras* can be quite finicky and has a relatively steep learning curve, perhaps because it can implement a wide range of RNNs (and other) tools. Communication with Python and *TensorFlow* has been problematic in the past.

A new and more limited competitor is *rnn*. It supports the basic RNN formulation, some deep learning structures, gated hidden layers, and LSTMs. Because it is written in R, it is quite accessible and is relatively easy to use. (But better documentation is needed.) It seems to perform reliably and new features are being added.

The final option is *mxnet* which currently falls between *keras* and *rnn* in flexibility, but lacks good documentation and can be tricky to install. All three are well worth trying—if they work!

The remarkable and growing array of options for RNNs is for most data analysts overwhelming. Mastery of even one RNN requires craft lore enriched by extensive hands-on experience. There seems to be nothing like widely accepted recipes, let alone compelling formal results. The various flavors of RNNs are typically built on sophisticated ideas that can be far ahead credible proofs of performance. A good option for data analysts may be to specialize in RNN variants that seem most appropriate for the kinds of data to be analyzed. There also may be for certain applications powerful options available from statistics and econometrics. Tools for the analysis of longitudinal data have been developed by these disciplines over the past several decades.

8.3.2.3 An RNN Application

We consider now an RNN example for longitudinal data in which for simplicity the single cross sectional unit is a city neighborhood. Ordinarily there are many cross-sectional units that can be people, families, schools, business establishments, or other entities. The response variable is the number of violent crimes reported per week in that neighborhood. There are two predictors: the number of nonviolent street crimes (e.g., trespassing, loitering) per week and a counter for the week itself. How well can one fit the number of violent crimes per week as a function of the number of street crimes and the week counter? The first addresses whether petty crime is related to serious crime. The second addresses trends and seasonal patterns. What makes these data appropriate for an RNN is that all three variables are longitudinal. The notion that petty crime is a harbinger of violent crime is a

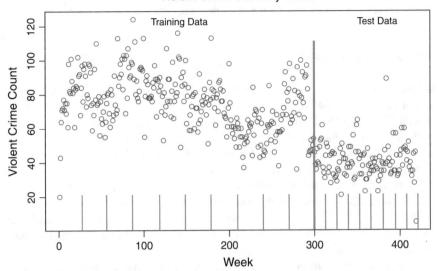

Fig. 8.12 Number of violent crimes by week with the training data, test data for which time segments are represented by short vertical lines, and the transition from training to test data represented by the tall vertical line

key feature of the "broken windows" hypothesis that has shaped crime prevention program in many major cities—"broken windows" is a stand-in for social disarray. These data were chosen because they raise several other important issues as well.

Figure 8.12 is a plot of the number of violent crimes by week. The first 300 weeks are used as training data. The last 119 weeks are used as test data. The training data and test data should be drawn from the same population to which inferences are being made. This follows if the training data and test data are random disjoint splits from the same initial dataset. But the split sample approach stumbles for temporal or spatial data because temporal order or spatial proximity must be maintained; random sampling violates this requirement.

For longitudinal data, researchers commonly use earlier observations for training and later observation for testing. But that can be problematic. In Fig. 8.12, the violent crime counts seem somewhat lower after week 300. We will soon see the consequences.

The 300 weeks of training data are segmented into ten 30 week intervals. Each of the ten intervals is analogous to the times when reinterviews might be undertaken in a panel survey. In effect, the training data has been organized by time into sequential temporal bins, each with an observed conditional mean to approximate using a recurrent neural net. Longitudinal associations between the fitted conditional means will be a direct consequence of longitudinal associations between the ten hidden layers. This follows from the RNN structure, which is a bit like a hidden Markov process. There is no particular substantive reason for how the panels are defined.

The main justification is to have a sufficient number of observations in each panel. In effect, one is using an RNN as a smoother.

There are also ten time intervals in the test data. The number of intervals in the training data and the number of intervals in the test data *must* be the same. Otherwise, the algorithmic structure developed from the training data would not apply to the test data. For this analysis, an important consequence is that the number of weeks included within each test data time interval is smaller than the number of weeks in each training data time interval. In that sense, the likely precision from the training data and test data differs; the test data are less dense.

Figure 8.13 shows the code used for the analysis. Getting the data into the right form constitutes much of the effort. This is common in deep learning applications. To start, one must subset the full data into training and test subsets. For each, the inputs must be separated from the response variable as well.

Then, conventional and sensible practice standardizes the training data.[23] Shown is the min/max transformation. Each variable is scaled so that its values can range from 0 to 1. Each transformed value measures how far that value is shifted from 0 to 1. It is a proportion of that 0–1 distance. One can also transform to z-scores. Without proper scaling, the RNN algorithm is far more difficult to tune and may not make much progress reducing the value of its loss function. Because the RNN weights will not be substantively interpreted, the scaling has no downside.

There are some differences of opinion about how to scale test data. Should the test data be scaled using its own summary statistics (e.g., its maximum and minimum) or should the test data be scaled using the summary statistics from the training data? Beysolow (2017: 92) favors the former. Chollet and Allaire (2018: 92–93) favor the latter. But, the issues can be subtle because a lot depends on the nature of the data (e.g., temporal or cross-sectional) and what kinds of generalizations are being sought. In this application, the reasoning is transparent. Using the training data summary statistics leads to test data values outside the 0–1 range.[24] Consequently, the test data are scaled using their own summary statistics.

Perhaps the most challenging task is to organize the training and test data into appropriate arrays. For *rnn*, there are three dimensions to consider. The first is the number of rows (i.e., cases) in the data. The second is the number of panels, or in this instance, time intervals. The third is the number of predictors. For the training data predictors, there are 30 rows, 10 panels, and 2 inputs. For our training data response variable, there are 30 rows, 10 panels, and 1 response variable. The same structure for rows and panels must be imposed on the test data. One can think of the data format as ten data matrices in ten different time periods with the rows for cases and columns for variables. A temporal structure *within* each time interval is uncommon, although with a bit of tweaking can be used in a conventional, time series, autoregression analysis with an RNN (Beysolow 2017: 120–124). Typically, the panel data will be cross-sectional within time intervals.

Figure 8.14 shows the reduction in L1 loss over epochs (i.e., passes through data). There is no real improvement until about epoch 1000, after which there is a rapid drop followed by gradual improvement. Sharp drops, sometimes called "cliffs" (Goodfellow et al. 2016: section 8.2.4), can cause problems when the very large

```
library(rnn)
## Get data in shape
setwd("~/Documents/R/LASweep")
load("~/Documents/R/LASweep/CrimeData120.rdata")
plot(Crimes[,1],xlab="Week",ylab="Violent Crime Count",
     main="Violent Crime Count by Week",col="blue", cex.main=1)
trainingData<-Crimes[1:300,]; testData<-Crimes[301:400,]
x<-trainingData[,c(2,3)]; y<-trainingData[,1]
xtest<-testData[,c(2,3)]; ytest<-testData[,1]
# MinMax Scale
minmax<-function(x) (x-min(x))/(max(x)-min(x))
# Training data
train_Street<-minmax(x[,1])
train_Streets<-matrix(train_Street,ncol=10,byrow=T)
train_Week<-minmax(x[,2])
train_Weeks<-matrix(train_Week,ncol=10,byrow=T)
train_Serious<-minmax(y)
train_Seriouss<-matrix(train_Serious,ncol=10,byrow=T)
# Test data (Standardized on itself)
test_Street<-minmax(xtest[,1])
test_Streets<-matrix(test_Street,ncol=10,byrow=T)
test_Week<-minmax(xtest[,2])
test_Weeks<-matrix(test_Week,ncol=10,byrow=T)
test_Serious<-minmax(ytest)
test_Seriouss<-matrix(test_Serious,ncol=10,byrow=T)
X<-array(c(train_Streets,train_Weeks),dim=c(30,10,2))
Y<-array(train_Seriouss,dim=c(30,10,1))
Xtest<-array(c(test_Streets,test_Weeks),dim=c(30,10,2))
Ytest<-array(test_Seriouss,dim=c(30,10,1))
## RNN
rnn1<-trainr(Y=Y,
             X=X, learningrate=.1,
             momentum=.5, use_bias = T, network_type = "rnn",
             numepochs = 20000, hidden_dim = c(5,3,1))
save(rnn1,file="rnn1.rdata")
plot(colMeans(rnn1$error),col="Blue",
     xlab="Epoch", ylab="Average L1 Loss",
     main="Average L1 Loss Over 1000 Epochs",cex=.5)
Yp<-predictr(rnn1,X)
plot(colMeans(Yp),ylim=c(.45,.60),type="b",col="blue",
     xlab="Time Period",cex.main=1,
     ylab="Mean Standardized Number of Violent Crimes",
     main="Fitted and Observed Conditional Means in
     The Training data Over 10 Time Intervals")
lines(colMeans(train_Seriouss),col="red",type="b")
text(5,.53,"Actual"); text(5,.50,"Fitted")
Tptest<-predictr(rnn1,Xtest)
plot(colMeans(Tptest),ylim=c(.20,.70),type="b",col="blue",
     xlab="Time Period",cex.main=1,
     ylab="Mean Standardized Number of Violent Crimes",
     main="Fitted and Observed Conditional Means in
     The Test data Over 10 Time Intervals")
lines(colMeans(test_Seriouss),col="red",type="b")
text(5,.33,"Actual");text(5,.58,"Fitted")
```

Fig. 8.13 R code for a recurrent neural network application

Fig. 8.14 Progress of L1 loss
over epochs

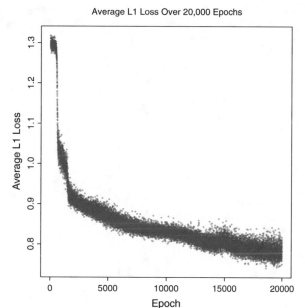

changes in weights move the optimizer far away from the global solution. In this case, the cliff was helpful.[25] But, it took an afternoon of trying different network structures and different tuning parameter values to arrive at instructive results.

Figure 8.15 shows with the training data how well the fitted conditional means track the actual conditional means. The tracking is quite good, although a little low by about 0.05 units on the average for the 0–1 scale. A look back at Fig. 8.10 provides a diagrammatic reminder of the RNN structure used.

Figure 8.16 shows how well the fitted conditional means track the actual conditional means in the test data. As expected, the fitted values are far too large. On the average, the gap is about 20 points on the 0–1 scale. There had been a downward shift in the number of violent crimes per week that was unanticipated in the analysis of the training data. The training data and test data probably are not from the same joint probability distribution. Perhaps that is the general lesson from the analysis.

For many applications, it would be important to have measures of predictor importance and partial dependence plots. Currently, neither are available for *rnn* or other software for recurrent neural nets. That will probably change soon. For this analysis, we cannot separate empirically the impact of street crime from the impact of seasonal patterns.

There will be no attempt to undertake statistical inference. Because of the downward offset in the test data, it is difficult to argue credibly that the data were generated from a single joint probability distribution. The temporal dependence introduces additional complications. We are returned to some issues raised in Chap. 2 when regression splines were applied to data on water use in Tokyo. Finally, even if these difficulties could be circumvented, obtaining a good approximation of

Fig. 8.15 Fitted and actual conditional mean for training data (actual in red and fitted in blue.)

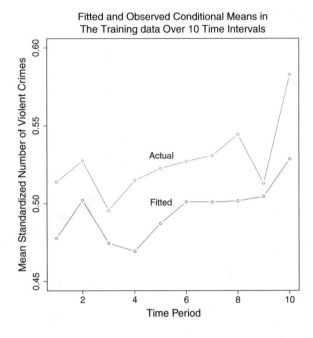

Fig. 8.16 Fitted and actual conditional mean for test data (actual in red and fitted in blue)

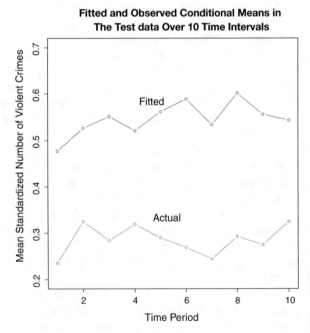

the sampling distributions for summary statistics for the fitted values (e.g., the MSE) is a major challenge. Given the temporal dependence in the data, the usual pairwise bootstrap is the wrong formulation.[26]

In summary, recurrent neural networks provides an interesting alternative to the many existing statistical procedure available for pooled cross section and time series data. However, arriving at satisfactory algorithmic performance requires a substantial time commitment guided primarily by still evolving craft lore. Moreover, new variants of RNNs appear on a regular basis, included in software that is too often of poorly documented and vulnerable to frustrating bugs. It will take at least a year or two before the application of recurrent neural networks becomes sufficiently routinized.[27]

8.3.3 Adversarial Neural Networks

It is commonly accepted in economics that competition is good. All of the competitors are motivated to improve their performance and at least in principle, various forms of optimality may be obtained. These ideas can be applied to learning algorithms. We are still concerned with the distribution of some outcome variable conditional on a set of predictors, but we make the fitting process competitive.

In outline form, there are two neural networks. One tries to solve some problem such as running an electrical power grid. The goal might be to keep the voltage over the grid at relatively a constant amplitude. Any gap between the desired voltage and the actual voltage goes into the loss function. The second algorithm tries to undermine the performance of the first by, for example, attempting to introduce misinformation about grid voltage. The first algorithm might respond by improving barriers to outside misinformation. The two algorithms iterate back and forth so that in the end, the power grid's neural network learns how to be more secure (Joseph et al. 2019).

There is a special form of adversarial learning whose details are beyond the scope of this book, but it is so intriguing that a brief discussion is unavoidable. Generative adversarial networks (GANs) are not only very effective adversarial procedures, but raise epistemological questions about the nature of synthetic data (Goodfellow et al. 2014).

There, again, are two neural networks. The discriminator network tries to determine which images of, say, cats are real and which are phony. The generator network tries to fool the discriminator by producing phony cat images and mixing them in with the true cat images in the training data. With each iteration, both networks will typically improve their performance. The discriminator gets better at distinguishing real images of cats from phony images of cats. The generators get better at producing phony images of cats that are more like real images of cats. The competition ends when the generator has produced phony images that the discriminator cannot distinguish from the real images. The discriminator can do no better than a coin flip because the real and phony images differ by just a bit of unstructured noise. Humans generally cannot tell the difference either.

A bit more abstractly, the discriminator tries to learn the decision boundaries between outcome classes from algorithmic inputs exploiting $f(Y|\mathbf{X})$. The generator tries to learn the inputs for the different outcome classes exploiting $g(\mathbf{X}|Y)$. Y is either real or phony images of cats. $\mathbf{X}$ is the pixels of the input images. There are, however, many important theoretical issues that have just begun to be explored (e.g., Ng and Jordan 2020). Like so many recent developments in machine learning, practice has gotten far in front of theory.

Some have suggested that when the competition ends, the generator has constructed a Platonic ideal of the real thing. One has, for example, the Platonic ideal of a cat from which much can be learned even though the image is synthetic. For example, the mathematical definition of triangle is a Platonic ideal. It does not empirically exist. Yet, one can learn a lot about empirical triangles from the Platonic ideal. This opens the door to constructing many different kinds of synthetic data that may have scientific and policy applications.[28] Use will be made of these ideas in the next chapter when genetic algorithms are introduced.

At the moment, there does not seem to be GANs software in R except for what can be done in *Keras*. There are coding examples that easily can be found on the internet (https://skymind.ai/wiki/generative-adversarial-network-gan). But training GANs is a major challenge. A neural network whisperer may be required.

8.4   Conclusions

As already noted, the advantages of conventional neural networks compared to random forests and gradient boosting are not apparent. For data analysts, there seems to be no need to deploy vanilla neural networks if these other options are available. In marked contrast, convolutional neural networks seems to be the dominant approach for analyses of image data.

The case for recurrent neural nets compared to procedures from statistics and econometrics also is unclear. It is too soon to tell. A lot depends on the kind of data to be analyzed. For, say, speech recognition, RNNs and extensions that include LSTM features are probably best tool. For social science and biomedical applications, such as analyzing panel survey data, conventional econometric methods may work best. And if explanation is the primary goal, RNNs are usually not helpful.

Complicating methods choices further, there are new developments appearing almost daily. GANs are perhaps a powerful example in which technical and philosophical issues are raised. Even for GANs, it can be difficult to separate the hype from the reality, and craft lore is in great flux. Perhaps the best advice is to make a substantial effort to keep current or to work with colleagues who do.

Demonstrations and Exercises

Working with image data is too demanding for exercises in this book. Given the data and available software, there is no easy way to provide hands-on experience. A prerequisite may be a commitment to become facile with *TensorFlow*. Readers who are interested in applying convolution neural networks, nevertheless, may be best served by looking for strong tutorials on the internet (e.g., https://tensorflow. rstudio.com/keras/). There will be some working with the *MNIST* data in particular, although the handwritten digits can be accurately classified with conventional neural networks. Better still would be to work through the Chollet and Allaire textbook (2018). Still, the following exercises are very instructive. Both probably will stretch you.

Set 1

There is an earlier example with code for a "vanilla" neural network with a single binary outcome. How about you try a "vanilla" neural network with two binary outcomes. These are not the two classes from a single binary outcome. They are two separate ("multi-label") binary outcomes.

Install and load the library *DAAG*. Then load the data *nassCDS* and the documentation in *nasshead*. This is a large dataset with information on automobile accidents. A wide variety of analyses could be undertaken, but a relatively simple one will turn out to be challenging enough. Your two binary outcome variables are to be "airbag" and "seatbelt." Your predictors will be "ageOFocc," "yearacc," and "sex." You will use the libraries *neuralnet, NeuralNetTools, and pdp*. These were all used in the earlier neural network illustration (with code). But with two outcome variables, some changes are necessary.

The formula takes the form of $Y_1 + Y_2 \sim X_1 + X_2 + X_3$. The fitted values for Y_1 and Y_2 will be stored in different columns. Take this into account when you construct your confusion tables. For the *olden* procedure in *NeuralNetTools* you will need to specify *out_var* $=$ to get the results for each of the outcomes. For *partial* in the *pdp* library, you will need to specify *out_var* $=$ as well as *pred.var* $=$.

Here are some suggestions. Work with about 1000 training observations and about 1000 test observations. Otherwise you will have to wait quite a while each time you try to tune and run the procedure. Start with a very simple network, and you may need to increase the number of steps. If that runs, try complicating it slightly. It seems to help if the final hidden layer has two nodes. If it runs in a second or two in real time, there is probably something wrong. Check to make sure the fitted values for each outcome vary. Once it runs properly, the confusion tables, Olden measures of importance, and one or more partial plots should look familiar and sensible. Good luck.

Set 2

You can use *rnn* to analyze a univariate time series. The data are a time series of observations of CO2 concentrations measured at Mauna Loa, Hawaii (*co2*, not *CO2*). Your job is to specify and estimate an AR1 model (an autoregression model with a one time period of lagged values of the response) using *rnn* in R. It will help if you begin by drawing the structure of a univariate time series within an RNN. That will help think about how to specify the "*hidden_dim* =" argument. (Hint: you can analogize to the vanilla RNN or the stacked RNN.) Then, if you look back at RNN code provided earlier, you should be able figure out how to proceed. But it will probably take some tinkering.

To get you started in the right direction, below is the code you need to set up the data for *rnn*. If you read the *rnn* documentation carefully you should be able to figure what comes next. Note that the min/max form of standardization is being used.

```
data(co2)
library(rnn)
Ylag<-as.matrix((co2[1:467]-min(co2[1:467])))/
(max(co2[1:467])-min(co2[1:467])))
Y<-as.matrix((co2[2:468]-min(co2[2:468])))/
(max(co2[2:468])-min(co2[2:468])))
```

Once you have acceptable results, compare them to the results from the same AR1 formulation using *lm*. You will need to figure out how to make fair comparisons between the performance of the two approaches to an AR1 model using the exact same data. Think through in practice which procedure would be preferable at least for analyses of univariate time series data. Again, good luck.

Endnotes

[1] The color coding of the arrows in Fig. 8.1 is meant to indicate that each hidden layer m has its own set of weights. These weights typically will differ from one another.

[2] The chain rule for three variables X, Y, and Z is $\frac{dz}{dx} = \frac{dz}{dy}\frac{dy}{dx}$.

[3] The operation of the chain rule is hidden within $\sum_{i=1}^{N} \frac{\partial L_i}{\partial \alpha'_{kl}}$.

[4] The integration functions are a form of regularization because they are a weighted average, much as in gradient boosting when fitted values are linearly combined.

[5] Operationally, the latent variables are just the output from the activation functions applied to the immediately preceding linear combinations. One standardizes output from each activation function for each of the latent variables.

[6] The software in R for neural networks and related tools is at the moment in considerable flux because in R coders are playing catch-up. There is also the major "disruptor" of Google's *TensorFlow 2.0* that implements various forms of deep learning with a user interface in the package *Keras* that makes the procedure reasonably accessible. If one chooses to go all in on deep learning, it probably makes good sense to learn *Keras* and *TensorFlow*. But that might be overkill for plain

vanilla neural networks. More will be said about software for deep learning shortly, but by the time you are reading this, the computing environment in R for neural networks may be quite different.

[7] Formally, the stagewise approach is less desirable. It is better to compute the weights for all layers at once. Better accuracy will usually result. But human time counts too, and small losses in accuracy often can be sensibly traded for large reductions in training time.

[8] A comparison of chapter 9 to chapter 11 in Goodfellow et al. (2016) is a very telling illustration.

[9] A validation dataset is the same as an evaluation dataset.

[10] "Grayscale" is defined differently in different disciplines and even within a single discipline can be numerically represented in different ways. For our purposes, a grayscale is just a numeric variable covering a range of shades from black to white.

[11] To take the next step into formal statistical inference remains a formidable conceptual and computational challenge for the same reasons that surfaced earlier for other learning procedures—but more so with all of the tuning. Still, with access to legitimate test data, uncertainty from newly realized IID data can be addressed taking as fixed the training data and the convolutional neural network structure resolved.

[12] In practice where would be many more pixels. 48 pixels likely are far too coarse.

[13] The mathematical operation to arrive at the sum is the dot product of each filter pixel and its overlaid image pixel.

[14] A convolution is a mathematical operation on two functions in which one function modifies the shape of the other function.

[15] $(3 \times 1) + (3 \times 1) + (3 \times 1) + (2 \times 0) + (2 \times 0) + (2 \times 0) + (1 \times -1) + (1 \times -1) + (1 \times -1) = 6.$

[16] Pixels located at the edges of an image are filtered less often than pixels located elsewhere. In that sense, they are treated as less important. Padding the image can correct for that.

[17] Another heads up on disciplinary differences. The term "tensor" is used to refer to data structures. A scaler is a tensor with 0 dimensions. The number 27 is an example. A vector is a tensor with one dimension. A single variable is an example. A matrix is a tensor with two dimensions. The datasets in earlier chapters are examples: one dimension for cases and another dimension for variables. A three-dimensional array is a tensor with three dimensions, sometimes called a three-dimensional matrix. Panel data from surveys is an example. One dimension is cases, another dimension is time, and another dimension is variables. Images can be represented in a four-dimensional (or more) tensor: rows of the image, columns of the image, the content of each pixel (e.g., color saturation) and case. (Each image is a case.)

[18] When this material was originally written, *Keras* was unable to execute tutorial examples in textbooks and posted on the internet. Even with the assistance for programmers from *GitHub*, there were apparently fundamental incompatibilities between *TensorFlow*, Python 3.7, and *Keras* in R. The problems could be easily reproduced, but not fixed. Such difficulties may occur in the future because as one component is updated, the other components must be updated as well. It is a bit like trying to herd cats. But with the recent release of *TensorFlow 2.0* (i.e., fall of 2019), all of the moving parts seem to be cooperating. Useful didactic material can be found at https://tensorflow.rstudio.com/keras/articles/tutorial_basic_classification.html. But to reiterate: *TensorFlow 2.0* earns its keep on important but very specialized applications. It is not a general purpose algorithmic learning platform and does not respond to many of the issues raised in earlier chapters. And tuning remains a major challenge.

[19] Broadly conceived, s_t is the state of some dynamical system that evolves over time and can be represented as difference equations long popular in economics (Chiang, 1984: chapter 16).

[20] If each time period had its own weights, one could not forecast. One would need to know that values of the new weights for the time period in which the forecasts were being sought. Such weights probably would not be known.

[21] For example, having an indicator variable for each case included as inputs might be helpful, especially if there are a substantial number of points in time for each case. In this instance, the dependence is caused by different levels for different cases.

[22] There has been some interest among deep learning researchers in employing deep learning with graphical models to characterize probability distributions. The issues are very familiar to

statisticians. For example, there have been deep learning applications to what statisticians have long called "multiple imputation" Little and Rubin (2020: chapter 10). The interest in probability distributions naturally leads to inference about posterior distributions from a Bayesian perspective. The work to date seems peripheral to the statistical inference as considered in this book (Cf. Goodfellow et al. 2016: chapters 16 and 19).

[23] The terms "scaling" or "normalizing" are often used instead.

[24] This follows from the drop in the number of reported violent crimes in the test data. Clearly there is a change in level. For the training data, the level can be captured in RNN bias nodes.

[25] For some other network structures and other tunings, a cliff proved fatal. The algorithm moved sharply away from a promising path and was unable to recover over several thousand additional epochs.

[26] There are other possible bootstrap options for temporal data (Kreiss and Paparoditis 2011).

[27] The author of rnn, Bastiaan Quast, is well aware of RNN's limitations and seems committed to providing more features and better documentation. Currently available are extensions to long short-term memory formulations and to gated recurrent units.

[28] This was first brought to my attention by colleagues Michael Kerns and Aaron Roth. It is also from them I first heard the term "neural net whisperers" to characterize people unusually skilled at training neural networks.

References

Beysolow, T. (2017). *Introduction to deep learning in R*. San Francisco: Apress.
Box, G. E. P., Jenkins, G. M., & Reinsel, G. (1994). *Time series analysis: Forecasting & control* (3rd ed.). New York: Prentice Hall.
Chiang, A. C. (1984) *Fundamental methods of mathematical economics* (3rd ed.). New York: McGraw Hill.
Chollet, F., & Allaire, J. J. (2018) *Deep learning with R*. Shelter Island: Manning Publications.
Ghatak, A. (2019). *Deep learning with R*. New York: Springer.
Goodfellow, I., Bengio, Y., & Courville, A. (2016). *Deep learning*. Cambridge: MIT Press.
Goodfellow, I., Pouget-Abadie, J., Mirza, M., Xu, B., Warde-Farley, D., Ozair, S., et al. (2014). Generative adversarial networks. In *Proceedings of the International Conference on Neural Information Processing Systems (NIPS 2014)* (pp. 2672–2680).
Greene, W. H. (2003). *Econometric analysis* (5th ed.). New York: Prentice Hall.
Günther, F., & Fritsch, S. (2010). neuralnet: Training in neural networks. *The R Journal, 2*(1), 30–39.
Hastie, T., Tibshirani, R., & Friedman, J. (2009). *The elements of statistical learning* (2nd ed.). New York: Springer-Verlag.
Hsiao, C. (1986). *Analysis of panel data*. New York: Cambridge University Press.
Islam, M. A., & Chowdhury, R. (2017). *Analysis of repeated measures data*. New York: Springer.
Joseph, A. D., Nelson, B., Rubinstein, P., & Tygar, J. D. (2019). *Adversarial machine learning*. Cambridge: Cambridge University.
Kedem, B., & Fokianos, K. (2002). *Regression models for time series analysis*. New York: Wiley.
Kreiss, J.-P., & Paparoditis, E. (2011). Bootstrap methods for dependent data. *Journal of the Korean Statistical Society, 40*(4), 357–378.
Lapan, M. (2018). *Deep reinforcement learning hands on*. Birmingham: Packt Publishing.
Little, R., & Rubin, D. (2020). *Statistical analysis with missing data* (3rd ed.). New York: John Wiley.
Neal, R., & Zhang, J. (2006). High dimensional classification with Bayesian neural networks and Dirichlet diffusion trees. In I. Guyon, S. Gunn, M. Nikravesh, & L. Zadeh (Eds.), *Feature extraction, foundations and applications*. New York: Springer.

Ng, A. Y., & Jordan, M. J. (2020). On discriminative vs. generative classifiers: A comparison of logistic regression and naive Bayes. In *NIPS*. https://papers.nips.cc/paper/2020-on-discriminative-vs-generative-classifiers-a-comparison-of-logistic-regression-and-naive-bayes.pdf

Pagan, A. (1980). Some identification and estimation results for regression models with stochastically varying coefficients. *Journal of Econometrics, 13*, 341–363.

Ripley, B. D. (1996). *Pattern recognition and neural networks*. Cambridge: Cambridge University Press.

Robinson, P. M. (1989). Nonparametric estimation of time-varying parameters. In P. Hackl (Ed.), *Statistical analysis and forecasting of economic structural change*. Berlin: Springer.

Rosenblatt, F. (1958). The Perceptron: A probabilistic model for information storage and organization of the brain. *Psychological Review, 65*, 386–408.

Rumelhart, D. E., Hinton, G. E., & Williams, R. J. (1986). Learning representations by back-propagating errors. *Nature, 323*, 533–536.

Tucci, M. P. (1995). Time-varying parameters: A critical introduction. *Structural Change and Economic Dynamics, 6*(2), 237–260.

Olden, J. D., Joy, M. K., & Death, R. G. (2004). An accurate comparison of methods for quantifying variable importance in artificial neural networks using simulated data. *Ecological Modeling, 178*, 389–397.

Olson, M., Wyner, A., & Berk, R. A. (2018). Modern neural networks generalize to small data set. In *NIPS Conference Proceedings*

Pascanu, R., Gulcehere, C., Cho, K., & Begio, Y. (2014). How to construct deep recurrent neural networks. arXiv: 13126026v5

Chapter 9
Reinforcement Learning and Genetic Algorithms

Summary There are a wide variety of empirical settings that do not easily fit within an optimization framework and for which results that are "good," but not necessarily the "best," are the only practical option. When business firms compete, for instance, a single firm can dominate a market by "just" being better than its competitors. Over the past decade, reinforcement learning has built on this perspective with considerable success. Although several features of reinforcement learning are some distance from our full regression approach, its promise motivates a brief discussion. Reinforcement learning also is sometimes included as a component of deep learning.

9.1 Introduction to Reinforcement Learning

The menagerie of statistical learning procedures continues to grow, typically in response to challenging empirical and policy problems. Although already a bit dated, curious readers might benefit from several chapters on deep learning in the textbook by Goodfellow et al. (2016). Rather than proceed here with several short sketches of some very recent and rather specialized tools, this chapter considers another and very different approach to machine learning that has broad and powerful applicability. We are still interested in the conditional distribution of some response variable given a set of predictors; we have not fully abandoned our regression perspective. But given all that has been discussed earlier, some mental gymnastics may be required.

Each of the algorithms examined in previous chapters had one or more clear response variables serving as fitting targets and a loss function to be minimized. Differences between the algorithms centered on how the fitted values were learned. The enterprise was optimization, ideally with a convex loss function. One important lesson was that quite often performance differences between the procedures were small.

© Springer Nature Switzerland AG 2020

R. A. Berk, *Statistical Learning from a Regression Perspective*,
Springer Texts in Statistics, https://doi.org/10.1007/978-3-030-40189-4_9

Suppose there is no fitting target defined before the analysis begins, and no loss function to optimize. Is there something useful that still might be produced by a learning algorithm? The resounding answer is yes. The goal is to accomplish some task well, even if not necessarily optimally, and some outcomes are "merely" better than others. In perhaps its simplest form, consider the "n-armed bandit problem" (Sutton and Barto 2018: 25–26). There are n slot machines and a motivated gambler. Each slot machine returns a jackpot with an unknown probability that differs across machines. The gambler seeks to maximize average returns. To do that, the gambler needs to play machines that pay well but also try other machines that might pay better. Exploration must be combined with exploitation in an effective manner. This tradeoff is guided substantially by the reinforcement received from each turn. The strategy employed is invented along the way.

Real world problems are often much messier. Imagine trying to get home from work and getting stuck in near gridlock, rush hour traffic. Your goal is to drive home quickly. Your normal route home is effectively impassable, and you start taking side streets. You know the general direction in which you need to go, but getting there necessarily involves lots of left and right turns down numerous side streets. Eventually you get home. You have learned an alternative route home you can use when your usual route is blocked. It is probably not the optimal alternative route, but if it works well enough, at least compared to your usual route that was effectively precluded.

But that is only a start. Suppose you suspect there are faster routes you could have taken. It would make sense to try some others that might be preferable when the next gridlock occurs. Perhaps some untaken, early turns that seemed to be poor choices would have allowed for later turns more than making up the lost time.

Ideally, you would try all possible routes to identify the route taking you home in the shortest time. That would be an optimization exercise. But a brute-force approach would be impractical and effectively impossible. One can imagine a decision tree representation starting from your place of work with branching sets of choices. If you had 10 choice points and 3 choices available at each (e.g., go left, go right, go straight), there would be nearly 60,000 possible routes. A means must be found to search more efficiently.

Several creative approaches have been proposed (Choudhary 2019), with perhaps the most successful a Monte Carlo Tree Search (Silver et al. 2016). Various branching paths can be followed until a leaf node is reached. These are analogous to the terminal nodes in a regression tree that here provide some amount of reinforcement. For this illustration, leaf nodes with smaller values are more rewarding because they represent shorter travel times; you always wind up at home, but each leaf node shows the time it took to get there.[1]

How is the subset of routes to be tested chosen? Perhaps the easiest method that can have good properties requires that each route to be tested is chosen independently and at random so that each route has the same probability of being selected. But this does not take advantage of information that is obtained sequentially as each route is evaluated. You might learn early, for instance, that starting out with two right turns seems for the subsequent routes tested to lead to shorter travel times than, say, starting out left/right. It would then make sense, therefore, to sample potential routes home more densely if their first two turns are right/right. However, you would not want to overlook routes that had yet to be evaluated. Perhaps they lead to even better outcomes. On occasion, therefore, you should take a randomly chosen gamble on a new route that had not been tested.

The same reasoning would be applied to all choice points. For example, after the initial left/left, you might again have the same choices: left/left, left/right, right/left, and right/right. At each branching choice point, you would balance decisions that have worked well in the past against exploring new paths that have been underexplored or even totally ignored. The balancing means favoring the most promising routes to the leaf nodes. Yet, some "long shots" are also examined. You would have undertaken an exploration–exploitation tradeoff.

There are many additional, artful details in how Monte Carlo Tree Search works that make for entertaining reading (Silver et al. 2016). A proper discussion would take us far afield. But, in the end, the best tree *among those explored* can be chosen for use. One has a very sophisticated and powerful form of reinforcement learning.

Early forms of reinforcement learning have been formalized and expanded in important ways so that, for example, certain forms of optimality can be reintroduced. A proper discussion is beyond our scope. Sutton and Barto (2018) provide excellent introduction. Lapan (2018) discusses a variety of current, deep learning applications in an accessible form. The R library *ReinforcementLearning* does not have the very latest bells and whistles, but is a very good way to apply effectively the foundational ideas (Proellochs 2019). For many analyses, the bells and whistles are at best a distraction.

Despite the many interesting advances, it appears that statistical inference has not yet garnered much attention in reinforcement learning circles, at least as statisticians would judge it. Lapan's (2018) book, for example, contains nothing that probably would qualify. Extensive data snooping built into reinforcement learning creates all of the usual complications. Once again, however, inferential tools capitalizing on training data and test data have some promise as a partial solution. Thinking that through has yet to be done. For example, what should be the estimand?

9.2 Genetic Algorithms

Sometimes computer code written to simulate some natural phenomenon turns out to be a potential data analysis tool. Neural networks seem to have morphed in this fashion. Genetic algorithms appear to be experiencing a similar transformation. Whereas neural networks were initially grounded in how neurons interact, genetic algorithms share the common framework of natural selection. When used to study evolution, they are not tasked with data analysis, either as a data summary tool or as a data generation model. Applied to learning problems, they can proceed as a variant on reinforcement learning.[2]

Suppose there is an optimization problem and an initial population of candidate solutions, each evaluated for their "fitness." Based on that fitness, an initial culling of the population follows; better fitness increases the chances of survival. The survivors "reproduce," but in the process, the algorithm introduces mutations, crossovers, and sometimes other alterations to some of the progeny. Crossovers, for example, produce offspring whose makeup is a combination of the features of two members of the population. Fitness is again evaluated, and the population is culled a second time. The process continues until population fitness attains a target level of fitness (Affenseller et al. 2009: Section 1.2). Thus, genetic algorithms are not "algorithmic" in Breiman's sense. They do not explicitly link inputs to outputs but can be a key component of how the linking gets done.

To illustrate how this can work, consider again neural networks and which links should be included between inputs, latent variables, and outputs. In a somewhat artificial fashion, one part of the fitting challenge can be isolated: what should be the structure of the neural network? The discussion that follows draws heavily from Mitchell's introductory application of genetic algorithms to neural network architecture (Mitchell 1998: 70–71).

Figure 9.1 is a matrix representation of a simple, feedforward, neural network with six inputs $(X1 \ldots X6)$, three latent variables $(Z1 \ldots Z3)$, and one numerical response (Y). There is no feedback. The 1's denote links, and the 0's denote the absence of links. Consistent with usual practice, there are no links between inputs. But there are potential links between inputs, latent variables, and the response that need to be specified. For example, $X5$ is connected to $Z3$, but not the other latent variables. $X6$ is connected to none of the latent variables but is connected directly to Y.

Network #1 is a vector of binary indicators consistent with the figure. The indicators are entered by row, excluding the fixed relationships, as one would read

Fig. 9.1 A matrix representation of simple neural network (A 1 denotes a link and a 0 denotes no link. The red entries can be either a 1 or a 0. The black entries are fixed. Two solution candidates are shown below the matrix.)

A Neural Network in Matrix Format

	X1	X2	X3	X4	X5	X6	Z1	Z2	Z3	Y
X1	—									
X2	0	—								
X3	0	0	—							
X4	0	0	0	—						
X5	0	0	0		—					
X6	0	0	0	0		—				
Z1	1	1	1	1	0	0	—			
Z2	1	0	0	1	0	0	0	—		
Z3	0	0	1	1	1	0	0	0	—	
Y	0	0	0	0	0	1	1	1	1	—

Network #1: 111100100100000111000000001111

Network #2: 110101100100001011000000100111

words in an English sentence. Network #2 is another vector of binary indicators that represents another structure for the six inputs, three latent variables, and one response. Both representations can be seen as candidate solutions for which fitness is measured by a loss function with Y and $\hat{Y}$ as arguments. The algorithm could begin with a substantial number of such candidate solutions. A neural network would be fit with each. The task is to find the neural network specification that minimizes the loss, and that loss will depend in part on the architecture of the network.

What about a brute-force solution? Just try all possible network specifications and find the one with the best fit. However, for all but relatively simple networks, the task may not be computationally feasible. Each possible network specification would require its own set of fitted values. We faced a similar problem earlier when we considered all possible classification trees for a given dataset. Much as a greedy algorithm can provide a method to arrive at a good tree, a genetic algorithm can provide a method to arrive at a good network specification. "Good" should not be read as "best."

One might proceed as follows:

1. Generate a population of N network specifications two of which are illustrated by network #1 and network #2 in Fig. 9.1. There would be some constraints, such as not allowing links between inputs and requiring at least one path from an input to the response. The population of specifications would not be exhaustive.[3]
2. Suppose Y is numeric. As a measure of fitness, compute the mean squared error for each candidate specification. Here, a neural network is applied to each candidate network structure. A smaller mean squared error means that the particular network structure is more fit.
3. Sample with replacement N candidate specifications with the probability proportional to fitness. This, on average, makes the population more fit.
4. Introduce crossovers. Using this new population of size N, choose pairs of candidate specifications with a specified probability (i.e., a tuning parameter). The probability can be small. For example, if there are 500 candidate solutions, perhaps 10 random pairs would be selected. For each selected pair, choose with equal probability a random location in the sequence of 1s and 0s. For example, suppose for network #1 and #2, the equivalent of a coin flip comes up heads. A crossover is required. There are 28 possible break point locations, and suppose the fifth possible break point (going left to right) is randomly selected. The values of 1,1,1,1,0 from network solution #1 would be swapped with values 1,1,0,1,0 from network #2 solution. Sometimes the number of values swapped by design is small (e.g., 6).
5. Introduce mutations. For each candidate solution in the new population, mutate a few of its values with a small probability. This means on occasion changing a 0 to a 1 and a 1 to a 0, where such changes are allowed (e.g., not between inputs).
6. Compute the mean squared error for each of progeny.
7. Repeat steps 2–7 and repeat until there have been a sufficient number of population generations (e.g., 100).

8. Select the network structure from the population of network structures that is most fit (i.e., has the smallest mean squared error).

There are many variations on this basic structure: compute fitness → sample proportional to fitness → crossovers → mutations → repeat from the top. The intent is to capitalize on chance variation that improves fitness.

A bit in the spirit of random forests, there are important chance mechanisms built into genetic algorithms. These, in turn, introduce uncertainty to the results. But just as in random forests, the uncertainty affects algorithmic reliability; are the results replicable?

One could empirically address algorithmic reliability by simply running the algorithm many times and studying the distribution of results. For example, an analogue of the usual 95% prediction interval might be computed for distribution of possible fitness values. A narrow interval could mean that each of the chance outcomes has about the same fitness and that the algorithm can reliably reproduce approximately the same level of fitness.

Such ideas could be expanded to support hypothesis testing. One might test the null hypothesis that two population fitness distribution have the same mean fitness even though their two mutation probabilities were 0.10 and 0.40, respectively. In short, statistical inference might facilitate research on the algorithm itself.

9.3 An Application

As noted several times above, a highly unbalanced distribution of a response variable can present a data analysis challenge for all classifiers. Parametric tools like logistic regression likely will fail miserably, and even powerful adaptive classification procedures, such as random forests, that can capitalize on asymmetric cost ratios, may not perform in a satisfactory manner. If the classification errors for the rare outcome class are given much greater weight, some progress can be made. The algorithm will disproportionately try to fit those cases. But no new information has been added. In effect, the same rare observations are just used over and over, and many important predictor configurations may not be present in the data. Should one have a strong interest in predictor importance or partial dependence associations, very little may be learned. In other words, if there is very accurate classification/forecasting from the marginal distribution of the outcome variable alone, no predictors can improve performance much, and none can be characterized as important. Sometimes genetic algorithms can help. Consider the following example.

For intimate partner violence, police often are soon called back to the same household. However, (thankfully) the chances that an IPV victim will be injured in subsequent incidents are quite small. We draw from data on 22,449 reported IPV incidents in 2013, from a major urban area. Police were dispatched again within that

Fig. 9.2 Risk probabilities
from a logistic regression for
a repeat IPV incident in
which the victim was injured

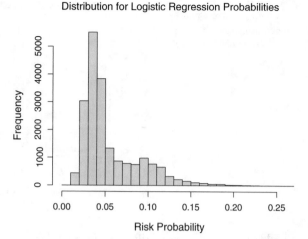

year to about 20% of the same households and in 5% of the repeat cases, injuries to
the victim by the same perpetrator were reported (Details can be found in Berk and
Sorenson (2019).) The forecasting challenge is to predict which perpetrators will
injure their victims in a repeat incident. Because special reporting forms had been
designed 2 years earlier, an unusually rich, and perhaps unique, set of predictors was
obtainable.[4]

For those predictors, Fig. 9.2 shows the distribution of fitted values from a logistic
regression using as the response of whether a given perpetrator committed a repeat
IPV crime in which the victim was injured. The other class was either (1) the
absence of any reported, repeat IPV incident, or (2) a reported, repeat IPV incident
in which the victim was uninjured. The mass of the fitted probabilities for a repeat
IPV incident with injuries is centered around 0.04, and none exceeds 0.30. Using
the standard .50 threshold, no perpetrator would be forecasted to commit a new IPV
crime in which the victim is injured. The unsatisfactory statistical performance was
anticipated (Berk and Bleich 2013).

When the misclassification errors for the rare outcome class were weighted
ten times more heavily, and stochastic gradient boosting, implemented with the
R library *gbm*, was employed as the classifier, Fig. 9.3 shows the results. The
distribution of risk probabilities is dramatically improved, and a substantial number
of perpetrators are forecasted to commit repeat IPV in which there are victim
injuries. However, because of the 10 to 1 weighting, many of those forecasted to
re-offend were false positives. In addition, there was little credible information
about predictor importance or about partial dependence associations with the
response. The algorithm worked harder to classify perpetrators who were violent
repeat offenders, but still had no new information on a wider range of predictor
configurations that might have improved forecasting accuracy.

We turned to a genetic algorithm *GA* in R, using the boosted algorithmic structure
learned from the training data as a fitness function.[5] Cases with larger probabilities

Fig. 9.3 Risk probabilities
for whether an IPV victim is
injured from test data using
stochastic gradient boosting

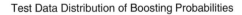

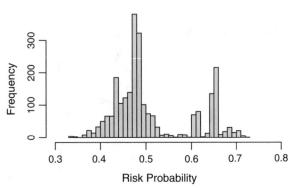

of committing a new IPV crime in which the victim was injured were defined as more fit. For the *GA* algorithm, all of the predictors were either originally indicator variables or were recoded to be indicator variables. A perpetrator could be over 30 years of age or not. A perpetrator could have a prior record of IPV incidents or not. Or there could be children present or not. It was then possible to proceed with essentially the same sequence of *GA* operations just described.

The probability that an indicator predictor would have its value mutated from 1 to 0 or from 0 to 1 was set to 0.10. Altering the probability to 0.05 or 0.25 made no meaningful difference except for sometimes increasing the number of populations needed before no further improvement was obtained. The probability of a crossover ("sexual reproduction") between a random pair of perpetrators was set to 0.80. Setting that value as low as 0.10 did not change the results in an important way, although again, sometimes the number of populations needed changed somewhat. The default crossover method was a "single point" procedure; for a single randomly chosen perpetrator, all predictor values for columns to the right of a randomly chosen column are interchanged with the values from the same columns for another randomly chosen perpetrator (Umbarkar and Sheth 2015: Section 2.1). By default, the fittest 5% of the cases automatically survived to the next generation with no changes. Otherwise, sampling was proportional to fitness. Many of the background details can be found in Scrucca (2014). In the end, we had a population of 500 very high risk perpetrators.

Figure 9.4 displays the distribution of risk probabilities in the final population of offenders selected by the genetic algorithm. Virtually all perpetrators are predicted to engage in a new IPV incident in which the victim is injured. The mass of the data falls a little above 0.70; the algorithm performed as hoped. Code for the application of the *GA* is shown in Fig. 9.5. It assumes access to the earlier stochastic gradient boosting output from *gbm*, which provided the fitness function.

Predictors were defined as important determinants of the fitted values if they had the *same* value (i.e., either a 1 or a 0) for all 500 perpetrators; their values were

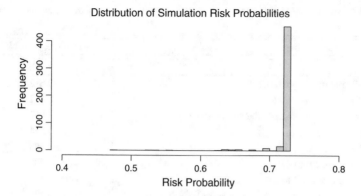

Fig. 9.4 Risk probabilities from the genetic algorithm

```
## Genetic Algorithm Application
load("gbm2.rdata") # Get the earlier gbm results
library(GA) # load GA library
library(gbm) # load gbm library

# The function f says for some data inputs x
# get the fitness value from gbm output.
# Fitness is the fitted probability.

f<-function(x, gbmMod) # To compute fitness function
{
  x <- matrix(x, nrow=1) # matrix with one row
  x <- data.frame(x) # make a data frame
  names(x) <- gbm2$var.names # give columns their names
  return( predict(gbmMod, newdata=x, n.trees=12,
          type="response") ) # embed usual predict function
}

## Initialize with all predictors set to 1
## set start values for all variable values
## use results from output gbm2.

f(rep(1,34), gbmMod=gbm2) # needed arguments
ga3<-ga(type="binary",fitness=f,lower=rep(0,34),
          upper=rep(1,34),pcrossover=.8,
          nBits=34,popSize = 500,gbmMod=gbm2,
          maxiter=100,pmutation = 0.1)
save(ga3,file="ga3.rdata")
```

Fig. 9.5 R code for genetic algorithm using earlier gbm output

Table 9.1 Mean risk probabilities computed by reverse coding with predictors in order of importance

Predictor reverse coding	Mean risk probability
None	0.718
Prior IPV reports: 1.0 to 0.0	0.612
Furniture in disarray: 0.0 to 1.0	0.642
Contact information given to the victim: 0.0 to 1.0	0.662
Victim strangled: 1.0 to 0.0	0.664
Offender polite: 0.0 to 1.0	0.683
Offender < 30: 1.0 to 0.0	0.700
Offender arrested: 1.0 to 0.0	0.701
A prior PFA (i.e., protection from abuse order): 1.0 to 0.0	0.709
Victim < 30: 1.0 to 0.0	0.712

universally shared. We could then measure their impact on the fitted probabilities with reverse coding. For each predictor, we changed either an existing 1 to a 0 or an existing 0 to a 1 and then computed how much the average risk probability declined. In effect, perpetrators were being made less fit. This is in the same spirit as the predictor shuffling methods for variable importance provided by random forests.

At the top of Table 9.1 is the baseline. When the values of the predictors are set as the genetic algorithm directed, the mean fitted probability of a repeat incident in which the victim was injured is 0.718. Then, each predictor in turn was reverse coded, and the mean probability computed again. The drop in the average risk probability is a very direct measure of each predictor's impact on the fitted values. For example, when the existence of prior IPV is reversed to no such prior, the average risk probability drops from 0.718 to 0.612 (i.e., a little more ten probability points).

How "real" are the perpetrators constructed by the genetic algorithm? Although none of the actual offenders had predictor values that were all identical to those of any members of the selective, very high risk population, a substantial number were close. The genetic algorithm constructed a population that was a little worse than all of the worst, real perpetrators, but not a collection of science fiction monsters. Alternatively, the synthetic population perhaps has use as Platonic ideal, IPV perpetrators from which one can learn. A more detailed discussion can be found in Berk and Sorenson (2019).

The analysis raises a number of problems for statistical inference. In contrast to earlier applications of stochastic gradient boosting, the analysis only used training data. More fundamentally, it is unclear what joint probability distribution is relevant for synthetic data or what is being estimated. As before, however, the uncertainty in the algorithm itself can be explored.

9.4 Conclusions

Genetic algorithms alter the distribution of a response variable conditional on a set of predictors. One also can see why genetic algorithms are said to "learn" and why there are connections to reinforcement learning. The algorithms discover what works. With steps that have parallels in natural selection, solutions that are more fit survive. In contrast to conventional optimization methods like gradient descent, there is no overall loss function being minimized. Still, a solution is likely to be good in part because of built-in random components that help to prevent a GA algorithm from getting mired in less desirable, local results. For these and other more technical reasons, genetic algorithms can be folded into discussions of machine learning. They can also be a key feature of recent developments in deep learning when conventional machine learning may be overmatched (Lapan 2018).

Demonstrations and Exercises

An important question for genetic algorithms is how much the results depend on the mutation and crossover probabilities. Although this is no doubt dataset and task specific, it can be productively examined. There is also a question about whether populations that are equally fit are the same or different in their other characteristics. Is there more than a way to be the most fit? At the very least, these exercises will provide lots of hands-on practice with the genetic algorithm *GA*.

Set 1

Load the *pima.te* in the *MASS* library and fit stochastic gradient boosting with diabetes coded 0 and no diabetes coded 1. The fitted probabilities can be used as a measure of fitness (i.e., those with higher probabilities of not having diabetes are more fit) and as such can be used as a fitness function. Apply the genetic algorithm *GA* trying various values for the crossover and mutation probabilities. You are aiming to construct a hypothetical population of individuals who have a very small chance of getting diabetes. What do you learn about the impact of those tuning parameters? Do they matter? If so, in what ways? (You will probably need to read Scrucca's 2013 paper to get some of the necessary details on *GA*'s tuning parameters.)

Set 2

From the preceding exercise select your most fit population. To do this, you will need to figure out a sensible way how to measure "most fit." If you have several populations that are effectively "most fit" pick any one.

You will now have a hypothetical low risk population (i.e., unlikely to get diabetes). What can you learn about the predictors that characterize this hypothetical population? There are several ways one might try to answer this question and no single right way. You will need to think this through and then probably write some code. It is not likely that an off-the-shelf procedure will be fully satisfactory. (Hint: Take a look at what information the algorithm retains in *ga-class*.)

Repeat this with the second most fit population or another hypothetical population that is equally fit. Are the predictors that characterize this population the same? What are the implications of what you learned?

Endnotes

[1] In our gridlock example, the set of possible decisions is fixed and does not depend on what choices you make. Among the most exciting applications of tree search algorithms involve playing against some opponent who reacts to your decisions and counters by changing the mix of choices you have available. The setting is adversarial. A game of checkers is a simple example. With each alternative move, the available decisions and their consequences can change. The most impressive performance to date is by Google's AlphaGo AI that beat the best Go player in the world. A discussion of adversarial reinforcement learning is beyond the scope of this book in part because the regression formulation is a stretch. The setting is a game. See Silver et al. (2016). It is very cool stuff.

[2] There is some disagreement about whether genetic algorithms should be seen as reinforcement learning, and there are indeed some important differences (Sutton and Barto 2018: 8–9). This section can be productively read even if genetic algorithms are at least a distant cousin to reinforcement learning.

[3] The manner in which the initial population is generated often does not matter a great deal. For example, an initial population of 500 could be composed of 500 identical network specifications. Variation in the population is introduced later.

[4] The new form was designed by Susan B. Sorenson in collaboration with the local police department (Berk and Sorenson 2019).

[5] GA is written by Luca Scrucca. It is rich in options and features that work well. The documentation in R is a little thin, but additional background material is available in Scrucca (2014, 2017). It has a substantial learning curve if one wants to master its many variants.

References

Affenseller, M., Winkler, S., Wagner, S., & Beham, A. (2009). *Genetic algorithms and genetic programming: Modern concepts and practical applications.* New York: Chapman & Hall.

Berk, R. A., & Bleich, J. (2013) Statistical procedures for forecasting criminal behavior: A comparative assessment. *Journal of Criminology and Public Policy, 12*(3), 515–544.

Berk, R. A., & Sorenson, S. (2019). An algorithmic approach to forecasting rare violent events: An illustration based on IPV perpetration. arXiv: 1903.00604v1.

Choudhary, A. (2019). Introduction to Monte Carlo tree search: The game-changing algorithm behind DeepMind's AlphaGo. *Analytics Vidhya*, Jan 23. https://www.analyticsvidhya.com/blog/2019/01/monte-carlo-tree-search-introduction-algorithm-deepmind-alphago/

Goodfellow, I., Bengio, Y., & Courville, A. (2016). *Deep learning*. Cambridge: MIT Press.

Lapan, M. (2018). *Deep reinforcement learning hands on*. Birmingham: Packt Publishing.

Mitchell, M. (1998). *An introduction to genetic algorithms*. Cambridge: MIT Press.

Proellochs, N. (2019). *Reinforcement learning in R*. https://cran.r-project.org/web/packages/ReinforcementLearning/vignettes/ReinforcementLearning.html

Scrucca, L. (2014). GA: A package for genetic algorithms in R. *Journal of Statistical Software, 53*(4), 1–37.

Scrucca, L. (2017). On some extensions to GA package: Hybrid optimisation, parallelisation and islands evolution. *The R Journal, 9*(1), 187–206.

Silver, D., Huang, A., Maddison, C.J., Guez, A., Sifre, L., van den Driessche, G., et al. (2016). Mastering the game of go with deep neural networks and tree search. *Nature, 529*(28), 484–489.

Sutton, R. S., & Barto, A. G. (2018). *Reinforcement learning* (2nd ed.). Cambridge: A Bradford Book.

Umbarkar, A. J., & Sheth, P. D. (2015). Crossover operators in genetic algorithms: A review. *ICTACT Journal of Soft Computing, 6*(1), 1083–1092.

Chapter 10
Integrating Themes and a Bit of Craft Lore

Summary By the time this chapter has been reached, a great deal of information has been provided. Thoughtful readers have no doubt been trying to extract some general themes beyond the technical details. The next two sections aim to provide some help.

10.1 Some Integrating Technical Themes

Over the past decade, the number of statistical learning procedures that can be viewed as a form of regression has grown rapidly. Typically, they are minor variants on or inconsequential extensions of the procedures discussed in earlier chapters. In contrast, augmentations of neural networks under the rubric of deep learning are major advances for particular kinds of data and the specialized analyses they require. There have also been important developments in formal theory in statistics and computer science, but unfortunately, the gap between theory and practice continues to grow. Much of the useful guidance that exist comes from craft lore and artful hand-waving.

The heterogeneity in concepts, language, and notation that learning algorithms bring can obscure several important commonalities.

1. Statistical learning can be organized into three frameworks: supervised learning, unsupervised learning, and semisupervised learning. We have focused exclusively on supervised learning. In statistical language, it has all been about regression analysis and $Y|X$. Within that structure, deep learning is an important special case.
2. Statistical learning is undertaken with algorithms, not models. Algorithms "merely" compute things. Models are statements about how the world works. A failure to act on that distinction can lead to all sorts of grief.

© Springer Nature Switzerland AG 2020   415
R. A. Berk, *Statistical Learning from a Regression Perspective*,
Springer Texts in Statistics, https://doi.org/10.1007/978-3-030-40189-4_10

3. The relevance is artificial intelligences is obscure because there is no agreement on how artificial intelligence is defined. For example, some define artificial intelligence as the ability of a machine to sense its environment and respond adaptively to that information. Yet, the thermostat in your place of work or residence does exactly that.

4. When seen as various forms of regression analysis, all of the learning algorithms we have considered attempt to adaptively construct complex sets of fitted values that are responsive to the data on hand. The means by which this is done can vary, but the quest is the same.

5. The pursuit of sufficiently complex fitted values makes the fitted values very vulnerable to overfitting. Regularization, therefore, is a necessary part of the fitting exercise. There is a dizzying array of regularization methods that can be used alone or in various combinations. But the aim for all is to counter overfitting.

6. Regularization does not address data snooping, and data snooping is nearly universal in statistical learning. Learning algorithms commonly automate the search for agreeable results and discard results that do not qualify. Tuning toward the same end is standard. Data snooping is a fundamental challenge to all Level II analyses and all statistical inference in particular. Test data can help, but the existing tools are not fully satisfactory.

7. The use of test data can promote valid estimation, statistical tests, and confidence/prediction intervals, but typically the training data and computed algorithmic structure is fixed. Because an important source of uncertainty is ignored, the estimation precision commonly is too optimistic. If nevertheless, confidence/prediction intervals are too wide or statistical tests have insufficient power, precision would likely be worse if it were possible to include all sources of uncertainty.

8. Although there are fallback options in certain circumstances, the common prerequisite for any statistical inference is IID data from a substantively relevant, joint probability distribution. Then an appropriate estimand must be defined, ideally justified by more than intuition. It is not likely to be a functional of the true response surface, but rather a functional of an acknowledged approximation.

9. The dance between complex fitted values and regularization to ameliorate overfitting leads to black box procedures. One can get fitted values that perform very well, but the role of the predictors responsible is typically obscure. There are auxiliary algorithms that can help (e.g., partial dependence plots), and more such advances are in the offing.

10. The black box problem underscores that statistical learning procedures depend on algorithms, not models, in which ends can justify means. If one's primary data analysis goal to explain, statistical learning is not likely to be helpful, and formal causal inference is typically off the table. When feasible, one then is better off doing experiments.

11. Statistical learning also is not properly used for feature selection or dimension reduction. There are far better statistical tools for such activities. Employing statistical learning instead can lead to very misleading results.

12. Subject-matter expertise and extensive knowledge about how the data were collected are under-appreciated contributors to statistical learning. To repeat a warning from Chap. 1, without such contributions, one risks building a statistical bridge to nowhere, or worse, to the wrong place.

10.2 Integrating Themes Addressing Ethics and Politics

In practice, there are at least as many challenges applying learning algorithms in real settings as in their technical content. This is not the venue to address the issues in any depth. But, it may be a good venue for a heads up.

There is so much new literature being produced that an internet search is probably the best way to begin a deep dive into the material. One can get a taste the challenges in criminal justice setting from the paper by Huq (2019) and in public health applications from papers by Mooney and Pejaver (2018) and Obermeyer et al. (2019).

To illustrate briefly, we focus on "fairness" in the criminal justice system. Risk assessments are commonly undertaken at various decision points and these risk assessments — forecasts of "future dangerousness" — are sometimes done with learning algorithms. A common complaint is that the assessments of risk are biased because the algorithms "bake-in" bias contained in criminal justice data. There certainly are legitimate concerns about how bias can be built into criminal justice risk assessments. But the issues are subtle and complicated.

Several different kinds of fairness have been defined, some of which are incompatible with one another (Berk et al. in press). For example, equality of outcome can be very difficult to reconcile with equality of treatment. Thus, men in the United States are vastly overrepresented in federal and state prisons compared to women. Gender is a legally protected class. One has, therefore, inequality of outcome about which one could litigate. But, there is no dispute that men commit the vast major of violent crimes. Men around the world have a higher base rate for violent crime. In part because in the United States a felony conviction for a crime of violence is likely yield a prison sentence, men are far more likely than women to be incarcerated.

It would be possible to reduce the overrepresentation of men in prison by discounting at charging and sentencing the seriousness of violent crimes committed by men. Inequality of outcome at least could be reduced. But to achieve a greater equality of outcome, one would have introduced inequality of treatment; male felons would be treated differently from female felons even if convicted for the very same kind of violent crime. By reducing one kind of unfairness, another kind of unfairness has been increased. In this instance, the tradeoff is created in part by the different base rates for violent crimes for men compared to women.

There are also tradeoffs with accuracy. If a learning algorithm is designed to optimize some loss function, constraints placed on the optimization will reduce accuracy. It is relatively easy to impose certain fairness requirements on risk assessment algorithms, but more forecasting errors will be made. There will be, for instance, a greater number of individual incarcerated unnecessarily because their forecasted risk was inaccurately too high. There will also be a greater number of dangerous felons inappropriately released on probation because their forecasted risk was inaccurately too low. In the extreme, everyone can be equally worse off.

These are the sorts of difficult tradeoffs inherent in criminal justice risk assessments. Some progress can be made if all parties understand that no risk algorithm will error free or totally fair. The benchmark should not be perfection. The proper and sensible aspiration is to improve on current practice. Sometimes that is very easy to do. Sometimes it is not.

Unfortunately, some stakeholders approach the issues with unbending ideological positions that cannot be changed by facts. Subtle consideration of the many tradeoffs cannot be undertaken. A political stalemate can follow or perhaps worse, an ill-considered set of policies remain in place or are introduced. One can hope that as algorithmic risk assessment becomes more common, coupled with proper oversight, and demonstrably improves practice, greater rationality will prevail. But one also should never underestimate the inertia inherent in large bureaucracies. Organizational self-interest matters too.

Equally vexing issues and conflicts apply to a wide range of algorithmic applications. Consider facial recognition algorithms, mortgage lending by algorithm, algorithm-targeted disinformation over the internet, and the new concerns about "deep fake" news. These illustrate the kinds of risks one often faces bringing algorithmic procedures into the market or the policy process. And typically there are no technical solutions. The solutions, assuming they can be found, will be determined by legal and political processes.

Perhaps most fundamentally, there is the John Henry problem: the understandable tensions between gains in efficiencies ceding human activities to machines and the loss of day-to-day activities that help anchor one's sense of self, the functioning of households, the structure of communities, and the performance of markets. As the John Henry legend underscores, this is not a new phenomenon, despite a doomsday scenarios popular in science fiction, mass media, and even from some very well informed commentators. The 2015 open letter on artificial intelligence is perhaps the best illustration of a balanced assessment (https://futureoflife.org/ai-open-letter/). There are surely important societal impacts that need to be anticipated and addressed, but whether the human condition is about to experience dramatic and rapid change should remain an open question.

10.3   Some Suggestions for Day-to-Day Practice

Sometimes it is best to focus on things that one can control. Because the day-to-day training and deploying of algorithms is usually in the hands of an analyst, we turn to some craft lore that can help.

10.3.1 Choose the Right Data Analysis Procedure

Recall Breiman's distinction between two cultures: a "data modeling culture" and an "algorithmic modeling culture" (2001b).[1] The data modeling culture favors the generalized linear model and its various extensions. A data analysis begins with a mathematical expression meant to represent the mechanisms by which nature works. Estimation serves to fill in the details. The algorithmic modeling culture is concerned solely with linking inputs to outputs. The subject-matter mechanisms connecting the two are not represented and there is, therefore, no a priori vehicle by which inputs are transformed into outputs. A data analysis is undertaken to assemble computational machinery that fits the data well. There is no requirement whatsoever that nature's machinery is revealed.

But, often there is in practice no clear distinction between procedures that belong in the data modeling culture and procedures that belong in the algorithmic modeling culture. In both cultures, information extracted from data is essential. Even for a correct regression model, parameters estimates are obtained from data. Rather, there is a continuum characterized by how much the results depend on substantively informed constraints imposed on the analysis. For conventional regression, at one extreme, there are extensive constraints meant to represent the means by which nature proceeds. At the other extreme, random forests and stochastic gradient boosting mine associations in the data with virtually no substantively informed restrictions. Many procedures, such as those within the generalized additive model, fall in between.

How then should data analysis tools be selected? As a first cut, the importance of explicitly representing nature's role should be determined. If explanation is the dominant data analysis motive, procedures from the data modeling culture should be favored. If prediction is the dominant data analysis motive, procedures from the algorithmic modeling culture should be favored. If neither is dominant, procedures should be used that are a compromise between the two extremes.

If one is working within the data modeling culture, the choice of procedures is determined primarily by the correspondence between subjective-matter information available and features of a candidate modeling approach. The correspondence should be substantial. For example, if nature is known to proceed through a linear combination of causal variables, a form of conventional regression may well be appropriate.

Working within the algorithmic modeling culture, the choice of procedures is primarily determined by out-of-sample performance. One might hope that through formal mathematics and forecasting contests, clear winners and losers could be identified. Unfortunately, the results are rarely definitive. One major problem is that the forecasting performance is typically dataset specific; accuracy depends on particular features of the data that can differ across datasets. A winner on one forecasting task will often be a loser on another forecasting task. Another major problem is how to tune the procedures so that each is performing as well as it can on a given dataset. Because the kinds and numbers of tuning parameters vary across algorithmic methods, there is usually no way to insure that fair comparisons are being made. Still another problem is that a lot depends on exactly how forecasting performance is measured. For example, the area under an ROC curve will often pick different winners from those evaluated by cost-weighted classification error.

However, most of the algorithmic methods emphasized in earlier chapters can perform well in a wide range of applications. In practice, perhaps the best strategy is for a data analyst to select a method that he or she adequately understands, that has features responding best to the application at hand, and that has the most instructive output. For example, only some of the procedures discussed can easily adapt to classification errors that have asymmetric costs, and some can handle very large datasets better than others. The procedures can also differ by whether there are, for example, partial dependence plots and how variable importance is measured.

There are also several practical attributes that can help a data analyst chose a preferred learner. Among these criteria are:

1. *ease of use*—A combination of the procedure itself and the software with which it is implemented[2];
2. *readily available software*—R usually a good place to start in part because commercial packages are often several years behind[3];
3. *good documentation*—for both the procedure and the software[4];
4. *adaptability*—favor procedures and their software that can be easily adapted to unanticipated circumstances such as the need for test data;
5. *processing speed*—a function of the procedure, the number of observations, the number of variables, quality of the code (e.g., parallelization), and the hardware available (e.g., GPUs versus CPUs)[5];
6. *ease of dissemination*—some procedures and some kinds of output are easier to explain to users of the results;
7. *special features of the procedure*—examples include the ability to handle classification with more than two classes, ways to introduce asymmetric costs from fitting errors, and tools for peering into the black box; and
8. *cost*—some commercial products can be quite pricey.

If there is no clear winner, it can always be useful to apply more than one procedure and report more than one set of results.

10.3.2   Get to Know Your Software

There is not yet, and not likely to be in the near future, a consensus on how any of the various statistical learning procedures should be implemented in software. For example, a recent check on software available for support vector machines found in R alone working code for over a half dozen procedures. There is, as well, near anarchy in naming conventions, and notation. Thus, the term "cost," for instance, can mean several different things and a symbol such as γ can be a tuning parameter in one derivation and a key distributional feature in another derivation.

One cannot assume that a description of a procedure in a textbook (including this one) or a journal article corresponds fully to software using the very same name, even by the same authors. Consequently, it is very important to work with software for which there is good technical documentation for the procedures and algorithms being used. There also needs to be clear information on how to structure inputs, obtain outputs, and tune. Descriptions of two computer programs can use the same name for different features, or use very different names for the same features. And in either case, the naming conventions may not correspond to the naming conventions in the technical literature.

Even when the documentation looks to be clear and complete, a healthy dose of skepticism is useful. There are sometimes errors in the documentation, or in the software, or in both. So, it is usually important to "shake down" any new software with data that have previously been analyzed properly to determine if the new results make sense. Moreover, it is usually helpful to experiment with various tuning parameters to see if the results make sense.

It is also very important keep abreast of software updates, which can come as often as five or six times a year. As a routine matter, new features are added, existing features are deleted, bugs fixed, and documentation rewritten. These changes are often far more than cosmetic. Working with an older version of statistical learning software can lead to unnecessary problems.

Finally, a key software decision is whether to work primarily with shareware such as found in R or Python, or with commercial products. The tradeoffs have been discussed earlier at various points. Cost is certainly an issue, but perhaps more important is the tension between having the most current software and having the most stable software and documentation. Shareware is more likely to be on the leading edge, but often lacks the convenience and stability of commercial products. One possible strategy for individuals who are unfamiliar with a certain class of procedures is to begin with a good commercial product, and then once some hands-on skill has been developed, migrate to shareware.[6]

10.3.3 Do Not Forget the Basics

It is very easy to get caught up in the razzle-dazzle of statistical learning and for any given data analysis, neglect the elementary fundamentals. All data explorations must start with an effort to get "close" to the data. This requires a careful inspection of elementary descriptive statistics: means, standard deviations, histograms, cross-tabulations, scatterplots, and the like. It also means understanding how the data were generated and how the variables were measured. Moving into a statistical learning procedure without this groundwork can lead to substantial grief. For example, sometimes numeric values are given to missing data (e.g., -99). Treating these entries as legitimate values can seriously distort any data analysis, including ones undertaken with statistical learning.

It will often be helpful to apply one or more forms of conventional regression analysis before moving to statistical learning. One then obtains an initial sense of how good the fit is likely to be, of the likely signs of key relationships between predictors and the response, and of problems that might be more difficult to spot later (e.g., does one really have a weak learner?). An important implication is that it will often be handy to undertake statistical learning within a software environment in which a variety of statistical tools can be applied to the same data. This can weigh against single-purpose statistical learning software. However, one must think through if data snooping is involved and what its consequences might be. Staying at a Level I analysis, for instance, will help a lot. So will limiting the data exploration to training data when for a Level II analysis there also are test data.

To take one simple example, a tuning parameter in random forests may require a distinct value for each response class. But the order in which those arguments are entered into the expression for the tuning parameter may be unclear. In the binary case, for example, which category comes first? Is it $\omega = c(1, 0)$ or $\omega = c(0, 1)$? A wrong choice is easily made. Random forests will run for either and generate sensible-looking output. But the analysis has not been tuned as it should have been. It can be difficult to spot such errors unless one knows the marginal distribution of the response variable and the likely sign of relationships between each predictor and the response. A few cross-tabulations and a preliminary regression analysis with training data can help enormously. Subject-matter knowledge will also be important.

10.3.4   Getting Good Data

As noted many times, there is no substitute for good data. The fact that boosting, for example, can make weak classifiers stronger, does not mean that boosting can make weak data stronger. There are no surprises in what properties good data should have: a large number of observations, little measurement error, a rich set of predictors, a reasonably well-balanced response variable distribution, and IID data from an appropriate joint probability distribution. It is very important to invest time and resources in data collection. One cannot count on statistical learning successfully coming to the rescue. Indeed, some forms of statistical learning can be quite fussy and easily pulled off course by noisy data, let alone data that have substantial and systematic measurement error. And when the response variable is highly unbalance or badly skewed, finding that needle in a haystack requires first having And when the response variable is highly unbalance or badly skewed, finding that needle in a haystack requires first having a very large haystack.

The case for having legitimate test data is very strong. That is, one needs IID test data from the joint probability distribution responsible for the training data. Sample splitting is also an option, especially if the number of observations is large. Algorithmic learning procedures that use out-of-bag data or the equivalent may not formally need a test dataset. The out-of-bag observations can serve that purpose. But most algorithmic learning procedures currently are not designed generate random samples of the data, even when that might make a lot of sense. Therefore, having access to test data is usually essential.

Even for random forests, test data beyond the out-of-bag observations can come in handy. Comparisons between how random forests perform and how other approaches (including conventional regression) perform are often very instructive. For example, one might learn that the key relationships are linear and that it is not worth losing degrees of freedom fitting more complex functions. Yet such comparisons cannot be undertaken unless there are test data shared by all of the statistical procedures likely to be used.

10.3.5 Match Your Goals to What You Can Credibly Do

Much of the early literature on statistical and machine learning was formulated around some $f(X)$. There is a real function, adopted by nature, through which the data were generated. An essential goal of a data analysis is to recover the data-generating function from a dataset. It can be very tempting, therefore, to frame all supervised learning in a similar manner.

But, one of the themes of this book has been that more modest goals are likely to be appropriate. Algorithmic learning is not built around a conventional model of the data generation process. Ideally, the data are realized IID from a joint probability distribution. But data analysts will usually not have access to all of the important predictors, let alone predictors that are all well measured. Various kinds of data snooping will often be impossible to avoid. For these and other reasons, a Level I analysis may be the primary enterprise. The generative $f(X)$ is irrelevant.

There will be circumstances when a Level II analysis can be justified and properly undertaken. These circumstances are addressed in various sections of the book. There are two major take-home messages. First, the algorithmic output will depend on an approximation of the true response surface or more abstractly, population functionals of interest. Second, assume-and-proceed statistics must be avoided. The case for a Level II analysis must be made.

Although causal thinking can be important as the research task is being formulated and the data are being collected, statistical learning is not designed for Level III analyses. It can be very tempting to use some forms of statistical learning output, such as variable importance plots, to make causal statements. But the various definitions of importance do not comport well with the canonical definition of a causal effect, and the output is not derived from a causal model. There is some very new work that proposes to use statistical learning for causal inference within the "doubly robust" framework introduced in the boosting chapter, but in that setting, statistical learning is just a fancy way to improve the usual covariance adjustments. Statistical learning is not deployed in a stand-alone manner.

An important implication of the difficulties with Level III analyses is that using algorithmic learning procedures to do variable selection can lead to a conceptual swamp. If the purpose is to screen for "important" causal variables, it is not apparent how the statistical learning output is properly used for that purpose. This does not preclude dimension reduction in service of other ends. For example, zeroing-out some weights when fitting a neural network can be a useful form of regularization.

In short, a Level I analysis is always an option. In some settings, a Level II analysis can work. But there will usually be substantial challenges. Prudence may dictate not undertaking statistical inference or at least to limit the Level II analysis to subsets of procedures that can be strongly defended. A Level III analysis is rarely appropriate, and interpreting statistical learning output in causal terms can be seductive. It is easy to forget that for statistical learning, there is no model.

10.4   Some Concluding Observations

Over the past decade statistical learning has become one of the more important tools available for applied statisticians and data analysts. But, the hype in which some procedures are wrapped can obscure important limitations and lead to analyses undertaken without sufficient care. Strong similarities to existing data analysis tools also can be obscured.

Statistical learning properly done will often require a major attitude adjustment. One of most difficult obstacles to effective applications is discarding premises from conventional modeling. This will especially difficult for experienced data analysts trained in traditional methods. One of the most common errors is to overlay algorithmic learning on top of model-based conceptions. Statistical learning is not just more of the same.

Finally, users of results from statistical learning must proceed with care. There is lots of money to be made, and professional reputations to be built, with statistical razzle-dazzle that is actually voodoo statistics. It can be very important from time to time to get technical advice from knowledgeable individuals who have no skin in the game.

Endnotes

[1] As emphasized throughout this book, current thinking makes "algorithmic modeling" an oxymoron. But in deference to Leo Breiman's insights, the term will be used in this section.

[2] For neural networks and its extensions, tuning time is a major consideration.

[3] There are excellent and free procedures available for Python users, but they are not discussed in this book;

[4] Be wary of commercial products that hide the details for their procedures by calling them proprietary.

[5] These days, even laptops will often perform well enough on most of the learning algorithms available in R.

[6] Comparisons between shareware and commercial software are becoming more difficult over time. There is big money to be made in "data analytics" being adopted by so many business firms and government agencies. Consequently, there is a race to bring the latest technology — or old technology labeled as new technology — to the market, packaged with slick advertising and polished user interfaces. The quality of the underlying analysis code and supporting documentation can suffer badly.

References

Berk, R. A., Heirdari, H., Jabbari, S., Kearns, M., & Roth, A. (in press). Fairness in criminal justice risk assessments: The state of the art. *Sociological Methods and Research.*

Breiman, L. (2001b) Statistical modeling: Two cultures (with discussion). *Statistical Science, 16,* 199–231.

Huq, A. Z. (2018) Racial equality in algorithmic criminal justice. *Duke Law Journal, 68,* 1043.

Mooney, S. J., & Pejaver, V. (2018) Big data in public health: Terminology, machine learning, and privacy. *Annual Review of Public Health, 39,* 95–112.

Obermeyer, Z., Powers, B., Vogeli, C., & Mullainathan, S. (2019). Dissecting racial bias in an algorithm used to manage the health of populations. *Science, 366*(646), 44–453.

Bibliography

Angrist, J. D., & Pischke, J. (2009). *Mostly harmless econometrics*. Princeton: Princeton University Press.

Baca-García, E., Perez-Rodriguez, M. M., Basurte-Villamor, I., Saiz-Ruiz, J., Leiva-Murillo, J. M., de Prado-Cumplido, M., et al. (2006). Using data mining to explore complex clinical decisions: A study of hospitalization after a suicide attempt. *Journal of Clinical Psychiatry, 67*(7), 1124–1132.

Berk, R. A., & Bleich, J. (2014). Forecast violence to inform sentencing decisions. *Journal of Quantitative Criminology, 30*, 79–96.

Berk, R. A., & Hyatt, J. (2015). Machine learning forecasts of risk to inform sentencing decisions. *Federal Sentencing Reporter, 27*(4), 222–228.

Berk, R. A., Olson, M., Buja, A., & Ouss, A. (2019). Using recursive partitioning to find and estimate heterogenous treatment effects in randomized clinical trials. arXiv: 1807.04164v1.

Berk, R. A., & Rothenberg, S. (2004). *Water Resource Dynamics in Asian Pacific Cities*. Statistics Department Preprint Series, UCLA.

Bühlmann, P. (2006). Boosting for high dimensional linear models. *The Annals of Statistics, 34*(2), 559–583.

Bühlmann, P., & Yu, B. (2006). Sparse boosting. *Journal of Machine Learning Research, 7*, 1001–1024.

Buja, A., & Rolke, W. (2007). *Calibration for Simultaneity: (Re) Sampling Methods for Simultaneous Inference with Application to Function Estimation and Functional Data*. Working paper at www-stat.wharton.upenn.edu/buja/

Buja, A., & Stuetzle, W. (2000). *Smoothing Effects of Bagging*. Working paper at www-stat.wharton.upenn.edu/buja/

Buja, A., Stuetzle, W., & Shen, Y. (2005). *Loss Functions for Binary Class Probability Estimation and Classification: Structure and Applications*. Unpublished manuscript, Department of Statistics, The Wharton School, University of Pennsylvania.

Candel, A., Parmar, V., LeDell, E., & Arora, A. (2016). *Deep learning with H2O*. Mountain View, CA: H2O.ai Inc.

Deng, L., & Yu, D. (2014). *Deep learning: Methods and applications*. Boston: Now Publishers, Inc.

Fan, J., & Gijbels, I. (1996a). *Local polynomial modeling and its applications*. New York: Chapman & Hall.

Fan, J., & Gijbels, I. (1996b). Variable bandwidth and local linear regression smoothers. *The Annals of Statistics, 20*(4), 2008–2036.

Fan, G., & Gray, B. (2005). Regression tree analysis using TARGET. *Journal of Computational and Graphical Statistics, 14*, 206–218.

Faraway, J. (2004). Human animation using nonparametric regression. *Journal of Computational and Graphical Statistics, 13*, 537–553.

Friedman, J. H. (1991). Multivariate adaptive regression splines (with discussion). *The Annals of Statistics, 19*, 1–82.

Friedman, J. H., & Hall, P. (2000). *On Bagging and Nonlinear Estimation*. Technical Report. Department of Statistics, Stanford University.

Gareth, M., & Zhu, J. (2007). *Functional Linear Regression That's Interpretable*. Working Paper, Department of Statistics, Marshall School of Business, University of California.

Ghosh, M., Reid, N., & Fraser, D. A. S. (2010). Ancillary statistics: A review. *Statistica Sinica, 20*, 1309–1332.

Good, P. I. (2004). *Permutation, parametric and bootstrap tests of hypotheses*. New York: Springer.

Hastie, T. J., & Tibshirani, R. J. (1996). Discriminant adaptive nearest neighbor classification. *IEEE Pattern Recognition and Machine Intelligence, 18*, 607–616.

Hothorn, T., & Lausen, B. (2003). Double-Bagging: Combining classifiers by bootstrap aggregation. *Pattern Recognition, 36*, 1303–1309.

Hurvich, C. M., & Tsai, C. (1989). Regression and time series model selection in small samples. *Biometrika, 76*(2), 297–307.

Jiu, J., Zhang, J., Jiang, X., & Liu, J. (2010). The group Dantzig selector. *Journal of Machine Learning Research, 9*, 461–468.

Kessler, R. C., Warner, C. H., Ivany, C., Petukhova, M. V., Rose, S., Bromet, E. J., et al. (2015). Predicting suicides after psychiatric hospitalization in US army soldiers: The army study to assess risk and resilience in service members (Army STARRS). *JAMA Psychiatry, 72*(1), 49–57.

Krieger, A., Long, C., & Wyner, A. (2001). Boosting noisy data. *Proceedings of the International Conference on Machine Learning*. Amsterdam: Mogan Kauffman.

Index

© Springer Nature Switzerland AG 2020
R. A. Berk, *Statistical Learning from a Regression Perspective*,
Springer Texts in Statistics, https://doi.org/10.1007/978-3-030-40189-4

Printed in the United States
by Baker & Taylor Publisher Services